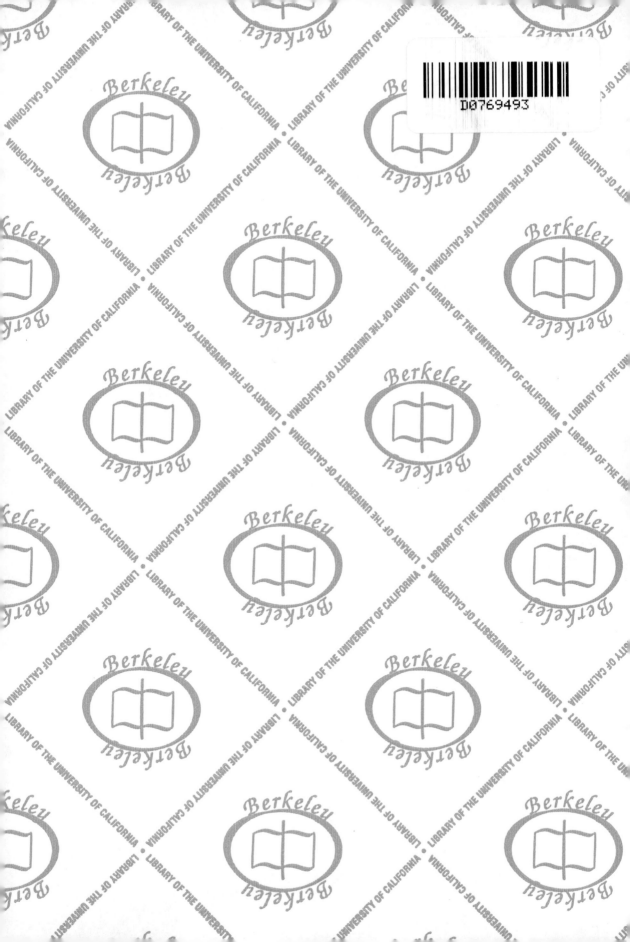

Visual Development

Second Edition

Nigel W. Daw

Yale University School of Medicine
New Haven, Connecticut

With 140 Illustrations

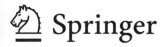 Springer

Nigel W. Daw
Department of Ophthalmology and Visual Sciences
Department of Neurobiology
Yale University School of Medicine
New Haven, CT 06520, USA

Library of Congress Control Number: 2005923440

ISBN 10: 0-387-25371-8
ISBN 13: 978-0387-25371-8

Printed on acid-free paper.

Printed in the United States of America.   (TB/EB)

9 8 7 6 5 4 3 2 1

springeronline.com

Preface to the Second Edition

It is ten years since the first edition of this book was written and considerable research has been done in that time. The development of vernier acuity and contour discrimination have been more carefully defined. Genes that play a role in myopia have been localized. New techniques using Gabor patches in various configurations have enabled scientists to define amblyopia in more careful terms, particularly the concept of spatial uncertainty, and whether it is due to undersampling or distorted sampling. Amblyopia was never simply a matter of a deficit in acuity, but it has taken careful experiments to show exactly what it is beyond that.

Ten years ago, the molecules that govern the crossing of the optic nerve fibers in the chiasm, and which project to the contralateral side and which to the ipsilateral side, were completely unknown. So were the molecules that govern the topography of the projections within the visual system. Today, we know some molecules involved in both these developmental events, as well as some that mark the boundaries of the visual cortex.

The technique of optical imaging of the visual cortex has enabled scientists to visualize the ocular dominance and orientation columns. Scientists can now use this technique to study the development of these columns, and the effect of various forms of visual deprivation on them, in a way that was not possible with single unit recordings.

It has also become increasingly apparent that there are many critical periods in the development of the visual system. The critical period for the effect of a particular form of visual deprivation in many cases lasts longer than the period of development of the property affected, and the period during which recovery can be obtained lasts longer still. Moreover, there are different critical periods for different properties. Properties handled at a higher level of the system have a later critical period. In addition, the critical period can be affected by the previous visual history of the animal, and by the technique used to evaluate it. For all these reasons, the chapter on critical periods has become much more involved.

Ten years ago, quite a lot was known about mechanisms of long-term potentiation and long-term depression, and not much about plasticity in the visual cortex resulting from monocular deprivation. Today, a considerable amount is known about mechanisms of ocular dominance plasticity, and it is also known that the mechanisms for long-term potentiation and long-term depression are not always the same. Thus, the order of the chapters on these two topics has been inverted and the balance between them altered.

The subject of the effect of out-of-focus images on the size of the eyeball has also been a very active area of research. We still do not know how the signal gets from the neural retina to the choroid and sclera, but there are a few molecules known that increase in response to plus lenses and decrease in response to minus lenses, or vice versa, which may be candidates for the signal.

For all these reasons, it is high time that this book should be revised. The aim of the book is the same as it was in the first edition—to provide a short summary of findings in the field that can be used by ophthalmology residents, optometry students, graduate students in neurobiology and psychology, senior undergraduates, and, since the field is so diverse, for experts to read chapters outside their area of expertise.

I am most grateful to Grace Gray for reading the whole book and providing a number of suggestions for clarification. I am also very grateful to Barbara Chapman, Velma Dobson, Maria Donoghue-Velleca, Quentin Fischer, Jane Gwiazda, Louise Hainline, Robert Hess, Arnold Heynen, Lynne Kiorpes, Dennis Levi, Anna Roe, Bill Stell, Josh Wallman, and Yupeng Yang, who provided comments on individual chapters and hopefully caught most of my errors. I also thank Sarah Gelo, supported by the Core Grant from the National Eye Institute to the Department of Ophthalmology and Visual Sciences at Yale University, for assistance.

Nigel W. Daw
New Haven, CT

Preface to the First Edition

Research in the area of visual development has become a multidisciplinary affair. Students who acquire an interest in the field therefore need to understand several different aspects of the subject. The development of acuity measured by psychophysicists is the concern of optometrists and ophthalmologists and depends on changes in the anatomy of the retina and the physiology of cells in the visual pathway. Scientists working on the cellular, molecular and biochemical mechanisms lean on anatomical studies, physiology and psychophysics in designing and interpreting their experiments. Indeed, the laboratories of the leading scientists working on the subject now all use a large variety of techniques in their studies.

Because the study of visual development is pursued by workers in many disciplines, from medicine to basic science, I have tried to write this book at a level at which it can be understood by a variety of students: graduate students in neurobiology and psychology, as well as optometry students and ophthalmology residents. The text assumes some knowledge of basic terms such as acuity, but a glossary is provided should the reader find some words that are unfamiliar. The emphasis is on facts and conclusions, rather than on methods and procedures. Many details are left out.

However, I hope that the experts will also read the book. The subject has become so wide-ranging that not many people have the time to read literature on all aspects of it. The book is also intended for experts in one area to get a grasp of the basics of the subject in other disciplines that are not their primary discipline.

To write a book covering such a wide variety of disciplines, I have had to simplify. The book does not go into controversies in detail. Instead, it provides my summary of what seems to me to be the best evidence. Not everybody will agree with my synthesis. Some experts will read it and be outraged at some of my statements. However, my outrageous statements were intended to be constructive: I hope that they will provoke thought and point the way to more experiments that will carry the field forward.

I am grateful to Colin Blakemore for inviting me to write this book. The process has been an educational one for me, and led to a number of insights which may have been apparent to others, but not to me. A number of friends and colleagues have helped me in the preparation of the book. Grace Gray in particular read the entire text twice, and improved it throughout. Robert Hess went through the whole section on Visual Deprivation, and made many valuable comments. John Lisman did the same for the section on Mechanisms. Janette Atkinson, Marty Banks, Oliver Braddick, Jan Naegele, Pasko Rakic, and Josh Wallman read individual chapters in their area of expertise and made many corrections and improvements. Several of my colleagues in the Department of Ophthalmology—Ethan Cohen, Jonathan Kirsch, Thomas Hughes, Colin Barnstable, Silvia Reid and Helen Flavin—gave comments on various portions of the text, and Marc Weitzman read two whole sections. I would like to thank them all. However, I did not adopt all of their suggestions, and the errors and omissions are mine. I would also like to thank Janet Hescock and Bob Brown for help in the preparation of the text and figures, together with support from the Core Grant to Yale University from the National Eye Institute.

Nigel W. Daw
New Haven, CT

Contents

Chapter 1

Introduction... 1

Chapter 2

Functional Organization of the Visual System

1. General Anatomical Organization.. 8
2. Function in the Retina... 10
3. Function in the Lateral Geniculate Nucleus............................ 16
4. Function in the Visual Cortex.. 18
   4.1. Columnar Organization of Cortex.................................. 19
5. Parallel Processing within the Visual System........................ 21
6. Hierarchical Processing within the Visual System.................... 22
7. Summary... 26

Part I

Development of the Visual System

Chapter 3

Development of Visual Capabilities

1. Methods for Studying Infant Vision.................................... 32
2. Development of Monocular Vision....................................... 34
   2.1. Acuity... 34
   2.2. Contrast Sensitivity.. 36
   2.3. Vernier Acuity.. 41
   2.4. Contour Integration... 43
   2.5. Summary... 47
3. Development of Binocular Vision....................................... 47
   3.1. Depth Perception.. 48
   3.2. Orthotropia... 49
   3.3. Stereopsis.. 50
   3.4. Correlation of the Onset of Stereopsis and Segregation
        of Ocular Dominance Columns..................................... 52
   3.5. The Pre- and Poststereoptic Periods............................. 54
   3.6. Summary... 55

4. Development of Eye Movements.. 56
   4.1. Fixation and Refixation.. 56
   4.2. Saccades.. 56
   4.3. Smooth Pursuit.. 58
   4.4. Vergence and Accommodation.. 59
   4.5. Optokinetic Nystagmus.. 60
   4.6. Summary... 61

Chapter 4

Anatomical Development of the Visual System

1. Development of the Retina and the Projections
   within It.. 66
2. Crossing in the Optic Chiasm 67
   2.1. Errors at the Chiasm in Albino Animals.. 68
3. Development of the Lateral Geniculate Nucleus.................................... 70
4. Topography of Projections.. 72
5. Development of Visual Cortex and Projections to It............................... 74
   5.1. Development of Geniculocortical Projections 75
   5.2. Formation of Layers in the Cortex 75
   5.3. Role of the Subplate Neurons... 77
   5.4. Tangential Projections.. 78
   5.5. Development of Connections to and from Layers in the
        Visual Cortex 79
6. Development of Clusters of Cells with Similar Properties....................... 81
   6.1. Formation of Ocular Dominance Columns..................................... 81
   6.2. Formation of Blobs and Pinwheels... 82
   6.3. Development of Lateral Connections 82
7. Other Events during Differentiation.. 82
8. Summary... 85

Chapter 5

Development of Receptive Field Properties

1. Development in the Retina and Lateral Geniculate
   Nucleus.. 93
2. Development in the Visual Cortex... 96
3. Development in the Absence of Light and Activity 103
4. Summary... 106

Part II
Amblyopia and the Effects of Visual Deprivation

Chapter 6

Modifications to the Visual Input that Lead to Nervous System Changes

1. Strabismus.. 113
2. Anisometropia.. 119
3. Astigmatism 119
4. Cataract... 121
5. Myopia... 123
6. Summary... 134

Chapter 7

Physiological and Anatomical Changes that Result from Optical and Motor Deficits

1. Monocular Deprivation.. 127
2. Orientation and Direction Deprivation.. 132
3. One Eye Out of Focus.. 134
4. Strabismus... 135
5. Summary.. 141

Chapter 8

What Is Amblyopia?

1. Amblyopia from Anisometropia... 145
2. Effect of Cataracts... 148
3. Amblyopia from Strabismus... 150
   3.1. Crowding... 153
   3.2. Vernier Acuity... 156
   3.3. Spatial Uncertainty... 156
   3.4. Suppression.. 160
4. Summary.. 164

Chapter 9

Critical Periods

1. General Principles from Experiments with Animals............................. 170
   1.1. The System Is Plastic between Eye Opening and Puberty.............. 170
   1.2. More Severe Deprivations Have a Larger Effect............................ 171
   1.3. Higher Levels of the System Have a Later Critical Period.............. 172
   1.4. Different Properties Have Different Critical Periods....................... 173
   1.5. The Critical Period Depends on the Previous Visual History
        of the Animal... 175
   1.6. Procedures Affect the Critical Period... 175
   1.7. The Periods of Development, Disruption, and Recovery
        May Be Different... 177
2. Critical Periods in Humans... 178
   2.1. Disruption of Acuity.. 178
   2.2. Recovery from Disruption of Acuity... 181
   2.3. Binocularity.. 183
   2.4. Stereopsis... 183
   2.5. Movement... 186
3. Summary.. 187

Part III

Mechanisms of Plasticity

Chapter 10

Concepts of Plasticity

1. The Hebb Postulate.. 198
2. How Electrical Activity Can Strengthen Some Synapses and
   Weaken Others... 199

3. Feedback from the Postsynaptic Cell to the
Presynaptic Terminal... 200
4. Criteria for Critical Factors in the Critical Period 201
5. Summary.. 205

Chapter 11
Mechanisms of Plasticity in the Visual Cortex

1. Electrical Activity 208
2. Polarization of the Postsynaptic Neuron 210
3. NMDA Receptors 211
4. Metabotropic Glutamate Receptors.. 224
5. GABA... 215
6. Brain Derived Neurotrophic Factor (BDNF)... 217
7. Calcium, α-Calcium/Calmodulin Kinase, and Calcineurin 219
8. cAMP and Protein Kinase A 221
9. A Kinase Anchoring Protein at the Postsynaptic Density 221
10. Other Protein Kinases.. 222
11. Cyclic AMP Response Binding Element (CREB)..................................... 223
12. Genes and Protein Synthesis.. 223
13. Modulatory Factors 225
14. Nerve Growth Factor (NGF)... 226
15. Immune System Molecules... 226
16. Different Mechanisms for Different Aspects of Plasticity 227
17. Summary... 227

Chapter 12

**Long-Term Potentiation and Long-Term Depression as
Early Steps in Ocular Dominance Plasticity** 235

Chapter 13

Deprivation Myopia and Emmetropization 243

Glossary.. 255

Index.. 265

1

Introduction

This book will discuss visual development, leading on to visual deprivation, where the development is disturbed by faults in the optics or motor control of the eye. Visual deprivation is an important and fascinating subject from several points of view: clinical, philosophical, historical, and scientific. Many general questions in these areas have been framed over the years in terms of the visual system. This is not surprising, because we are visual animals. If dogs ruled the world, the title of this book would be *Olfactory Development*. As it is, vision is our most important sense, and the first that we think of in discussing scientific and philosophical questions.

A large number of people have personally experienced some form of visual deprivation. Anything that affects the images on the retinas of young children can have lasting effects on the part of the brain that processes visual signals. This can occur if one eye is in focus, but the other is not; if vertical lines are in focus, but horizontal lines are not; if the two eyes look in different directions (strabismus); if the lens of one or both eyes is cloudy (cataract); or if the eyeball grows so much that objects can no longer be focused on the retina. Frequently these conditions lead to poor vision in one or both eyes as a result of changes that have occurred in the central visual system, even after the images on the retinas are made clear and coordinated. After the Greeks, this is named *amblyopia*, meaning blunt vision or dull vision. The colloquial term for amblyopia is *lazy eye*. Between 2% and 4% of the population may become amblyopic from visual deprivation.

Philosophers became interested in the subject of visual deprivation when William Molyneux posed his famous question in the late 17th century. After his wife became blind, Molyneux wrote to John Locke, saying "Suppose a man born blind, and now adult, and taught by his touch to distinguish between a cube and a sphere of the same metal.... Suppose then the cube and sphere placed on a table and the blind man made to see; query, Whether by his sight, before he touched them, he could now distinguish and tell which is the globe, and which the cube? To which the acute and judicious proposer answers: not. For though he has obtained the experience of how a globe, how a cube, affects his touch, yet he has not yet attained the experience that what affects his touch so or so, must affect his sight so or so."

Locke's comment in 1690 was "I agree with this thinking gentleman, whom I am proud to call my friend, in his answer to this his problem, and am of opinion that the blind man, at first sight, would not be able with certainty to say which was the globe, which the cube whilst he only saw them; though he could unerringly name them by his touch, and certainly distinguish them by the difference of their figures felt" (see Locke, 1846).

Some material to test Molyneux's question was available during his time. Congenital cataract was quite common, and an operation for it, called *couching*, had been invented in either Arabia or India at least 1000 years before (Hirschberg, 1982). A sharp needle was used to make a hole in the sclera, a blunt needle was inserted, and the lens gently pushed downward out of the line of sight. Occasionally the lens was removed altogether with a hollow needle, but not many surgeons were expert enough to do this well. Thus the operation was often not successful. Moreover, vision was not fully restored because of lack of adequate correction for the absent lens. Consequently, the topic of Molyneux's question remained an armchair discussion for another half century.

Only when doctors finally realized that the cataract is in the lens was the vision of substantial numbers of patients restored. At this time, Daviel promulgated a cleaner operation for cataract by removing the lens through a flap in the cornea. Generally speaking, the results of this operation were successful in producing a clear image on the retina when spectacles were worn, but were disappointing to the patients in terms of their visual perception. Daviel stated in 1762 after 22 cases, "I can assert, indeed, with absolute assurance, that not a single one of these patients has recognized the objects shown to him after the operation, without the use of touch, unless they have been many times shown to him and named. . . . If it has been said that some such patients can distinguish objects exactly and completely immediately after the operation, then this shows that they were not really blind from birth, for the latter have no real idea at all of even the meanest objects" (Von Senden, 1960, p. 106).

Numerous cases were reported following Daviel's report, and the results were generally the same. Von Senden collected them in a summary in 1932 (von Senden, 1960). Where vision was tested soon after the operation, patients could distinguish color, but they had little idea of form or shape, no idea of distance, no idea of depth, and very little idea of solidity. Their problem was not just a matter of transferring the recognition of objects by touch to the recognition of objects by sight. Their visual perception was itself defective. Frequently patients became depressed because the gift of sight was confusing for them (von Senden, 1960; Gregory, 1974). They could not, in fact, see like normal people, and their previous tactual and auditory world was not easily correlated with their new visual world.

Locke was the apostle of empiricism. He believed that everything is learned. The opposing point of view is that everything is innate. The debate between the two points of view raged for many years under various headings, such as *nature versus nurture* (for the belief that properties are with us at birth, versus the idea that properties are learned from experience after birth). One might think, from the cases discussed by von Senden, that Locke's point of view is correct. As we will discuss, neither is strictly correct. While

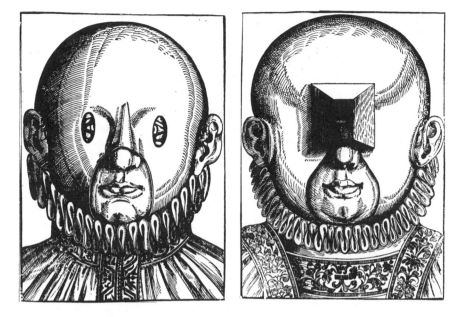

FIG. 1.1. Masks for squinters. On the left is a mask for a convergent squinter with holes placed to try and force the eyes to look outward. On the right is a mask for divergent squinters containing two prisms that will make the images converge. (From Bartisch, 1583.)

some properties are learned, others are there at birth. Moreover (an answer to Molyneux's question that Locke did not consider) properties can be present at birth and then degenerate.

The history of strabismus (i.e., being cross-eyed or squinting) is as venerable as that of cataract. Hippocrates (460–375 BC) believed that there was a genetic component, saying, "If, therefore, bald persons have for the most part bald children, grey-eyed parents grey-eyed children, squinting parents squinting children, and so on . . . " (see Hippocrates, 1923). Paulus of Aegina (625–690) recommended wearing a mask with "an opening for each eye so placed as to induce the eyes to assume direct positions in order to see through these openings." Georg Bartisch (1535–1606) illustrates such a mask for convergent strabismus, together with a mask containing prisms for divergent strabismus (Fig. 1.1).

Surgery for strabismus was initially tried by Chevalier John Taylor in the 18th century (Albert, 1992). It is not clear exactly what he did. Many of his operations were not successful: he treated Johann Sebastian Bach twice, and Bach went blind afterward. However, Taylor was a colorful personality who gave great publicity to the possibility of surgery for the problem. The first successful surgery is attributed to Johann Freidrich Dieffenbach (1792–1847), although others attempted it, some successfully, around the same date. In the early days, the operation was performed as much for cosmetic as for visual effect. From ancient times strabismus was associated with an "evil eye" and people who had it were frequently treated with suspicion and contempt, much like the village idiot. They were more concerned about the ridicule and shame from their crooked eye than any visual problems caused by it.

Indeed, surgery for strabismus, like surgery for cataract, can be a disappointment to the patient. If the crooked eye has established a compensating point of fixation away from the fovea that is coordinated with the normal point of fixation at the fovea in the good eye, then the operation can lead to double vision. The double vision can be much more disturbing than the amblyopia in the lazy eye that was there before the operation.

If treatment is to be successful for cataract or strabismus acquired early in life, and disappointment is to be avoided, the treatment must be started early. This point was not fully appreciated until the middle of the 20th century. A nonsurgical treatment for amblyopia in strabismus (patching of the good eye) was recommended by Buffon in 1743. However, this treatment fell into disrepute, and it was not until almost 200 years later that it became apparent that it could be successful in young children, but not older children (Von Noorden, 1990). Slowly ophthalmologists turned from the idea that strabismus is a congenital defect to the idea that it is also a developmental defect (Von Noorden, 1990; Tychsen, 1993). This latter idea led to the recognition of the importance of early intervention, and to the concept of a critical period after which intervention would be unsuccessful.

The modern period in the investigation of visual deprivation started with the work of Torsten Wiesel and David Hubel in the early 1960s, for which they were awarded the Nobel Prize in 1981 (Wiesel, 1982). It was this work that enabled the behavioral observations made in the clinic to be correlated with physiological and anatomical changes that occur in the central visual system. Several technical advances contributed to this work. First, there was the invention of the microelectrode, which allowed investigation of the properties of single cells in the visual system. Second, there was the development of an anatomical method for demonstrating the endings of axons projecting from the eyes to the visual cortex. Third, there was the development of techniques for visualizing how cells in the cortex that have similar properties are grouped together.

These techniques were employed to demonstrate that the main site for changes occurring after visual deprivation is the primary visual cortex. Projections to the primary visual cortex change. Properties of cells in the visual cortex change. Connections between cells in the visual cortex change. In other words, sensory signals carried from the eye to the brain have a dramatic effect on the structure and physiological properties of the brain.

More recently, research focus has moved to the biochemical steps occurring in these events. Many suggestions as to what these steps might be comes from work on *long-term potentiation*. This is a phenomenon that has been studied in the hippocampus as well as the visual cortex, and is believed to underlie memory, primarily because it occurs in the hippocampus at all ages, and lesions of the hippocampus are known to disrupt memory.

This book will trace the main themes in this story. The first section will summarize the psychophysical properties, the anatomy, and the physiology of normal development of the visual system. An important component of this section will be to point out which aspects of development depend on sensory signals, and which do not. There is considerable development after birth. Indeed, acuity in an infant is sufficiently poor (less than 10% of normal adult acuity) that a newborn infant is legally blind by adult criteria. Thus the effects of visual deprivation will depend on when in development the deprivation occurs.

The second section will cover the behavioral, physiological, and anatomical effects of visual deprivation. This section will present a summary of the clinical literature on the subject, and will also summarize the basic science literature from experiments on animals. Next, the clinical and basic research findings will be correlated with each other to provide insights into the basic mechanisms of human pathology resulting from visual deprivation.

The third section will cover mechanisms of visual deprivation. Here we are addressing our understanding of deprivation as it unfolds. The sensory signals that reach the visual cortex have long-term effects that eventually lead to anatomical changes. There must be a number of intermediate steps between the sensory signals and the anatomical changes. The steps are beginning to be understood. Moreover, some of the steps are present in young animals and relatively absent in adults, and these steps are the ones that make the visual cortex of young animals more able to adapt to the signals coming in. However, there is a lot more to be discovered and this is a very active area of research at the moment. In fact, this section of the book was the first to go out of date after the first edition was published, and will be again after publication of this edition.

The story has come a long way since Molyneux set down his question. There have been both philosophical and practical developments. The realization that there are innate properties in the visual cortex that can degenerate in the absence of proper visual input has led ophthalmologists to intervene earlier and earlier. The knowledge of ophthalmologists that treatment of cataract is much less likely to be successful than treatment of strabismus, and that treatment of strabismus may bring back acuity but not stereopsis, has led basic scientists to measure the critical periods for the development of these features more accurately. There have been few books that bring together the various aspects of the story, and none at the level of this one, so I hope that the publication of this book will foster yet more interactions in the field.

References

Albert, D. M. (1992). Introduction. In L. Howe (Ed.), *The muscles of the eye* (pp. 3–30). Delran, N.J.: Gryphon Editions.

Bartisch, G. (1583). *Ophthalmodouleia, das ist augendienst*. Dresden: Stockel.

Buffon, M. de (1743). Dissertation sur la cause du strabisme ou les yeux louches. *Hist. Acad. R. Sci.*, 231–248.

Gregory, R. L. (1974). *Concepts and mechanisms of perception* (pp. 65–129). New York: Scribners.

Hippocrates. (1923). Air, water and Places. In W. H. S. Jones (Ed.), *Collected works* (p. 111). London: William Heinemann.

Hirschberg, J. (1982). *History of ophthalmology, Vol. 1*. (F. C. Blodi, Trans.). Bonn: J. P. Wayenborgh Verlag.

Locke, J. (1846). *An essay concerning human understanding* (30th ed.) (p. 84). London: Thomas Tegg.

Tychsen, L. (1993). Motion sensitivity and the origins of infantile strabismus. In K. Simins, (Ed.), *Early visual development, normal and abnormal* (pp. 384–386). New York: Oxford University Press.

Von Noorden, G. K. (1990). *Binocular vision and ocular motility.* St. Louis: Mosby.

von Senden, M. (1960). *Space and sight* (P. Heath, Trans.). Glencoe, Ill.: The Free Press.

Wiesel, T. N. (1982). Postnatal development of the visual cortex and the influence of environment. *Nature,* 299:583–591.

2

Functional Organization of the Visual System

The visual system must convert the pattern of light that falls on the retina into perception. This involves a transformation of the visual image in several dimensions. Take, for example, depth perception: There are several cues to depth perception, including disparity, vergence, perspective, shading, texture gradients, interposition, motion parallax, size, and accommodation. For complete perception, all of these must be analyzed. Where some cues conflict with others (see Kaufman, 1974), the system must resolve the conflicts and come to a decision. Where the cues agree with each other, the system produces a perception of the distance of an object from the subject, its position in relation to other objects nearby, and the three-dimensional shape of the object.

As another example, consider color vision: The most important property of color, for the survival of the species, is not the pleasurable sensations that it gives, but the fact that it helps to recognize objects. The visual system has evolved so that the color of an object remains constant when lighted by different sources of illumination, and against different backgrounds. This is known as *object color constancy*. What the brain recognizes is a property of the object, namely the percentage of each wavelength that is reflected by the object (reflection spectrum). The composition of the wavelengths reaching the eye from the object is the product of the reflection spectrum and the illumination falling on the object—what the visual system does, as Helmholtz put it, is to "discount the source of illumination." This is a complicated calculation, as shown by numerous attempts in the last century to provide a mathematical formula for it.

One could provide a number of other examples, including shape perception, pattern perception, and control of eye movements, if space permitted. In all cases, the basic job of the visual system is to recognize objects and their position in space. Sometimes this leads to illusions such as the Ponzo illusion (Fig. 2.1). In this illusion the two cylinders are the same length, but the bottom one appears to be shorter because of the presence of the converging lines. However, this is not so much an illusion as the visual system

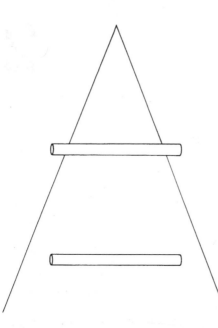

FIG. 2.1. Ponzo illusion. The two cylinders are the same length, but the converging lines make the top cylinder appear longer because of the effects of perspective.

operating in a sensible way to recognize distance. As another example, the brightness of an object, as well as its color, is influenced by the surroundings (Fig. 2.2). In this illustration, the ball on the top reflects the same amount of light as the ball on the bottom, but because the top one is seen against a dark background, it appears to be lighter than the bottom one. What this chapter is designed to do is to give a broad idea, to the extent that current knowledge permits, of how the visual system is organized to provide these constancies and perceptions.

1. General Anatomical Organization

The initial processing of the image takes place in the retina. The retina projects to four nuclei, with different functions: the lateral geniculate nucleus, for perception of objects; the superior colliculus, for control of eye movements; the pretectum, for control of the pupil; and the suprachiasmatic nucleus, for control of diurnal rhythms and hormonal changes (Fig. 2.3). In most of these areas, and in higher areas of the visual system, there is a topographic organization. That is, the retina maps to the nucleus in an organized fashion. Neighboring parts of the retina project to neighboring parts of the nucleus, so that there is a map of the field of view within the nucleus.

The lateral geniculate nucleus has several layers, and the two eyes project to separate layers. The lateral geniculate projects on to primary visual cortex (V1), which is also known as striate cortex because the input layer can be seen as a stripe without magnification. Primary visual cortex is where the signals from the two eyes come together. There are also projections to the cortex

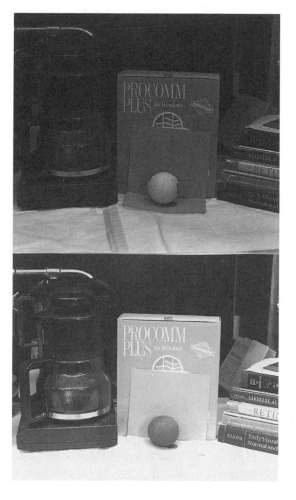

FIG. 2.2. How the brightness of an object depends on the background. Two photographs were taken of a scene with a light ball in the top scene and a dark ball in the bottom scene. Then the whole of the top scene was darkened, so that the amount of light coming from the two balls is identical. Because of contrast with the immediate background, the top ball looks lighter than the bottom one.

from the superior colliculus through the pulvinar, known as the extrastriate pathway to cortex.

Cortex in general has six layers (I, II, III, IV, V, and VI). Signals come in to layer IV. Layer IV projects to layers II and III, which send signals to other areas of cortex. Layers II and III project to layer V, which sends signals back to the superior colliculus. Layers II, III, and V project to layer VI, which sends signals back to the lateral geniculate nucleus. The complete story is far more complicated than this, but these are the predominant projections.

A large number of areas in the cerebral cortex deal with vision—at least 32 in the macaque monkey (Van Essen, Anderson, & Felleman, 1992) and 13 in the cat (Rosenquist, 1985). These have been best described in the monkey (Fig. 2.4). The large number of areas, and the even larger number of connections between them—305 at last count in the macaque—is bewildering. Broadly speaking, these areas can be thought of as lying along two pathways (Ungerleider & Pasternak, 2004). One goes through V1 and the secondary visual cortex (V2), then on to the temporal cortex. This pathway deals primarily

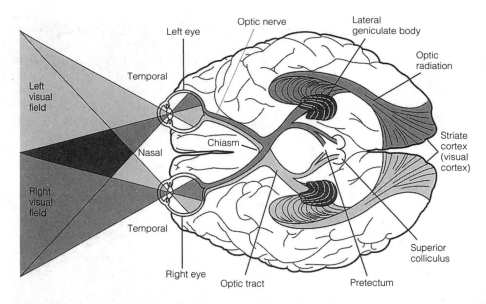

FIG. 2.3. Overall view of the visual system as seen from below. The retina projects to the lateral geniculate body, the superior colliculus, the pretectal area, and the suprachiasmatic nucleus (not shown). The lateral geniculate nucleus projects to the visual cortex. Axons from the nasal retina cross in the chiasm and axons from the temporal retina do not. Consequently, the left cortex deals with the right field of view and vice versa.

with what an object is, that is, its shape, form, and color. The other also goes through V1 and V2, and then on to the parietal cortex. This pathway deals primarily with where an object is and with the control of eye movements. In addition signals from different senses converge in the parietal pathway. Although the multiplicity of interconnections between areas in the parietal pathway and areas in the temporal pathway shows that this is an oversimplification, it is a useful one.

Different areas handle different properties of the visual stimulus. For example, V4 contains many cells that respond to color and shape, while V5 (also called MT) contains many cells that respond to movement (Zeki, 1978; Pasupathy & Connor, 2002). What specific properties are dealt with in the other 30 or so areas is currently a topic of active research. It will be many years before the differences between the various areas are completely characterized.

2. Function in the Retina

The main function of the retina is to convert information about brightness (speaking more correctly, luminance) into information about contrast (Kuffler, 1953). Generally speaking, the visual system is concerned with relative quantities—the luminance of an object in relation to the luminance of objects around it, the long wavelengths coming from an object in relation to medium and short wavelengths, and so on. Many of these relative comparisons are made in the retina. Just about the only function in the visual system

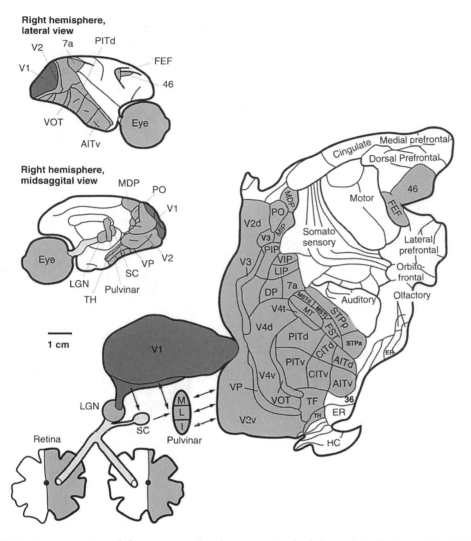

FIG. 2.4. An overview of the macaque visual system. On the left is a lateral view of the right cortex (top) and a midsaggital view looking at the medial surface with the left hemisphere removed (middle). Projections from the retina are summarized at the bottom: the geniculostriate pathway goes from the retina to the lateral geniculate nucleus (LGN) to V1; the extrastriate pathway goes from the retina to the superior colliculus (SC) to the pulvinar to V2 and other areas. On the right is shown a flattened view of the cortex with sulci and gyri smoothed out and with a cut between V1 and V2, which are in reality next to each other, to permit this illustration. Visual areas on the temporal pathway dealing with form and color are V4 and inferotemporal areas (PITd, PITv, CITd, CITv, AITd, AITv); visual areas on the parietal pathway dealing with location and eye movements are PO, VIP, LIP, and 7a; MT and MST, which deal with movement and disparity, feed into both of these pathways. MIP and VIP receive somatosensory as well as visual input. The function of many areas is not yet defined. [Reprinted with permission from Van Essen, D. C., et al. (1992). *Science*, *255*, 419–423. Copyright 1992 AAAS.]

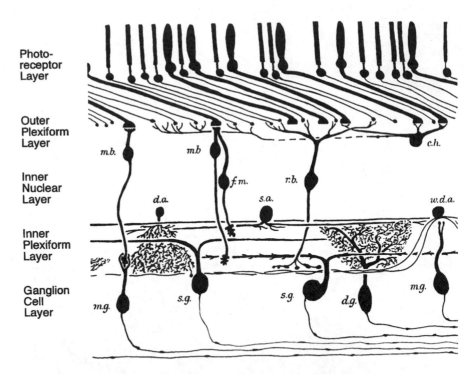

FIG. 2.5. Diagram of various cell types found in the macaque monkey and human retinas. Some ganglion cells have small dendritic arborizations (e.g., midget ganglion cells, m.g.) and others have large arborizations (e.g., stratified ganglion cells, s.g.). Abbreviations: m.b., midget bipolar cell; f.m., flat midget bipolar cell; r.b., rod bipolar cell; r.h., rod horizontal cell; d.a., diffuse amacrine cell; w.d.a., wide diffuse amacrine cell; m.g., midget ganglion cell; s.g., stratified ganglion cell; d.g., diffuse ganglion cell. [Reprinted with permission from Boycott, B.B., & Dowling, J.E. (1969). Organization of the primate retina: light microscopy. *Philosphical Transaction of the Royal Society of London. Series B. Biological sciences, 255*, 109–184. Figure 98. (Royal Society, London)].

that needs luminance information is control of the pupil, and this is dealt with by a special class of cells that projects only to the pretectum.

The retina has five main layers (Fig. 2.5). Light is absorbed by the photoreceptors (rods and cones) that send signals to bipolar cells in the inner nuclear layer, which in turn connect to ganglion cells in the ganglion cell layer. The ganglion cells project to the lateral geniculate nucleus. Then there are two sets of cells, also with cell bodies in the inner nuclear layer, that make lateral connections. Horizontal cells make lateral connections between one photoreceptor terminal and another in the outer plexiform layer. Amacrine cells make lateral connections between one bipolar cell terminal and another in the inner plexiform layer. These lateral connections are used to compare signals from light falling on one part of the retina with signals from another part of the retina.

To understand how these comparisons are made, consider recordings from a bipolar cell, for example, the depolarizing cone bipolar cell (Fig. 2.6). The bipolar cell has a *receptive field*. The receptive field is defined as the region of visual space in which changes in luminance will affect the activity

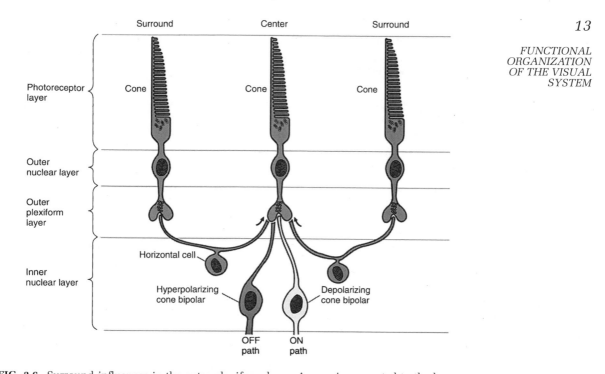

FIG. 2.6. Surround influences in the outer plexiform layer. A cone is connected to the hyperpolarizing cone bipolar cell with a sign-conserving synapse and to the depolarizing cone bipolar cell with a sign-reversing synapse (see Glossary). At the same time, cones in the surround connect to horizontal cells, which contact the cone in the center and decrease the release of transmitter from it, and consequently antagonize signals going to both types of bipolar cell. Thus, the depolarizing cone bipolar cell is depolarized by light falling on the central cone and its response is reduced when light also falls on the surround. Similarly, the hyperpolarizing cone bipolar cell is hyperpolarized by light falling on the central cone and its response is also reduced when light also falls on the surround.

of the cell. Such changes are mediated by all the parts of the retina that affect activity in the bipolar cell. Light falling on photoreceptors that are directly connected to the depolarizing cone bipolar cell will depolarize it. Light falling on photoreceptors that are connected indirectly through horizontal cells will oppose or antagonize this influence. Direct connections form the center of the receptive field, and indirect ones form the surround. Thus the bipolar cell will respond to objects falling on the center of its receptive field that are lighter than the background. In contrast, the hyperpolarizing bipolar cell responds to objects that are darker than the background through a similar process—it is hyperpolarized by light falling in the center of its receptive field and depolarized by light falling on the surround (Werblin & Dowling, 1969).

Two other properties are handled by the retina. First, a distinction is made between fine detail and movement. Second, the signals from the rods, which handle vision in dim light, and the cones, which deal with vision in bright light, are combined.

The distinction between fine detail and movement is made in the connections between bipolar cells and ganglion cells (Fig. 2.5). Some ganglion cells receive input from a limited number of bipolar cells and a limited number of photoreceptors (Polyak, 1941). They have small dendritic arborizations, small cell bodies, and give sustained responses. Thus, they have small receptive fields; that is, the area from which photoreceptors feed into them is small, and this is what gives them the ability to analyze fine detail. Examples are the midget ganglion cells in Figure 2.5. Other ganglion cells receive input from bipolar cells and photoreceptors over a wider area. They have larger dendritic arborizations, larger cell bodies, and give transient responses. Examples are the stratified ganglion cells in Figure 2.5. It is the transient nature of their response that enables them to respond to movement within their receptive field (De Monasterio & Gouras, 1975).

Bipolar cells and ganglion cells connect to each other in the inner plexiform layer with additional local and lateral connections through amacrine cells. The inner plexiform layer is divided into two sublaminae (Famiglietti & Kolb, 1976; also see Fig. 2.7). Sublamina b deals with signals for objects brighter than the background; cone bipolar cells that depolarize for such objects connect to ganglion cells that increase their firing rate when a light is turned on and are thus said to have ON responses. Sublamina a handles signals for objects that are darker than the background; cone bipolar cells that depolarize for such objects connect to ganglion cells that decrease their firing rate when a light is turned on and increase it when a light is turned off and are said to have OFF responses. Signals from the rod photoreceptors feed into this same network through rod amacrine cells, so that the ganglion cells respond in a similar fashion to both rod and cone signals.

It is the action of these bipolar and ganglion cells that is responsible for our perception of the balls in Figure 2.2. Depolarizing bipolar cells and ON center ganglion cells that receive the image of the left ball on the center of their receptive fields will fire, signaling that this ball is brighter than the background. Hyperpolarizing bipolar cells and OFF center ganglion cells that have the image of the right ball on the center of their receptive fields will fire, signaling that the right ball is darker than the background. Of course, the connections of the bipolar and ganglion cells are fairly short-range—other cells that are higher in the system, and have long-range connections, will compare the left ball with the right one, but the comparison of an object with its immediately neighboring objects is done in the retina.

The first stage of color processing also takes place within the retina. There are three types of cone photoreceptors, which absorb long-wavelength light (L), medium-wavelength light (M), and short-wavelength light (S). A class of ganglion cell called the *small bistratified ganglion cell* receives input from S cones in the ON sublamina via a blue cone bipolar cell, and input from L and M cones in the OFF sublamina via a diffuse bipolar cell. The summation of these inputs produces an ON response from blue light and an OFF response from yellow light (Dacey, 2000). The circuitry for red/green responses is not as clear, but there are ganglion cells with ON responses to red light and OFF responses to green light and vice versa (see Dacey, 2000).

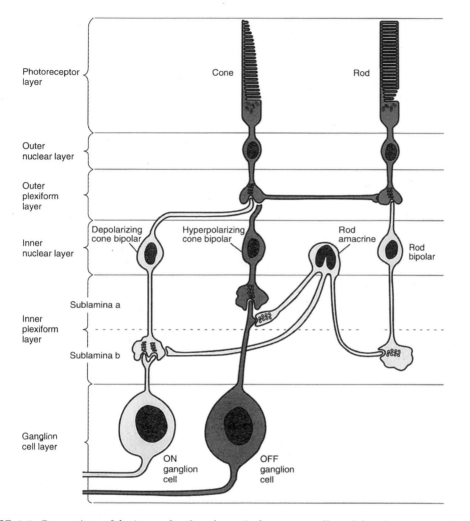

FIG. 2.7. Connections of the inner plexiform layer. Rod amacrine cells and depolarizing cone bipolar cells converge in sublamina b onto ON center ganglion cells. Hyperpolarizing bipolar cells connect to OFF center ganglion cells with a sign-conserving synapse and rod amacrine cells with a sign reversing synapse in sublamina a. Cells that depolarize in response to light are pale, and cells that hyperpolarize are shaded. Synapses between two pale cells or two shaded cells are sign conserving or excitatory; synapses between a shaded cell and a pale cell are sign reversing, or inhibitory.

The animal models that have been used to study the effects of visual deprivation are cat and monkey. This general picture is similar in the two species, except the cat has less color vision. Most of the cones in the cat are M cones; there are a few S cones but no L cones, and the percentage of color-coded cells is small. Also, the distinction between fine detail and movement is less pronounced in the cat than in the monkey. The fine detail ganglion cells are called P cells in the monkey and X cells in the cat (Enroth-Cugell & Robson, 1966), and the movement ganglion cells are called M cells in the monkey and Y cells in the cat.

Another class of ganglion cell found in the cat is called W or sluggish cells. This is a heterogeneous class of cells with a variety of different properties (Cleland & Levick, 1974; Stone & Fukuda, 1974). It includes cells that respond to brightness rather than contrast and project to the pretectum (sustained ON W cells). The main W cell projection is to the superior colliculus, the pretectum, and the suprachiasmatic nucleus. Some project to the lateral geniculate but the information from most of these cells is not sent to the primary visual cortex from there; therefore, the W cells are not part of the geniculostriate pathway. Although W cells comprise 50% of the ganglion cell population, they have small cell bodies and are not recorded very frequently in physiological experiments; therefore less is known about them. There is a class of rarely encountered cells found in the monkey that may correspond to the W cells, but their properties have not received a lot of attention (Schiller & Malpeli, 1977). Partly for this reason, and partly because most of the effects of visual deprivation are found in the geniculostriate pathway, W cells will not get much more mention in this book.

3. Function in the Lateral Geniculate Nucleus

The lateral geniculate nucleus (LGN) receives signals from the retina and transmits them on to the cortex without much processing. Signals from the left and right eyes remain segregated in different layers in the lateral geniculate (Fig. 2.8). In the macaque there are six layers: four dorsal with small cells, called the parvocellular layers (P), and two ventral with large cells called magnocellular (M). The fine detail cells project from the retina to the P layers, and the movement cells to the M layers, as reflected in the terminology for these two groups of cells (see Fig. 2.8). Counting from the bottom, layers 1, 4, and 6 receive input from the contralateral eye, and layers 2, 3, and 5 from the ipsilateral eye.

The properties of cells in the lateral geniculate are very like those of the cells in the retina that project to them (Wiesel & Hubel, 1966). There are cells that are excited by light in the center of their receptive field and inhibited by light in the surrounding area; these are ON center cells, just as in the retina. There are cells whose activity is reduced by light in the center and increased by light in the surround; these are OFF center cells. There are red/green and yellow/blue color-coded cells. There does not seem to be much convergence from different cell types in the retina onto single cells in the lateral geniculate. The main difference between the LGN and retinal cells that has been noted is that LGN cells give less response to white light illuminating the whole receptive field uniformly. This occurs because there are additional inhibitory interneurons in the lateral geniculate, so that antagonism from the surround of the receptive field of a cell more closely balances the center.

The lateral geniculate receives input from the various modulatory pathways located in the brainstem: noradrenaline input from the locus coeruleus, serotonin input from the raphe nuclei, and acetylcholine input from the parabrachial region (Sherman & Koch, 1986). It also receives some input from the eye movement system. These inputs modulate signals reaching the cortex

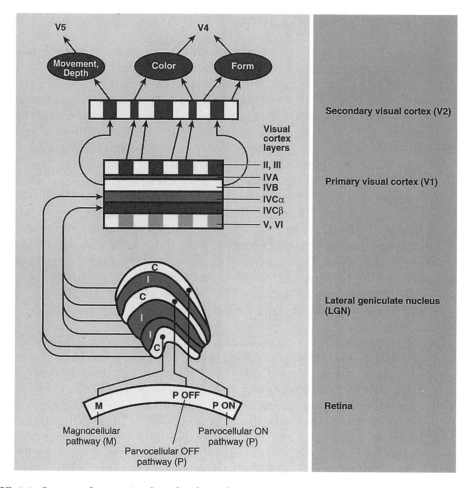

FIG. 2.8. Streams of processing for color, form, disparity, and movement between the retina and the visual cortex. The M pathway projects to the two lower layers of the lateral geniculate nucleus, next to layer IVC and then to layer IVB in the primary visual cortex. The signal is then passed to area V5 and the thick stripes in the secondary visual cortex. The P pathway projects to the upper four layers of the lateral geniculate nucleus with a preponderance of ON center cells in the upper two layers and OFF center cells in the middle two layers, and then to layer IVCß. The pathway splits into two streams; one deals with color, projecting from the blobs in layers II and III of the primary visual cortex to the thin stripes in the secondary visual cortex, and then to V4. The other deals with form, projecting from the interblob areas to the pale stripes in V2 and an area near V4. Input from the contralateral (C) retina is shown. Input from the ipsilateral (I) retina projects to the neighboring layers in the LGN.

by affecting attention and by directly inhibiting signals while saccadic eye movements are being made. The modulatory signals, and interactions between the visual cortex and lateral geniculate, are also responsible for the depolarization of lateral geniculate neurons that characterizes the transition from a state of sleep to a state of arousal (McCormick & Bal, 1997). Essentially, the function of the lateral geniculate nucleus is to gate signals going from the retina to the cortex, rather than to process them.

4. Function in the Visual Cortex

The visual cortex is the place where objects in and out of their visual context are analyzed in detail. For the analysis of form, there are cells that respond to the edges, curvature, and corners of objects. For the analysis of movement, there are cells that respond to the direction of movement, and to the direction of movement in relation to the background. For the analysis of color, there are cells that respond to wavelengths coming from an object in relation to wavelengths coming from objects nearby and to an average of the wavelengths from objects in other parts of the field of view.

The visual cortex is the first location in which signals from the two eyes converge onto a single cell. Signals from each eye in layer IV are kept largely separate in the adult, but the monocular cells in layer IV converge onto binocular cells in layers II, III, V, and VI. This is a statistical matter rather than an absolute matter—there are some binocular cells in layer IV and some monocular cells in layers II, III, V, and VI—but the tendency is clear. Consequently, visual cortex is the first location where one finds cells sensitive to disparity, that is, cells responding to objects nearer than the point of fixation and cells responding to objects further than the point of fixation (Poggio, Gonzalez, & Krause, 1988).

To a certain extent, form, color, movement, and disparity are dealt with by separate groups of cells. Because of this, layer IV, which is the input layer for the cortex, is more complicated in visual cortex than in any other area of cortex (Fig. 2.8). It is divided into sublayers IVA, IVB, IVCα, and IVCß. Projections from the movement cells in the magnocellular layers of the lateral geniculate come into layer IVCα, which projects to layer IVB. Layer IVB projects to secondary visual cortex (V2 and V5), and is therefore an output layer rather than an input layer. Cells in V2 that handle disparity also project on to V5, alias MT, which consequently deals with movement, disparity, and movement in depth (Zeki, 1978; Britten, 2004).

The cells in the parvocellular layers of the lateral geniculate, dealing with color and fine detail, project to layers IVCß and IVA (Fig. 2.8). These signals are analyzed further in other layers of the primary visual cortex. If one makes a horizontal section through primary visual cortex in layers III and II, and stains it for cytochrome oxidase, a mitochondrial enzyme that is found in areas of high metabolic activity, one finds patches of stain known as blobs. Color-coded cells without orientation selectivity are concentrated in the blobs, while the cells in the areas between the blobs respond to the orientation of an edge, and have less color selectivity (Livingstone & Hubel, 1984).

In the secondary visual cortex (V2), cells dealing with color, form, and disparity are also kept somewhat separate. If one stains V2 with cytochrome oxidase and cuts a horizontal section, one finds three sets of stripes: thick, thin, and pale stripes. The thin stripes process surface properties such as color and brightness, cells specific for disparity are concentrated in the thick stripes, and cells specific for orientation are concentrated in the pale stripes (Hubel & Livingstone, 1987; Roe, 2003). The thin stripes project to an area called V4, which deals particularly with color and form, and the thick stripes project to V5 and MST (DeYoe & van Essen, 1985). However, it should be emphasized that these concentrations of cells that process similar information and the projections described here are the predominant ones; there are also interconnections between the pathways for color, form, disparity, and movement (see Sincich & Horton, 2002; Ts'o, Roe, & Gilbert, 2001; Xiao & Felleman, 2004). This is to be expected because one can see, for example, depth, form, and movement in equiluminant color boundaries, although less easily than in luminance boundaries.

4.1. Columnar Organization of Cortex

The cerebral cortex is a two-dimensional sheet, 2 mm thick and with enough area to cover a large room. Within the 2-mm thickness, cells located above and below each other in the cortex tend to have similar properties. This is true in all parts of cortex, and was noticed first in the somatosensory cortex (Mountcastle, 1957), and later in the visual cortex of the cat (Hubel & Wiesel, 1962). Consequently the cortex is said to be organized into columns. The similar properties of the cells within a cortical column are most likely due to the arrangement of anatomical connections, which run primarily in a vertical direction.

In the monkey, there are columns for ocular dominance, color, and the orientation of edges (Livingstone & Hubel, 1984). While the cells in layers II, III, V, and VI tend to be binocular, they also tend to be dominated by one eye. A cell dominated by the left eye in layer II will tend to lie above axon terminals from the left eye in layer IV, and a cell dominated by the right eye in layer VI will tend to be below axon terminals from the right eye in layer IV, and so on. Color-coded cells in layer V or VI tend to lie under the blobs, which are located in layers III and II. When it comes to orientation, there are cells specific for vertical edges, for horizontal edges, and for a variety of orientations in between. Again, cells that lie in layers V and VI and are specific for vertical edges tend to be positioned below cells in layers II and III that are also specific for vertical edges. These cells are organized into *orientation columns.*

Every point in the field of view of each eye has to be analyzed for color and orientation, so the sets of columns overlap. The cytochrome oxidase blobs are lined up in the centers of the ocular dominance columns (Horton & Hubel, 1981; Fig. 2.9). The orientation columns are arranged around features, called pinwheels, which also tend to lie in the center of ocular dominance columns in both cat and monkey (Fig. 2.10). However, the centers of the pinwheels do not necessarily line up with the cytochrome oxidase blobs seen in the macaque (Bartfeld & Grinvald, 1992). The organization in the cat primary visual cortex is very like that of the macaque, except that color cells are absent (color-coded cells are mostly in the W cell projection, in the extrastriate pathway), so there are just two sets of overlapping columns for orientation and ocular dominance. The movement system, in area 17 of the primate, is an exception to the general rule of columnar processing; signals come in to layer IVCα, project to layer IVB, and then out of the primary visual cortex. However, this is the only known exception; in all other parts of cortex, processing is

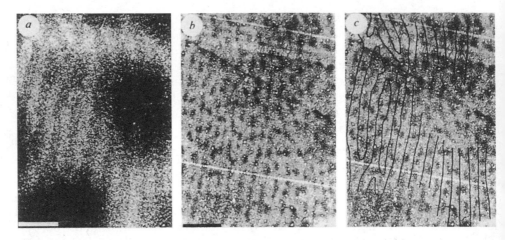

FIG. 2.9. (A) Dark-field autoradiograph of the striate cortex in a normal macaque showing ocular dominance columns. Section is tangential, grazing layer V (*dark ovals*) but passing mainly through layer IVC. (B) More superficial section from the same tissue block showing cytochrome oxidase patches. (C) Borders of the columns from (A) superimposed on (B). [Reprinted with permission from Horton, J. C., & Hubel, D. H. (1981). *Nature, 292*, 762.]

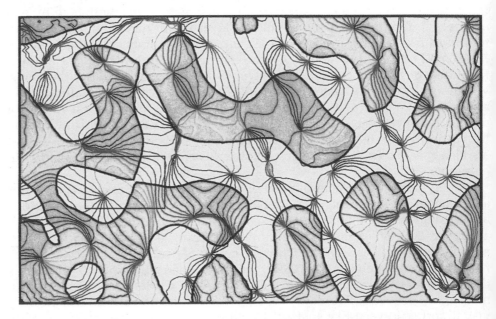

FIG. 2.10. Relationship between ocular dominance and orientation maps in the cat. Thick lines show the outlines of the ocular dominance columns. Thin lines join cells with the same orientation specificity. The pinwheels formed by these lines coming together tend to be centered on the ocular dominance columns. [Reprinted with permission from Hubener, M., et al. (1997). *Journal of Neuroscience, 17*, 9270–9284. Copyright 1997 Society for Neuroscience.]

columnar. A patch of cortex that contains the machinery to represent a single location in space (i.e., that analyzes signals in terms of ocular dominance, all colors, and all orientations) is known as a *hypercolumn*.

The visual properties dealt with in columns in V2 are not too different from the columnar properties of V1. As mentioned above, the thin stripes of cytochrome oxidase staining handle the surface properties of color and brightness, the pale stripes deal with orientation and form, and the thick stripes deal with disparity and movement. Most cells are driven binocularly—indeed a number can only be driven binocularly—so that in V2 ocular dominance is no longer a factor (Hubel & Livingstone, 1987). The thin stripes contain patches within which all colors are represented, arranged as they are in the spectrum (Xiao, Wang, & Felleman, 2003). The thick stripes contain columns for disparity, and both thick and pale stripes contain columns for orientation (Ts'o et al., 2001). Further details will undoubtedly emerge as more experiments are done.

Beyond V2, the parameters of the stimulus handled within columns is less clear. Obviously the parameters will change with the visual area because different visual areas deal with different properties of the stimulus. In V4, there may be separate columns for red, green, and blue (Zeki, 1977) although this is no longer certain. In V5, there are columns for direction of movement (Albright, Desimone, & Gross, 1984), for movement of objects in relation to the background as opposed to movement of the whole field of view (Born & Tootell, 1992), and for disparity (DeAngelis & Newsome, 1999). Further physiological details remain to be worked out in areas V4 and V5 and are completely unknown for the other 30 areas of the visual cortex, but every anatomical experiment that has been done shows punctate projections from one area to another, strongly suggesting the existence of columns everywhere.

5. Parallel Processing within the Visual System

It should be clear by now that different features of the visual stimulus are dealt with in parallel in the visual system. Signals for objects brighter than the background and signals for objects darker than the background are kept separate through four levels of processing—the bipolar cell, ganglion cell, lateral geniculate cell, and the first stage within V1—before being combined to analyze the orientation and direction of movement, independent of contrast (Fig. 2.8). Signals for color and for movement are partially separate through at least five levels of processing: the ganglion cell, lateral geniculate, V1, V2, and V4/V5. Signals for color and for form are partially separate through at least three levels of processing: V1, V2, and V4 (the area for processing form in the macaque at the level of V4 is still being identified, but it seems likely from deficits found in humans that there are separate areas for color and form at this level).

Very likely, parallel processing will continue to be found as higher levels of the cortex are analyzed. Depth perception remains to be worked out. Helmholtz listed a number of cues to depth perception, including disparity, convergence, accommodation, size, haze, interposition, and motion parallax. How the various cues to depth perception are analyzed and brought together is largely unknown. Cells sensitive for disparity are found in V1, in the thick stripes of V2, and in V3, V4, and V5. There are separate columns for near and far cells in V2, but how these are brought together with the other cues is largely unknown. Whatever the final details, it seems extremely likely that depth perception will be analyzed by columns in a parallel fashion because of the variety of cues that have to be evaluated and then combined.

6. Hierarchical Processing within the Visual System

What happens to the signals as they get transmitted within these parallel pathways and are processed along the way? The first experiments were done by Hubel and Wiesel (1962) and concerned the analysis of form in the cat. They recorded single cells in the visual cortex with a microelectrode in anesthetized paralyzed animals. Interestingly, the cells responded much more vigorously to bars and edges, particularly moving ones, than to lights turned on and off. There were cells that responded to orientation, with separate cells responding to lines brighter than the background and lines darker than the background. They called these *simple cells*, because their properties could be explained simply by input from a series of lateral geniculate cells lined up along the axis of the orientation (Fig. 2.11). They also found cells that responded to orientation independent of contrast, which they called *complex cells*, and proposed that they receive input from simple cells. The simple and complex cells responded to long bars, but other cells responded to short ones due to the influence of inhibitory signals, and these were called *hypercomplex*. Subsequently, investigators have found that the complex cells actually receive direct input from the lateral geniculate (see Stone, 1983), but the basic idea of a hierarchical organization in these cell types is nonetheless probably true.

Clearer evidence for a hierarchy of cell types comes from the color system (Daw, 1984). Photoreceptors converge onto the opponent color cells which

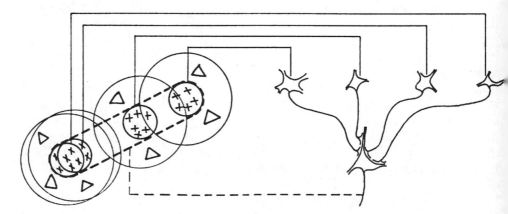

FIG. 2.11. Scheme for producing simple cells from the lateral geniculate input to the cortex. Four lateral geniculate cells with ON centers, positioned along a line, make excitatory connections with a cell in the cortex. The cortical cell will then respond to a line oriented along the 2 o'clock/8 o'clock axis. [Reprinted with permission from Hubel, D. H., & Wiesel, T. N. (1962). *Journal of Physiology*, *160*, 106–154. Blackwell Publishing.]

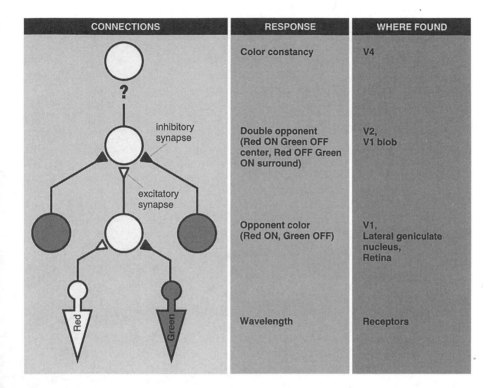

CONNECTIONS	RESPONSE	WHERE FOUND
	Color constancy	V4
inhibitory synapse	Double opponent (Red ON Green OFF center, Red OFF Green ON surround)	V2, V1 blob
excitatory synapse	Opponent color (Red ON, Green OFF)	V1, Lateral geniculate nucleus, Retina
Red Green	Wavelength	Receptors

FIG. 2.12. The first three stages in the processing of color vision. Red-absorbing cones excite bipolar cells and green cones inhibit them, to produce bipolar cells, ganglion cells, lateral geniculate cells, and cells in layer IVCß that give an ON response to red and an OFF response to green. Red ON, green OFF cells in the center of the receptive field excite the double opponent cell and red ON/green OFF cells in the surround inhibit it. This produces a cell that has an ON response to red and OFF response to green in the center, with an OFF response to red and ON response to green in the surround, because the sign of the response is reversed in the surround by the inhibitory synapse. Double opponent cells do not respond to uniform illumination (in the example illustrated, excitation from red in the center will be cancelled by inhibition from red in the periphery, and excitation from green in the periphery will be cancelled by inhibition from green in the center). Double opponent cells also do not respond to white light, because the input from the red receptors will be cancelled by the input from the green receptors. The synaptic organization between V1, V2, and V4 is not known, but the cells in V4 give a response that corresponds to object color constancy. *Open triangles* represent excitatory synapses, *solid triangles* inhibitory synapses.

respond positively to some wavelengths and negatively to others (see Fig. 2.12). Within the color system, bipolar cells, ganglion cells, lateral geniculate cells, and cells within layer IVCß of the cortex all include opponent color cells. At the next stage, in the blobs in V1, opponent color cells converge to form double opponent cells. These are cells that are opponent for color and also for space so that they respond to color contrasts and some spatial contrasts, but not to uniform illumination (see caption to Fig. 2.12). The response of a red/green double opponent cell to a grey spot in a green surround is the same as its response to a red spot in a grey surround; grey will activate both red and green receptors, with responses that will cancel each other, while red in the center and green in the surround will both excite the cell. Because a grey spot in a green surround appears reddish (this is called

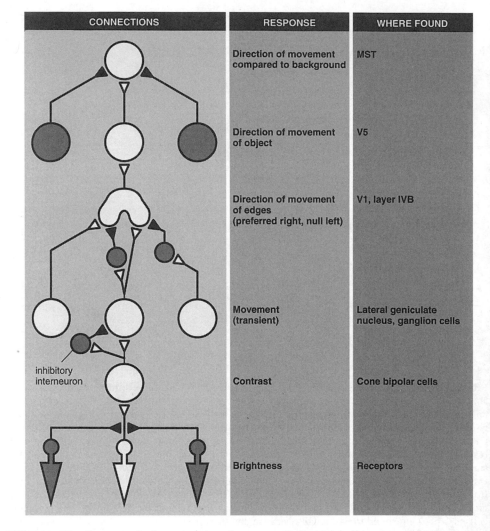

CONNECTIONS	RESPONSE	WHERE FOUND
	Direction of movement compared to background	MST
	Direction of movement of object	V5
	Direction of movement of edges (preferred right, null left)	V1, layer IVB
	Movement (transient)	Lateral geniculate nucleus, ganglion cells
inhibitory interneuron	Contrast	Cone bipolar cells
	Brightness	Receptors

FIG. 2.13. First five stages in the processing of movement information. Receptors respond to brightness and bipolar cells to contrast. Some circuit, perhaps a local inhibitory circuit, makes the response of the movement ganglion cells transient, and consequently the response of the movement lateral geniculate cells that follow them is also transient. Lateral inhibitory connections within the visual cortex reduce the response in one direction to produce direction-selective cells. The synaptic circuitry that produces a cell specific for the movement of the object, as opposed to the movement of the contours within the object, is not known, and is therefore left out. Presumably the direction of movement of the object in relation to its background is produced by excitatory connections from the direction-selective cells that process the object, and inhibitory connections from the direction-selective cells that process the background. *Open triangles* represent excitatory synapses, *solid triangles* inhibitory synapses.

simultaneous color contrast) double opponent cells explain the phenomenon of simultaneous color contrast (Daw, 1967).

Simultaneous color contrast is a local phenomenon, whereas object color constancy involves comparisons over a large part of the field of view. Cells in V1 have small receptive fields, whereas cells in V4 have large ones. Cells in V4 are affected by an average of the wavelengths coming from objects in a wide area of the field of view. Thus it seems likely that the double opponent cells in V1 converge onto cells in V2, and these converge again onto cells in V4 to give object color constancy (Zeki, 1983).

Evidence for a hierarchy of cell types is also clear in the movement system (Fig. 2.13). Cells in the magnocellular pathway in the retina and lateral geniculate respond to movement. In the primary visual cortex, one finds cells that respond to *direction* of movement; this response is generated because of lateral inhibitory connections that prevent the cell from responding to inappropriate directional movement. In V5, there are cells that respond to movement of the complete object, as opposed to movement of the individual contours of the object (Movshon, Adelson, Gizzi, & Newsome, 1985). There are also cells that respond to movement of an object in relation to the background, rather than movement of the object itself (Tanaka, Hikosaka, Saito, Yukie, Fukada, & Iwai, 1986; see Fig. 2.14). One can also distinguish first-order movement, defined by luminance, from second-order movement, defined by contrast. Functional magnetic resonance imaging (fMRI) studies in humans and data from brain lesions have demonstrated that first-order movement is computed in V1, whereas second-order movement is computed in higher visual areas (see Dumoulin, Baker, Hess, & Evans, 2003).

Stereoscopic depth perception is also arranged in a hierarchical fashion. The cells in V1 that are sensitive to disparity respond to absolute disparity. Cells in V2 and V5, on the other hand, respond to relative disparity (see Parker, 2004). Various behavioral and stimulation experiments show that V5 is involved in depth perception and in movement in depth. It seems likely, therefore, that V5 is the area where disparity cues and movement cues are brought together to produce a perception of the trajectory in space. However, the differences in receptive field properties between V2 and V5/MT and also between V5/MT and the areas that it projects to (MST and FST) remain to be detailed.

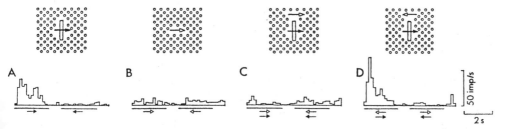

FIG. 2.14. Cell that responds to the movement of an object against the background. (A) Response to movement of bar. (B) Response to movement of background. (C) Response to movement of bar and background together in the same direction. (D) Response to movement of bar and background in opposite directions. Notice that movement of the bar against the background gives the largest response, and movement of the bar with the background gives little response. [Reprinted with permission from Tanaka, K., et al. (1986). *Journal of Neuroscience, 6,* 134–144. Copyright 1986, Society for Neuroscience.]

7. Summary

It is hoped that this brief summary will give an idea of how the visual system is organized. There are signal streams processed by cells that handle broad aspects of the visual input, with the details analyzed in parallel within the streams.

In the color stream, red/green, yellow/blue, and black/white aspects are processed in parallel. As one goes up the system, a comparison is first made between the long, medium, and short wavelength bands coming from a small area in the field of view. This is then compared with the wavelengths from the area in the immediate surround, and then with those from a large part of the field of view to create the perception of object color constancy.

In the form stream, objects lighter than the background and darker than the background are distinguished first. The orientation of edges and lines is analyzed, then the length of segments of the edges and lines. Finally, this analysis of an object's components has to be integrated into the perception of the object's form and shape.

In the movement stream, the response within the retina is transient, enabling movement to be detected. Lateral inhibitory connections operate on signals from the brighter-than-background pathway and from the darker-than-background pathway to give the direction of movement; these signals are then brought together to create the perception of direction of movement independent of contrast. Next, signals for the direction of movement of contours are combined to give the direction of movement of the whole object. Then the direction of movement of the object in relation to the background is distinguished from direction of movement of the object by itself.

In the depth system, disparity is detected immediately after signals from the two eyes come together in the cortex. There are cells specific for objects nearer than the fixation point and for objects further away than the fixation point. Disparity is actually a relative phenomenon, like brightness and color, and cells specific for relative disparity have been described in V2. However, how disparity is related to other cues about depth perception is unknown.

The concentration on streams of processing in this description is an oversimplification. For example, edges can be detected between two colored objects of equal luminance, showing that color signals enter the form pathway. Although some displays of stereopsis fail when one object is seen in relation to another of equal luminance, other displays succeed. Consequently, perception experiments suggest that there must be connections between the various streams and the anatomy proves that there are. However, the division of the visual system into streams of signal processing is a useful concept for understanding the overall organization.

References

Albright, T. D., Desimone, R., & Gross, C. G. (1984). Columnar organization of directionally selective cells in visual area MT of the macaque. *Journal of Neurophysiology, 51*, 16–31.

Bartfeld, E., & Grinvald, A. (1992). Relationships between orientation-preference pinwheels, cytochrome oxidase blobs, and ocular dominance columns in primate striate cortex. *Proceedings of the National Academy of Sciences of the United States of America, 89,* 11905–11909.

Born, R. T., & Tootell, R. H. (1992). Segregation of global and local motion processing in primate middle temporal visual area. *Nature, 357,* 497–499.

Boycott, B. B., & Dowling, J. E. (1969). Organization of the primate retina: light microscopy. *Philosophical Transaction of the Royal Society of London. Series B. Biological sciences, 255,* 109–184.

Britten, K. H. (2004). The middle temporal area: motion processing and the link to perception. In L. M. Chalupa & J. S. Werner (Eds.), *The Visual Neurosciences* (pp. 1203–1216). Cambridge, MA: MIT Press.

Cleland, B. G., & Levick, W. R. (1974). Properties of rarely encountered types of ganglion cells in the cat's retina and an overall classification. *Journal of Physiology, 240,* 457–492.

Dacey, D. M. (2000). Parallel pathways for spectral coding in primate retina. *Annual Review of Neuroscience, 23,* 743–775.

Daw, N. W. (1967). Goldfish retina: organization for simultaneous color contrast. *Science, 158,* 942–944.

Daw, N. W. (1984). The psychology and physiology of colour vision. *Trends in Neurosciences, 7,* 330–336.

DeAngelis, G. C., & Newsome, W. T. (1999). Organization of disparity-selective neurons in macaque area MT. *Journal of Neuroscience, 19,* 1398–1415.

De Monasterio, F. M., & Gouras, P. (1975). Functional properties of ganglion cells of the rhesus monkey retina. *Journal of Physiology, 251,* 167–195.

DeYoe, E. A., & Van Essen, D. C. (1985). Segregation of efferent connections and receptive field properties in visual area V2 of the macaque. *Nature, 317,* 58–61.

Dumoulin, S. O., Baker, C. L., Hess, R. F., & Evans, A. C. (2003). Cortical specialization for processing first- and second-order motion. *Cerebral Cortex, 13,* 1375–1385.

Enroth-Cugell, C., & Robson, J. G. (1966). The contrast sensitivity of retinal ganglion cells of the cat. *Journal of Physiology, 187,* 517–552.

Famiglietti, E. V., & Kolb, H. (1976). Structural basis for ON- and OFF-center responses in retinal ganglion cells. *Science, 194,* 193–195.

Horton, J. C., & Hubel, D. H. (1981). Regular patchy distribution of cytochrome oxidase staining in primary visual cortex of macaque monkey. *Nature, 292,* 762–764.

Hubel, D. H., & Wiesel, T. N. (1962). Receptive fields, binocular interaction and functional architecture in the cat's visual cortex. *Journal of Physiology, 160,* 106–154.

Hubel, D. H., & Livingstone, M. S. (1987). Segregation of form, color, and stereopsis in primate area 18. *Journal of Neuroscience, 7,* 3378–3415.

Hubener, M., Shoham, D., Grinvald, A., & Bonhoeffer, T. (1997). Spatial relationships among three columnar systems in cat area 17. *Journal of Neuroscience, 17,* 9270–9284.

Kaufman, L. (1974). *Sight and mind.* New York: Oxford University Press.

Kuffler, S. W. (1953). Discharge patterns and functional organization of mammalian retina. *Journal of Neurophysiology, 16,* 37–68.

Livingstone, M. S., & Hubel, D. H. (1984). Anatomy and physiology of a color system in the primate visual cortex. *Journal of Neuroscience, 4,* 309–356.

McCormick, D. A., & Bal, T. (1997). Sleep and arousal: thalamocortical mechanisms. *Annual Review of Neuroscience, 20,* 185–215.

Mountcastle, V. B. (1957). Modality and topographic properties of single neurons of cat's somatic sensory cortex. *Journal of Neurophysiology, 20,* 408–434.

Movshon, J. A., Adelson, E. H., Gizzi, M. S., & Newsome, W. T. (1985). The analysis of moving visual patterns. In C. Chaga, R. Gattass, & C. Gross (Eds.), *Pattern recognition mechanisms* (pp. 117–151). Vatican City: Pontifical Academy of Sciences.

Parker, A. J. (2004). From binocular disparity to the perception of stereoscopic depth. In L. M. Chalupa, & J. S. Werner (Eds.), *The visual neurosciences* (pp. 779–792). Cambridge, MA: MIT Press.

Pasupathy, A., & Connor, C. E. (2002). Population coding of shape in area V4. *Nature Neuroscience, 5,* 1332–1338.

Poggio, G. F., Gonzalez, F., & Krause, F. (1988). Stereoscopic mechanisms in monkey visual cortex: binocular correlation and disparity selectivity. *Journal of Neuroscience, 8,* 4531–4550.

Polyak, S. L. (1941). *The retina.* Chicago: University of Chicago Press.

Roe, A. W. (2003). Modular complexity of area V2 in the macaque monkey. In C. Collins, & J. H. Kaas (Eds.), *The primate visual system* (pp. 109–138). New York: CRC Press.

Rosenquist, A. C. (1985). Connections of visual cortical areas in the cat. In A. Peters, & E. G. Jones (eds.), *Cerebral cortex* (pp. 81–117). New York: Plenum.

Schiller, P. H., & Malpeli, J. G. (1977). Properties and tectal projections of monkey ganglion cells. *Journal of Neurophysiology, 40,* 428–445.

Sherman, S. M., & Koch, C. (1986). The control of retinogeniculate transmission in the mammalian lateral geniculate nucleus. *Experimental Brain Research, 63,* 1–20.

Sincich, L. C., & Horton, J. C. (2002). Divided by cytochrome oxidase: a map of the projections from V1 to V2 in macaques. *Science, 295,* 1734–1737.

Stone, J. (1983). *Parallel processing in the visual system.* New York: Plenum Press.

Stone, J., & Fukuda, Y. (1974). Properties of cat retinal ganglion cells: a comparison of W-cells with X- and Y-cells. *Journal of Neurophysiology, 37,* 722–748.

Tanaka, K., Hikosaka, K., Saito, H. E., Yukie, M., Fukada, Y., & Iwai, E. (1986). Analysis of local and wide-field movements in the superior temporal visual areas of the macaque monkey. *Journal of Neuroscience, 6,* 134–144.

Ts'o, D. Y., Roe, A. W., & Gilbert, C. D. (2001). A hierarchy of the functional organization for color, form and disparity in primate visual area V2. *Vision Research, 41,* 1333–1349.

Ungerleider, L. G., & Pasternak, T. (2004). Ventral and dorsal cortical processing streams. In L. M. Chalupa, & J. S. Werner (Eds.), *The visual neurosciences* (pp. 541–562). Cambridge, MA: MIT Press.

Van Essen, D. C., Anderson, C. H., & Felleman, D. J. (1992). Information processing in the primate visual system: an integrated systems perspective. *Science, 255,* 419–423.

Werblin, F. S., & Dowling, J. E. (1969). Organization of the retina of the mudpuppy, *Necturus maculosus.* II. Intracellular recording. *Journal of Neurophysiology, 32,* 339–355.

Wiesel, T. N., & Hubel, D. H. (1966). Spatial and chromatic interactions in the lateral geniculate body of the rhesus monkey. *Journal of Neurophysiology, 29,* 1115–1156.

Xiao, Y. P., Wang, Y., & Felleman, D. J. (2003). A spatially organized representation of colour in macaque cortical area V2. *Nature, 421,* 535–539.

Xiao, Y. P., & Felleman, D. J. (2004). Projections from primary visual cortex to cytochrome oxidase thin stripes and interstripes of macaque visual area 2. *Proceedings of the National Academy of Sciences of the United States of America, 101,* 7147–7151.

Zeki, S. M. (1977). Colour coding in the superior temporal sulcus of the rhesus monkey visual cortex. *Proceedings of the Royal Society of London. Series B. Biological sciences, 197,* 195–223.

Zeki, S. M. (1978). Uniformity and diversity of structure and function in rhesus monkey prestriate visual cortex. *Journal of Physiology, 277,* 273–290.

Zeki, S. M. (1983). Colour coding in the cerebral cortex: the reaction of cells in monkey visual cortex to wavelengths and colours. *Neuroscience, 9,* 741–765.

I

Development of the Visual System

3

Development of Visual Capabilities

Infants can see at birth. They can imitate mouth opening, as opposed to tongue protrusion, within a few hours (Salapatek & Cohen, 1987). While they may not discriminate their mother's face reliably from a stranger's face unless voice is present, they do look at their mother for longer than the stranger. They may not look their mother in the eye until 2 months of age, but this is because they are inspecting the external features of the face, such as the chin and hairline, rather than internal features, such as the eyes. All of this shows a substantial amount of visual perception at birth, and some control of eye movements. What develops after birth is a refinement of these properties.

The development of visual capabilities over the first few months is a coordinated matter involving sensory and motor aspects. Indeed, looking at objects is very much a sensory–motor activity. To put it briefly, the adult visual system can be thought of as three systems—noticing, moving the eyes, and inspecting. We notice objects in the peripheral field of view, and move the eyes with a saccadic movement to look at them if they demand attention. We converge the eyes to look at nearby objects, and diverge them to look at objects far away, so that the images in the two eyes can be fused into a single perception. Then we use the central part of the field of view to inspect objects and analyze their form, color, and distance in relation to other objects. Even the inspection of an object involves some eye movements because images that remain stationary on the retina fade away. To avoid this, the eyes drift slowly across the object, interspersed with small jerks called *microsaccades*. Fixation of one's gaze on an object is therefore an active process rather than a passive one.

Thus, improvement of the ability to see fine detail in an object depends on the ability to keep one's eyes tightly fixated on it. Likewise, improvement in binocular function goes hand-in-hand with the ability to converge or diverge one's eyes to look at the object. There is a cycle in the system: better sensory capability leads to more accurate eye movements leads to better sensory capability and so on.

Before dealing with the development of responses to visual stimuli, we need to ask: is the image on the infant retina a clear one? Is the limiting step in the analysis of the image its clarity, or its processing within the nervous system? The infant retina can be seen clearly with an ophthalmoscope. There do not appear to be any optical aberrations in the cornea or lens that would degrade the image substantially. The surfaces of the lens and cornea grow along with the eye, so that objects remain in focus for most children (Howland, 1993). Most infants have astigmatism—a cylindrical component to the focusing of the image on the retina—so that lines along one axis are in focus while lines along the perpendicular axis are not. However, this effect is probably too small in most cases to have perceptual consequences and is greatly reduced in amount or eliminated in the first year.

At 2 weeks of age, infants have some ability to focus their eyes on objects at different distances, and this ability increases during their first 3 months (Banks, 1980). There are several cues that adults use for accommodation, for example, blur, vergence (see Glossary), chromatic aberration, and disparity (see Glossary). We do not know which ones are used by young infants, except that disparity cannot be used soon after birth because it does not develop until later. The need for infants to accommodate is much less than that of adults. Their acuity is less than one tenth that of adults, so that they cannot detect whether an object is in or out of focus as well as an adult can. The fact that they do not make large accommodative efforts is due to lack of need as much as to lack of ability.

Thus, with the exception of some astigmatism, the image that falls on the infant retina is a clear one, and the infant can make adjustments for objects at different distances. Therefore, as vision develops, it is not the optics of the eyeball that develop as much as it is the properties of the photoreceptors, the retina, and the central visual system.

1. Methods for Studying Infant Vision

The history of the investigation of infant vision is a history of techniques as much as a history of discoveries. Infants cannot talk and are often inattentive. Two types of response have been monitored: gross electrophysiological responses, such as the visual evoked potential (VEP) and the electroretinogram (ERG), and eye movement responses, such as fixation on an object of interest and optokinetic nystagmus (OKN). As pointed out above, sensory and motor capabilities develop in tandem, so that an infant may not look at an object even though s/he sees it. In the case of electrophysiological responses, gross measurements represent the average of the firing of all the neurons involved. As a result, these measurements may underestimate the infant's real visual capabilities. It is a tribute to the care and skill of the investigators that the results from the various techniques, each with their own inherent limitations, agree quite well with each other. Modeling has also shown that some results are close to a theoretical limit for infant vision, suggesting that the results obtained are close to the actual visual capabilities.

In studying infant vision, psychologists have been concerned with a quantitative or psychophysical measurement of what infants see. As an example, consider acuity: This is measured in the eye doctor's office by looking at letters of the alphabet. If a person sees a letter at 6 meters that a normal person could see at 12 meters, they are said to have an acuity of 6/12 (Snellen acuity). Infants cannot read letters, so a grating (a pattern of black and white lines) is presented instead, and a technique is used to detect whether the infant can discriminate the grating from a uniform grey stimulus. The investigator then varies the spatial frequency of the grating, which is measured in cycles/degree (a measure of the number of lines in the grating that fit into 1° of visual angle as seen by the observer). 6/6 vision corresponds to 30 cycles per degree.

The technique most frequently used is called the *forced-choice preferential looking procedure* (FPL). This depends on the propensity of infants to look at an interesting display more often than a less interesting display. An infant is seated looking at two displays with a peephole between them (Teller, 1977). An observer, who does not know which display is which, decides whether the infant looks more at the left display or the right display (Fig. 3.1). The

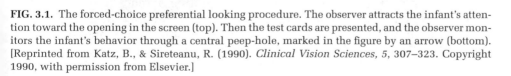

FIG. 3.1. The forced-choice preferential looking procedure. The observer attracts the infant's attention toward the opening in the screen (top). Then the test cards are presented, and the observer monitors the infant's behavior through a central peep-hole, marked in the figure by an arrow (bottom). [Reprinted from Katz, B., & Sireteanu, R. (1990). *Clinical Vision Sciences, 5*, 307–323. Copyright 1990, with permission from Elsevier.]

position of the interesting display is changed to left or right in a random order. A positive result (the records from the observer show that the infant is looking at the interesting display more often than the other more than 75% of the time) is significant, but a negative result could be due to inattentiveness on the part of the infant or inexperience on the part of the observer rather than failure of the infant to discriminate the displays.

Also used quite frequently is the VEP. This is an electrical potential recorded from the scalp of the infant by electrodes placed over the visual cortex. The infant does not have to be paying attention for this technique to work, but does need to fixate and accommodate, and the stimulus has to be one that will activate enough neurons in the cortex in synchrony that their combined activity shows up as an electrical change on the surface. Some investigators have been quite ingenious in devising stimuli that get good results with this technique.

Other methods have been used for particular studies. The ERG is a potential recorded between the cornea and the skin that represents the summed activity of cells in the retina. Thus, it can only be used to study properties of the retina, such as dark adaptation (see below). Optokinetic nystagmus is an oscillation of the eyes produced when looking at a stimulus slowly moving in one direction. The eyes follow the stimulus, and then flick back in the reverse direction with a saccadelike movement. Optokinetic nystagmus is believed to be primarily a subcortical phenomenon and needs a large stimulus covering a substantial amount of the visual field. Both these procedures are therefore of limited utility.

All these techniques have been primarily useful in testing discriminative ability and demonstrating changes in properties that can be quantified, such as acuity and stereopsis. When it comes to what the infant sees, we are still often at a loss. We can study wavelength discrimination but not very much about color vision. If, as seems likely, a child can recognize the faces of its mother and father long before it can say "Mama" and "Dada," we can only guess at many aspects of infant visual perception.

2. Development of Monocular Vision

In spite of all the problems with the techniques that are listed above, many visual properties have been studied successfully. For monocular vision, this includes acuity, contrast sensitivity, increment thresholds, adaptation, spectral sensitivity, perception of direction and orientation, and vernier acuity (see Glossary).

2.1. Acuity

This property is usually studied with a grating of black and white lines. When FPL is used, the infant is presented with a choice of a grating (the interesting stimulus) or a uniform stimulus of the same luminance (see stimuli in Fig. 3.1). The limit of acuity is represented by the finest grating that can be distinguished reliably from the uniform stimulus. When the VEP is measured,

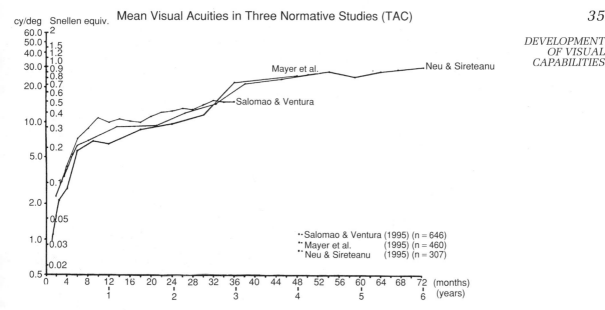

cy/deg Snellen equiv. Mean Visual Acuities in Three Normative Studies (TAC)

Salomao & Ventura (1995) (n = 646)
Mayer et al.   (1995) (n = 460)
Neu & Sireteanu (1995) (n = 307)

FIG. 3.2. Improvement of acuity with age, with comparison of data from three studies covering birth to 6 years of age, using Teller acuity cards as in Figure 3.1. [Reprinted with permission from Sireteanu, R. (2000). In *Handbook of brain and behaviour in human development* (pp. 629–652.)]

the most successful stimulus is a sweep stimulus (Norcia & Tyler, 1985). The contrast of the grating is reversed at 12 cycles/s, and the spatial frequency is incremented (swept) every 0.5 s, so that several spatial frequencies can be recorded in a short period of time.

There are some differences between the numbers generated by different experimenters and different techniques, but the agreement is actually quite remarkable. There is a large improvement found in all cases between birth and 6 months of age, from 1 to 3 cycles/degree (less than 20/200) to about 10 cycles/degree (20/60), and some further improvement after that (Teller, 1997; Sireteanu, 2000; Fig. 3.2).

A large part of the development of acuity can be explained by changes that occur in the retina in the size, shape, and distribution of photoreceptors and in the optics of the eye (Banks & Bennett, 1988). The eye is shorter, back to front, in the newborn, and the pupil is smaller; consequently, the image on the retina falls on a smaller area. The photoreceptors—and here we are concerned with the cone photoreceptors in the fovea, which is the region of highest acuity— are wider in the newborn (more than 6 μm, compared to 1.9 μm in the adult; see Fig. 3.3), so that they are spaced further apart (Yuodelis & Hendrickson, 1986). The outer segment of each individual photoreceptor is shorter and absorbs less light. These factors combine to predict a substantial improvement in acuity with age, as the percentage of the light falling on the photoreceptor that is absorbed increases and the width of an object that is covered by a single photoreceptor is reduced. However, the prediction is incomplete. Whereas acuity in the adult is close to the theoretical limit imposed by the properties of the eye and its photoreceptors, acuity in the newborn is not. There must be,

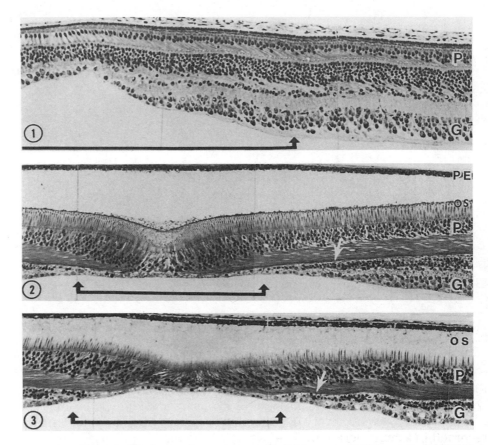

FIG. 3.3. Development of the human fovea. Ages are: birth (1); 45 months (2), and 72 years (3). Note that the rod-free area, marked by the *black arrows*, becomes smaller, and the cone outer segments in the fovea become narrower and longer. [Reprinted from Yuodelis, C., & Henrickson, A. E. (1986). *Vision Research, 26*, 847–855. Copyright 1986, with permission from Elsevier.]

in addition, some factors in the neural networks beyond the photoreceptors that restrict newborn acuity to a value less than the theoretical limit. These will be discussed in Chapter 5.

Acuity can also be measured with letters in a line, which is known as Snellen acuity. Such letters are less distinguishable than letters seen by themselves because the neighboring letters interfere with each other's visibility—a phenomenon known as crowding (Irvine, 1948). Snellen acuity continues to develop after 5 years of age (Simons, 1983). With a separation between the letters of 2.6′ of arc, acuity does not reach adult levels until 10 years of age (Hohmann & Haase, 1982).

2.2. Contrast Sensitivity

Sensitivity to contrast is a property that has been used to analyze several different aspects of the visual system. How sensitivity to contrast varies with spatial frequency can be seen in a display of sinusoidal stripes that vary in

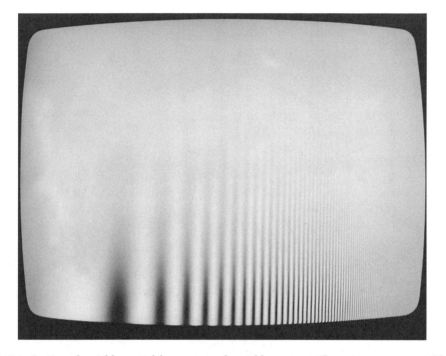

FIG. 3.4. Grating of variable spatial frequency and variable contrast. The stripes are most visible in the middle, less visible on the left edge, and invisible on the right edge. (Photograph provided by John Robson.)

spatial frequency along one axis and in contrast along the orthogonal axis (Fig. 3.4). At high spatial frequencies, the stripes cannot be seen, no matter how high the contrast. At medium spatial frequencies, quite low contrasts can be seen—less than 1% of the overall luminance. At low spatial frequencies, a larger contrast is needed for visibility than at medium spatial frequencies (this is called *low frequency fall-off*).

In experiments with infants, the subject is presented with a grating of uniform spatial frequency and contrast and observed to see if the stripes are being detected. The lowest contrast that can be seen at each spatial frequency is recorded and a curve is generated (Fig. 3.5). This curve is an accurate measurement of the positions where the stripes become invisible in Figure 3.4, which can be seen and traced approximately by hand. Needless to say, the actual experimental procedure is time consuming and getting the results is a slow process, particularly when working with infants.

The place where the curve meets the horizontal axis represents the finest grating that can be seen in any circumstances. This reading therefore corresponds to grating acuity. The peak of the curve shows the lowest contrast that can be detected at any spatial frequency. The fact that the curve drops at low spatial frequencies can be attributed to neural mechanisms that are designed to sharpen the response to pattern, such as inhibitory lateral influences, because a stripe that is wide enough to activate lateral inhibition will produce a reduced response. Consequently, the position of the peak of the curve on

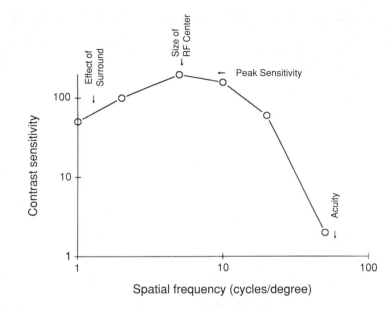

FIG. 3.5. Contrast sensitivity curve. For the significance of the various points on the curve, see the text.

the horizontal axis gives a reading of how wide a stripe has to be to induce the summation of excitatory influences without activating significant lateral inhibition as well.

All parts of the contrast sensitivity curve change with age (Atkinson, Braddick, & Moar, 1977; see Fig. 3.6). The high frequency cut-off changes as predicted from acuity measurements. The contrast that can be detected gets lower as the infant gets older for all spatial frequencies. The low frequency fall-off becomes more pronounced with age. Also, the position of the peak of the curve shifts to higher spatial frequency with age. Use of the VEP, combined with a sweep stimulus that reduces the time required to accumulate data, gives higher sensitivity in young subjects, but the tendencies are the same (Norcia, Tyler, & Hamer, 1990).

Many of these changes can be predicted, as can acuity changes, by the development of the cones in the fovea (Banks & Bennett, 1988; Wilson, 1988). The cones become longer with age, as well as narrower (Yuodelis & Hendrickson, 1986). In addition, the efficiency with which the inner segment funnels light into the outer segment increases. Both these morphological alterations increase the efficiency of the cones' light catching ability, and consequently increase the contrast sensitivity.

There are three processes at work in the development of contrast sensitivity, each with a different time course: overall contrast sensitivity, contrast sensitivity at high spatial frequencies, and the low frequency fall-off. Between birth and 10 weeks of age, contrast sensitivity improves at all spatial frequencies (Norcia et al., 1990). Improvement at high spatial frequencies is rapid, continuing until 4 years of age (Adams & Courage, 2002). Improvement at

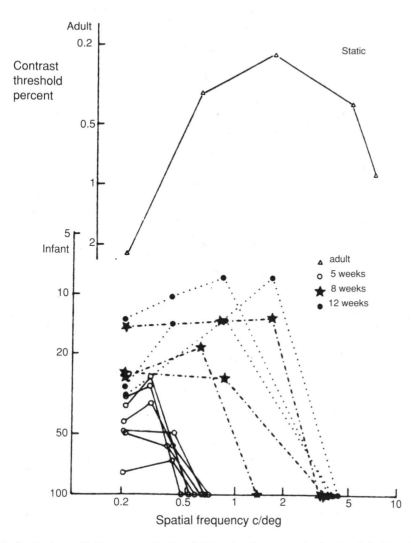

FIG. 3.6. Contrast sensitivity curves at 5, 8, and 12 weeks of age compared with adult. Data obtained from individual subjects by VEP. [Reprinted from Atkinson, J., et al. (1977), *Vision Research, 17,* 1037–1044. Copyright 1977, with permission from Elsevier.]

low spatial frequencies is slower, but goes on for longer, until 9 years of age (Adams & Courage, 2002).

These three processes can be attributed to different mechanisms (Wilson, 1988). Overall sensitivity is due largely to the increase in the length of the photoreceptors and the increase in funneling capacity. Increased sensitivity at high spatial frequencies is due to packing of the foveal cones closer together as well as the increase in the percentage of the photons caught. The psychophysical results therefore suggest that the increase in the length of the cones should be over around 10 weeks of age, and the increase in their packing density should continue after that. Unfortunately the number of human retinas that have been studied is few, so that further work is needed to establish whether the time course of the development of the two relevant morphological properties matches the psychophysical properties appropriately. The lateral inhibitory mechanisms that explain the low frequency fall-off and their development will be discussed in Chapter 5.

2.2.1. Spatial Frequency Channels

The overall contrast sensitivity curve in the adult is made up of several channels that are sensitive to different spatial frequencies. These channels presumably correspond to cells that are tuned to different spatial frequencies. For example, cells in the P pathway respond to finer spatial frequencies than cells in the M pathway. The existence of spatial frequency channels can be revealed by adaptation or masking experiments. In a typical adaptation experiment, the subject looks at a particular spatial frequency for a period of time, and afterward the sensitivity for that spatial frequency and ones near it is reduced, while the sensitivity for higher and lower spatial frequencies is not. The experiment is similar to a color adaptation experiment where the cones are tuned to different wavelengths; stimulation of the red cones makes them less sensitive, so the blue and green ones become relatively more sensitive. Spatial frequency adaptation experiments done in infants suggest that spatial frequency channels exist at an early age. This can be demonstrated at 6 weeks of age (Fiorentini, Pirchio, & Spinelli, 1983) with a larger effect at 12 weeks (Banks, Stephens, & Hartmann, 1985). Whether all spatial frequency channels are there at birth and whether some develop faster than others is not known, which is not surprising because we do not know precisely how many spatial frequency channels there are in the adult.

2.2.2. Spectral Sensitivity and Wavelength Discrimination

Spectral sensitivity is affected by the growth in the length of the photoreceptors which, as we have discussed, results in an increase in the percentage of photons absorbed. Rod photoreceptors show a threefold increase in their length (Drucker & Hendrickson, 1989). As a result, sensitivity in dim light is 1.7 log units below adult at 1 month of age, and one log unit below adult at 3 months of age, as measured by the preferential-looking technique (Teller & Bornstein, 1987). Cone photoreceptors grow in length similarly, so spectral sensitivity in the light-adapted state for the two-month infant is also about 10 times less than for an adult (Teller & Bornstein, 1987). The shape of the curve is approximately the same in infants and adults, but there is a greater contribution at short wavelengths in some infants. This may be due to optical properties of the eye rather than to an increased contribution from the blue cones (Teller & Bornstein, 1987).

Infants can distinguish red from white at 2 months of age. They have both red and green cone pigments, as shown by Rayleigh matches, where a spectral yellow is matched to a mixture of spectral red and green (when both red and green pigments are present, a specific ratio of spectral red to spectral green is required; when only one pigment is present, a wide variety of ratios is acceptable). The blue cone pigment is also present; discriminations that use the blue cone pigment can be made, but are poor. Wavelength discrimination and saturation discrimination are poor compared with the adult (Teller & Bornstein, 1987), and this can also be explained by the smaller percentage of photons caught by the photoreceptors (Banks & Bennett, 1988). Thus infants have red-, green-, and blue-absorbing cone pigments and a normal pigment in the rods just as in the adult, but their discriminative ability and sensitivity are poorer due to the shorter length of the photoreceptors.

2.2.3. Dark Adaptation

It takes over half an hour for adults to get used to very dim light, and this is due to the long time required for the rod pigment to regenerate. This adaptation to the dark can be measured by changes in the diameter of the pupil, and by measuring the threshold for a criterion level of ERG. The time course in infants is the same as in the adult—about 400 s (Hansen & Fulton, 1986, Fulton & Hansen, 1987), so one concludes that the kinetics of the infant rod pigment are the same as in the adult.

2.3. Vernier Acuity

Vernier acuity is the ability to detect breaks in a line. In the adult, vernier acuity is about 10 times better than grating acuity; that is, if the grating itself can be detected with lines spaced x minutes apart, the break will be detected with a displacement of $x/10$ min. Shimojo and Held (1987) investigated vernier acuity in 2- and 3-month old infants, and found that whereas vernier acuity is better than grating acuity in the adult, it is worse than grating acuity in the infant before 11 to 12 weeks of age (for their stimulus, see Fig. 3.7). Thus, vernier acuity develops more rapidly than grating acuity with a crossover at this age.

This rapid change may seem surprising, but there is an explanation. Vernier acuity increases faster than grating acuity with luminance, as predicted by Banks and Bennett (1988) from theoretical considerations. One would therefore expect infant vernier acuity to improve faster than grating acuity as the percentage of photons absorbed by the photoreceptors increases with age. In addition, vernier acuity is processed by modules of neurons that are located in the cortex. Vernier acuity falls off faster than grating acuity as one moves the stimulus away from the fovea. Both retinal (Banks, Sekuler, & Anderson, 1991) and cortical (Levi, Klein, & Aitsebaomo, 1985) factors contribute to this. Poor sampling by cortical neurons in infants could therefore contribute to poor vernier acuity (Shimojo & Held, 1987). Thus, there are two factors involved—improvement in the sensitivity of the photoreceptors and maturation of the visual cortex—and they both contribute to the rapid increase of vernier acuity compared with grating acuity.

Skoczenski and Norcia (2002) have measured vernier acuity and grating acuity over a wide range of ages using the VEP. They show, in agreement with previous authors (Carkeet, Levi, & Manny, 1997), that vernier acuity continues to develop for some time after grating acuity has reached a steady level

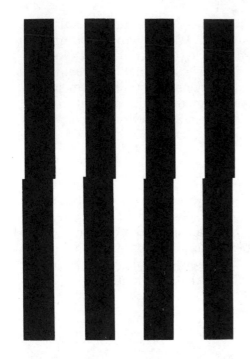

FIG. 3.7. Stimulus used to test vernier acuity in infants. [Reprinted from Shimojo, S., & Held, R. (1987). *Vision Research, 27*, 77–86. Copyright 1987, with permission from Elsevier.]

(Fig. 3.8). They used stationary gratings to avoid any confusion with movement. On the other hand, the level of acuity reached in teenagers was less than that seen in other studies, perhaps due to the use of VEPs. In any case, it is clear that there are processes, probably in the visual cortex, that allow vernier acuity to become finer for several years after grating acuity has obtained adult values.

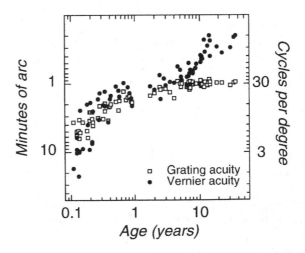

FIG. 3.8. Individual grating acuity and vernier acuity thresholds as a function of age. Each observer contributed a pair of measurements. The ordinate plots acuity in arc minutes (left axis) or in cycles per degree (right axis). [Reprinted from Skoczenski, A. M., & Norcia, A. M. (2002). *Psychological Science, 13*, 537–541. Copyright 2002 Blackwell Publishing Ltd.]

2.3.1. Orientation, Direction, and Movement Sensitivity

Orientation discrimination depends very much on the stimulus and technique used. Newborn infants can discriminate the orientation of a stimulus if they are habituated to one orientation, then presented with a choice of two orientations side by side (Slater, Morison, & Summers, 1988). The discrimination is not made if the test orientations are presented sequentially. Results with a dynamic stimulus and the VEP show some development after birth (Braddick, Wattam-Bell, & Atkinson, 1986). The dynamic stimulus consisted of a grating jittering 25 times per second in one orientation, followed by the same jitter in the perpendicular orientation. Three reversals of orientation per second give a noticeable response at 3 weeks of age, and eight reversals of orientation at 6 weeks of age. Clearly the infant has the cortical apparatus to detect orientations at birth, but this needs to mature before it can be seen clearly in a gross response such as the VEP.

Direction-specific responses must also be present at birth, because the newborn exhibits OKN. To detect the direction of movement to generate OKN, direction-specific cells are needed. However, like orientation-specific responses, they do not show up in the VEP until later on. Numerous different stimuli and procedures have been used to measure the development of movement responses. A summary as of 1996 is shown in Figure 3.9, which plots the threshold velocity in various experiments as a function of age from 6 to

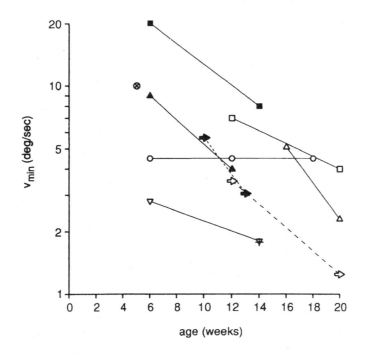

FIG. 3.9. Decrease in velocity threshold with age. Data with *arrows* and *broken lines* involved tasks that required direction discrimination, while the remainder involved discrimination between moving and static patterns. [Reprinted from Wattam-Bell, J. (1996). *Infant vision* (pp. 79–94). Copyright 1996 Blackwell Publishing Ltd.]

20 weeks of age (Wattam-Bell, 1996). Almost no studies have followed the responses of both infants and children to show the entire developmental time course, and at what age development is complete. Giaschi and Regan (1997) measured responses to movement of dots in a letter and found development of the sensitivity complete at 7 to 8 years of age, but did not test ages earlier than 3 to 4 years. Part of the problem is that different techniques and procedures are appropriate at different ages. In macaque monkeys, sensitivity to motion continues to develop for some time after contrast sensitivity has reached a plateau, so a similar result might be expected from humans (Kiorpes & Movshon, 2004).

It is interesting to compare responses to an OKN stimulus with responses to movement by preferential looking procedures (Mason, Braddick, & Wattam-Bell, 2003). Thresholds for the OKN response did not vary between 8 and 26 weeks of age, but there was a significant drop in adult levels. Thresholds for the preferential looking response dropped between 8 and 26 weeks of age followed by a smaller drop between 26 weeks and adult. Thresholds for OKN were lower than those for preferential looking at all ages. The hypothesis from these results is that OKN reflects a subcortical response and preferential looking a cortical response and these have different mechanisms and different time courses of development.

2.4. Contour Integration

Contour integration is a task in which the observer is asked to detect a circle of Gabor patches (see Glossary) in a display of patches of all orientations (Fig. 3.10). The circle is presented with varying amounts of noise, and the measurement is the amount of noise that can be tolerated while the discrimination can still be made. There is significant improvement in this task between 5 and 14 years of age (Kovacs, Kozma, Feher, & Benedek, 1999). Experiments in macaque monkeys show that the discrimination cannot be made at all before 20 weeks of age, when acuity is close to adult levels, and discrimination continues to improve after acuity has reached adult levels (Kiorpes & Bassin, 2003; see Fig. 3.11). This is clearly a phenomenon that matures late.

2.4.1. Vision in the Periphery of the Visual Field

Infants do not see very well in the periphery of their visual fields. The extent of the visual field is measured by perimetry, and results with three different methods are shown in Figure 3.12 (Dobson, Brown, Harvey, & Narter, 1998). The method that gives the widest results is white sphere kinetic perimetry (WSKP), where a white sphere is moved slowly from peripheral to central vision, and jiggled perpendicular to the path as it is moved. At 3 months of age, infants do not notice the sphere until it is 40° from the fovea in the temporal field. This is true whether or not there is a central stimulus to engage the infant's attention. Their fields widen until they reach close to the adult value of around 80° at 10 months of age. Nasal fields lag behind temporal fields in development. Some authors have suggested that acuity near the fovea may be

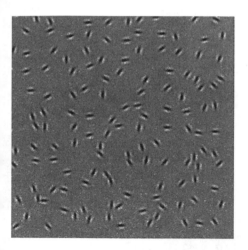

Jitter = 0 °

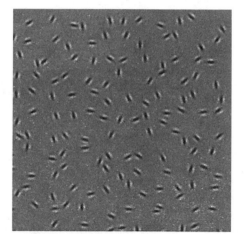

Jitter = +/- 30 °

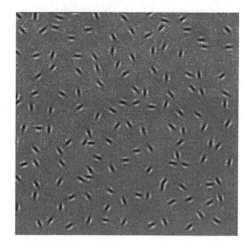

Jitter = +/- 60 °

FIG. 3.10. Display for a test of contour integration. The task is to detect the circular contour defined by a series of Gabor patches in the lower half of the display to the right of center. [Reprinted with permission of Cambridge University Press from Kiorpes, L., & Bassin, S. A. (2003). *Visual Neuroscience, 20*, 567–575.]

better than acuity at the fovea in the first few months of life because the fovea has not yet matured, but this appears not to be true.

2.4.2. Pattern Perception

There is a considerable literature on pattern perception in infants, which has been reviewed in several volumes (see Banks & Salapatek, 1983; Salapatek & Cohen, 1987; Weiss & Zelazo, 1991). It will not be reviewed in this book, because the prime purpose is to correlate behavioral and

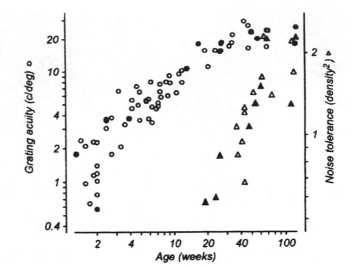

FIG. 3.11. Development of contour integration (*triangles*) compared to development of acuity (*circles*) in macaque monkeys. Open and closed symbols represent data from two different subjects. [Reprinted with the permission of Cambridge University Press from Kiorpes, L., & Bassin, S. A. (2003). *Visual Neuroscience, 20*, 567–575.]

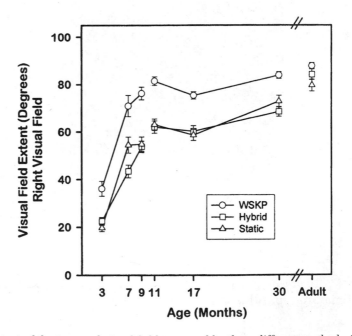

FIG. 3.12. Extent of the temporal visual field measured by three different methods. White sphere kinetic perimetry (WSKP) gives the widest results. [Reprinted from Dobson, V., et al. (1998). *Vision Research, 38*, 2743–2760. Copyright 1998, with permission from Elsevier.]

psychophysical properties with anatomy and physiology during development, and to show how these properties are disrupted by the effects of visual deprivation. Unfortunately, our understanding of the anatomy and physiology of the visual system has not yet reached the point where the more complicated aspects of pattern perception are understood in a detailed way. It is our hope that another book like this one will be able to address pattern perception, as well as the psychophysical properties dealt with above, in 10 to 20 years.

2.5. Summary

Some visual properties are present at birth. Rhodopsin in the rod photoreceptors has a spectral sensitivity curve with the same shape as the adult and regenerates with the same time course. All three cone pigments are present, and the light-adapted spectral sensitivity curve is close to that of the adult.

However, there are a number of properties that develop after birth. Several of these can be traced to the development of the cone photoreceptors in the fovea, which get longer and more tightly packed as the infant ages, and to the development of the rod photoreceptors around the fovea, which also get longer with age. These morphological changes play a large part between birth and a year of age in the improvement of acuity, contrast sensitivity, vernier acuity, and wavelength and saturation discrimination.

Other properties are present at birth but mature in a quantitative way as the retina and cortex develop. This includes specificity for orientation and direction of movement and, perhaps, also specificity of channels for different spatial frequencies. How this relates to the properties of the neurons in the central visual system will be discussed in Chapter 5.

3. Development of Binocular Vision

Getting the two eyes to work together is a complicated process. They must be able to converge or diverge so that the two images of an object fall on corresponding parts of the two retinas. For this to occur accurately requires good acuity in both eyes, good control of eye movements, and the ability to tell whether an object is closer or further away than the point of fixation. There must be good vision in both eyes, good connections between sensory and motor systems, and some depth perception.

Thus, there is a definite dependence of the various components of the system on each other during development. Vergence movements initially depend on cues other than stereopsis. Binocular function matures as the acuity in the retina matures and the vergence movements become more accurate. The development of stereopsis, which is required for the fine tuning of depth perception, awaits the development of some binocular coordination. Stereopsis then enables yet more accurate vergence movements. When one thinks about it, logic virtually dictates that this must be the sequence of events.

3.1. Depth Perception

Helmholtz listed several cues to depth perception, some monocular, such as perspective, size, superposition, motion parallax, accommodation, and haze, and some binocular, such as stereopsis and convergence. To these can be added the gradients of texture studied by Gibson and his colleagues (1950), where coarse textures are seen as being closer than fine ones.

Unfortunately it is extremely hard to study depth perception in very young infants. One of the first experiments on depth perception in infants was the visual cliff, studied by Walk and Gibson (1961). Here the infant is placed at the center of a glass table which is arranged so that half of the table has a pattern immediately beneath the glass and appears solid, and half is transparent, allowing a view of the same pattern on the floor, suggesting a precipitous drop (Fig. 3.13). The observer studies whether the infant avoids the cliff when it moves away from the center. The test requires crawling, and therefore cannot be done until several months of age although some results can be obtained based on heart rate. At that stage many but not all infants make the discrimination.

Yonas and his colleagues studied the response of infants to a number of different cues to depth perception (Yonas & Granrud, 1985). Much of their work was based on reaching by the infant with its hand to touch the object, which does not start until about 5 months of age. Their generalization was

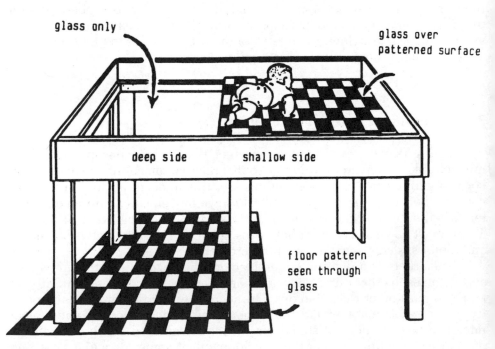

FIG. 3.13. The visual cliff. Infant is placed on divider and coaxed to go to a parent on either the deep or shallow side. Fewer excursions to the deep side are taken as an indicator of depth perception. [Reprinted with permission from Walk, R. D., & Gibson, E. J. (1961). *Psychological Monographs, 75,* 1–44.]

that infants respond to kinetic cues at 1 to 3 months of age, binocular cues at 3 to 5 months of age, and pictorial cues at 5 to 7 months of age. However, the only kinetic cue that they studied before the infant started to reach was an object expanding explosively, as though it would hit the infant. This elicited a blink reflex and head retraction. By binocular cues they meant stereopsis and convergence, which will be discussed below. Pictorial cues included size, texture gradient, shading, and interposition. It was clear that 7-month-old infants could respond to these as individual cues to depth perception.

There may be truth to the Yonas generalization. However, one wonders if infants might detect depth from some cues at an earlier age than they can physically respond to it with reaching responses. The crucial question from the developmental point of view is: what cues drive vergence movements early in life to give good binocular coordination? Is this simply avoidance of diplopia by some maximization of the response in binocular neurons? Or are cues to depth perception other than stereopsis involved? This remains to be tested thoroughly.

3.2. Orthotropia

Orthotropia is the ability of the eyes to look together at an object, to give a single visual image. It can be measured by the Hirschberg test, in which reflections from the cornea are noted in relation to the position of the pupil. For the results to be evaluated, one has to know the displacement of the corneal reflection from the optic axis or pupillary center (angle kappa), as well as the angle between the optic axis and the visual axis, which goes through the fovea.

Although this sounds like a straightforward procedure, results have been rather difficult to obtain and vary with different authors. However, the angle kappa varies with age, and when this is taken into account, the overall conclusion is that most infants are orthotropic, with some having an eye turned outward a little, which is called *exotropia* (Thorn, Gwiazda, Cruz, Bauer, & Held, 1994).

If infants were severely exotropic or esotropic (one eye turned inward), they would have double vision (diplopia). This would obviously be a severe handicap. However, there are two factors that make diplopia less likely in an infant. The adult does not get diplopia unless the images in the eyes are separated by a certain amount—15′ of arc along the horizontal axis near the fixation point. The area giving single vision is called *Panum's fusional area*. Panum's fusional area has not been measured in the young infant, but from everything that we have discussed about the development of acuity and the eyeball, one would expect it to be larger than in the adult. The second factor relates to the development of the fovea. The fovea is not well developed at birth, and nobody really knows whether infants fixate with the center of their rod-free area, or some point nearby. In any case, from observations of the morphology it is likely that the area of finest vision is not clearly positioned until the fovea develops, and the cones in the fovea have become densely packed. Consequently a small degree of esotropia or exotropia can be tolerated in the infant, whereas it would not be in the adult.

3.3. Stereopsis

The most precise cue to depth perception depends on disparity and is called *stereopsis*. Disparity occurs when the two images fall on noncorresponding parts of the two retinas. For objects closer than the fixation point, the disparity is called crossed because the lines of sight cross each other between the eyes and the surface on which the eyes are focused. Conversely, the disparity is called uncrossed for objects further away than the fixation point. As discussed in Chapter 2, there are cells in the adult visual cortex that respond to crossed disparity (near cells) and cells that respond to uncrossed disparity (far cells). Stereoscopic acuity in the adult, like vernier acuity, is better than grating acuity by a factor of approximately 10; stereoscopic acuity permits the detection of a disparity of several seconds of arc, whereas lines in a grating must be 1′ or 2′ of arc apart before they are seen. Therefore it seems likely that some fineness of tuning in the retina, in the form of a certain level of grating acuity, would be required before such fine-tuning can occur in the cortex.

The development of stereopsis has been given a great deal of attention for several reasons. It can be assayed by a variety of techniques. There is a quantity, stereoscopic acuity, that can be measured. Moreover, it represents the onset of fine-tuning in binocular function, and this onset is correlated with a number of other events.

Stereopsis can be measured using FPL and a pair of line displays. One display is arranged so that, for an adult, some lines appear to stand out in front of the others (Fig. 3.14). The other display is flat. The display with apparent depth becomes more interesting to the infant very suddenly around

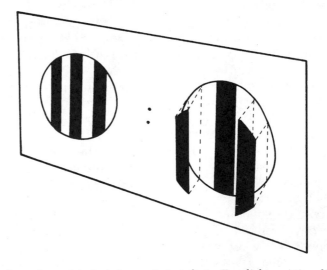

FIG. 3.14. Stimulus pair used to test stereopsis in infants. Two light-emitting diodes are in the center, with a flat display on the left, and a display with crossed disparity on the right (the *dashed lines* are there to demonstrate the effect). [Reprinted with permission from Held, R., et al. (1980). *Proceedings of the National Academy of Sciences of the United States of America, 77,* 5572–5574. Copyright 1980 National Academy of Sciences, USA.]

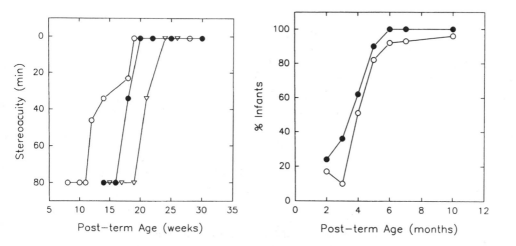

FIG. 3.15. (Left) Development of stereoacuity in three individuals. (Right) Percentage of infants who reached criterion for stereopsis when tested with crossed (•) or uncrossed (O) disparity. [Reprinted from Birch, E. E. (1993). *Early visual development, normal and abnormal* (pp. 224–236). Figures 13.4 and 13.3 by permission of Oxford University Press.]

16 weeks of age (Held, Birch, & Gwiazda, 1980). When the infant makes the discrimination, stereoscopic acuity can be measured, and it increases from more than 80′ of arc to less than 1′ of arc in a few weeks [Birch, Gwiazda, & Held, 1982; see Fig. 3.15(a)]. Interestingly, crossed disparity develops earlier than uncrossed disparity [Fig. 3.15(b)].

Stereopsis can also be measured with random-dot stereograms. In these, there is a pattern of dots around the edge of the display that is identical for the left and right eyes, and a pattern of dots in the center that is the same, but with a crossed or uncrossed displacement. For an adult, the center appears to stand out in front of or behind the plane of the edge pattern. A computer can be used to change the individual dots in a random way (dynamic stereogram) while keeping the left/right eye correlation, or to change the central display so that it appears to move. Forced-choice preferential looking measurement of stereopsis, using a moving random dot stereogram, also shows that stereopsis emerges at 3.5 to 6 months of age (Fox, Aslin, Shea, & Dumais, 1980). A similar time course is found with both stationary and dynamic random-dot stereograms using the VEP (Braddick, Atkinson, Julesz, Kropfl, Bodis-Wollner, & Raab, 1980; Petrig, Julesz, Kropfl, Baumgartner, & Anliker, 1981). Interestingly, although stereoacuity and vernier acuity are both examples of hyperacuity, vernier acuity does not show the rapid change between 3.5 and 6 months of age, implying that they have different mechanisms (Brown, 1997). After the initial rapid rise in stereoacuity, there is a slower rise to adult levels. The values depend on the stimuli and procedures used, but there is general agreement that there is little development after 10 years of age (Birch & Hale, 1989; Ciner, Schanelklitsch, & Herzberg, 1996; Leat, St Pierre, Hassan-Abadi, & Faubert, 2001).

Why does stereopsis appear so suddenly at a few months of age? Although the acuity and vergence movements that are needed to produce orthotropia obviously must reach a certain level of maturity before stereopsis can occur, improvement in grating acuity is small over the period during which stereopsis develops (compare Figs. 3.2 and 3.15), and the ability to converge develops before this time. Moreover, nothing in the development of the retina or the eye movement system would predict a different time of onset for crossed and uncrossed stereopsis. Schor (1985) argues that certain factors in monocular vision need to develop before stereopsis; small disparities are processed in the adult in spatial frequency channels tuned above 2.5 cycles/degree, and larger disparities are processed by lower spatial frequency channels. These channels may not be tuned adequately until 3 months of age. However, Schor's arguments aside, the most distinct correlation between the onset of stereopsis and another factor is with the segregation of ocular dominance columns.

3.4. Correlation of the Onset of Stereopsis and Segregation of Ocular Dominance Columns

This correlation was first pointed out by Held and his colleagues (for review, see Held, 1993). The correlation has not been pinned down very well in the human, so we will have to anticipate Chapters 4 and 5, and present some evidence from the macaque monkey and the cat.

The segregation of ocular dominance columns occurs at the input layer of the visual cortex, which is layer IV. At birth, the afferents from the left and right eyes overlap, and synapse on to the same neurons in layer IV. Then, at a time that varies with the species, they segregate into separate left and right eye columns within layer IV, synapsing onto separate neurons. The convergence of the signals from the two eyes then occurs at the next level, which may be layers II and III, or layers V and VI. Thus, there is binocular convergence within primary visual cortex in both the neonate and the adult, but the layer and level at which it occurs is different.

Stereopsis in cats has been studied with a variation of the FPL technique and an apparatus similar to the visual cliff (Timney, 1981). The kitten looks down on a pair of displays on the far side of a Plexiglas® surface and is made to jump down onto one side or the other (Fig. 3.16). There are monocular cues as well as binocular cues in this display, but most monocular cues are hidden by a mask. The disparity that can be detected with binocular viewing rises rapidly between 5 and 6 weeks of age due to stereoscopic mechanisms (Fig. 3.17). This is the same period of time over which the afferents to the cortex from the left and right eyes are segregating (LeVay, Stryker, & Shatz, 1978).

As we will see in Chapter 9, this occurs after orientation and direction selectivity have lost their plasticity and while the connections for ocular dominance are still plastic (Daw, 1994). For stereopsis to be accurate one needs to coordinate signals of the same orientation and direction specificity, and ocular dominance may need to be mutable while disparity and stereopsis are being organized.

Stereopsis in the macaque monkey has been studied with FPL and random-dot stereograms (O'Dell, Quick, & Boothe, 1991). Stereopsis appears at a mean age of 4 weeks and improves between then and 8 weeks of age.

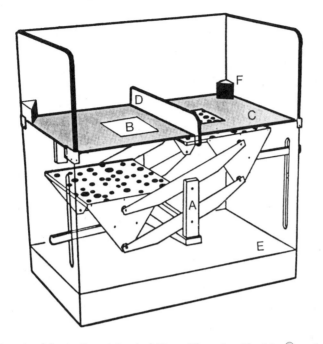

FIG. 3.16. Jumping stand for testing vision in kittens. There is a Plexiglas® surface (B) with two masks on it. Below it, a display of dots can be moved to vary the relative distance of the left and right sides from the Plexiglas® (A). A divider (D) forces the kitten to jump to one side or the other. Small speakers provide an audible indication of an incorrect choice. [Reprinted from Timney, B. N. (1981). *Investigative Opthalmology, 35,* 544–553, with permission from Association for Research in Vision and Ophthalmology.]

Again, this is the period of time over which the left and right eye afferents are segregating (LeVay, Wiesel, & Hubel, 1980).

Unfortunately, the time at which geniculocortical afferents segregate in the human is not well established. However, in a preliminary report, Hickey and Hitchcock found well-formed columns in a 6-month human infant and poorly formed columns in a 4-month infant (Hickey and Peduzzi, 1987). Thus there is a two-month window during which the segregation of afferents probably occurs. Because the experiments described above show that stereopsis emerges between 3 and 6 months, there is a reasonable correlation between development of stereopsis and segregation of ocular dominance columns in humans as well.

There are theoretical reasons to think that some binocular coordination of signals is required before cells sensitive to disparity develop. Sejnowski and his colleagues have modeled the conditions required (Berns, Dayan, & Sejnowski, 1993). Their model shows that if there is a correlation of activity within each eye but not between eyes, only monocular cells develop. If there is a small amount of correlation between the two eyes, only binocular zero-disparity cells develop. If there is a two-phase model, starting with a period of correlations within each eye, followed by a period that includes correlations between the eyes, the model produces binocular cells sensitive for zero disparity and monocular cells selective for non-zero disparity. The

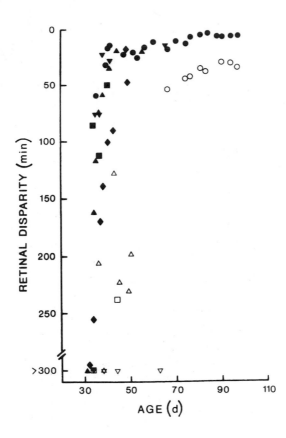

FIG. 3.17. Depth thresholds plotted as a function of age for kittens. Closed symbols, binocular thresholds; open symbols, monocular thresholds. [Reprinted from Timney, B. N. (1981). *Investigative Opthalmology, 35,* 544–553, with permission from Association for Research in Vision and Ophthalmology.]

model thus supports the notion that a two-phase process is required for the development of stereopsis.

When a correlation like this one between the development of stereopsis and ocular dominance segregation has been found in three separate species, it indicates a significant general developmental process. This observation has led Held and his colleagues to look for other properties that might vary between the pre- and poststereoptic periods (Held, 1993).

3.5. The Pre- and Poststereoptic Periods

Two aspects of binocular summation differ between the pre- and poststereoptic periods. The effects of signals from the left and right eyes on the pupil are summed in the adult. This can be seen by covering the left eye, observing the size of the pupil in the right eye, and observing whether the pupil contracts when the left eye is opened. Signals from the left eye start to have an effect on the size of the pupil in the right eye at 3 months of age, and the effect increases until adult summation is reached at 6 months of age (Birch & Held, 1983; see Fig. 3.18).

The effects of signals from the left and right eyes on acuity are also summed in the adult. Acuity is better by a factor of approximately $\sqrt{2}$ when both eyes are illuminated. This form of binocular summation occurs in the

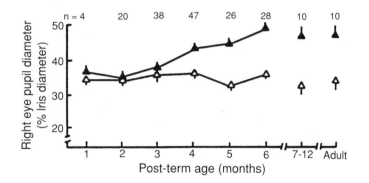

FIG. 3.18. Difference in pupil diameter in right eye with left eye occluded (▲) and with left eye open (△). The number of infants tested at each age is indicated along the top of the figure. [Reprinted from Birch, E. E., & Held, R. (1983). *Investigative Opthamology, 24*, 1103–1107, with permission from Association for Research in Vision and Ophthalmology.]

poststereoptic period but not in the prestereoptic period (Birch & Swanson, 1992).

Although these two forms of binocular summation correlate with the onset of stereopsis, the mechanism is unclear. According to signal/noise theory, detectability improves with summation of two signals if they have separate sources of noise but not if they have a common form of noise. Birch and her colleagues have used this point as an explanation for their findings. However, most noise in the visual system comes from the retina and there are separate sources of noise from the left and right eyes both before and after stereopsis occurs. What changes is the level at which the signals and their noise are combined, not the nature of the noise. Whatever the explanation, the correlation of binocular summation with stereopsis is most intriguing.

More important than summation for the function of the visual system are vergence movements and orthotropia. Although both vergence movements and orthotropia are present before stereopsis, orthotropia shows some improvement, and vergence movements show considerable quantitative improvement with the onset of stereopsis. Full convergence, as judged by the ability of the infant to follow a toy to within 12 cm of its face, appears between 8 and 16 weeks of age (Thorn et al., 1994). Orthotropia, as judged by some observers, is not complete until 12 weeks of age. Measurements of both orthotropia and vergence movements are subject to experimental inaccuracies, which are larger than the stereoscopic signals that can drive them when stereoscopic acuity reaches 1′ of arc. Consequently, it seems likely that the accuracy with which an infant can focus on an object improves beyond the limits of experimental error when stereoscopic acuity reaches its finest level of tuning.

3.6. Summary

These results show that the order in which events occur in the development of binocular vision is a logical one. At birth, the fovea is immature and grating acuity is poor, but the eyes look in approximately the same direction. The neonatal infant presumably does not have diplopia, but the eyes do not have to be as precisely aligned as they do in the adult to avoid it. Soon after birth, there is some binocular coordination and there is consequently some ability to make vergence movements.

Over the first 3 months the fovea matures, grating acuity improves, and the eyes become more able to fixate together on an object. Presumably cells in layer IV of the cortex are acquiring characteristics that will enable them to act as an appropriate input to near and far cells after stereopsis occurs.

Then, between 3 and 6 months of age, dramatic alterations occur in the visual cortex and in the ability of the eyes to work together. Stereopsis becomes detectable, followed by a rapid increase in stereoscopic acuity. The eyes develop the ability to make full convergence movements. Orthotropia is mature. Binocular summation occurs.

After 6 months of age there is further development in some visual properties. Grating acuity, for example, continues to improve. However, the main aspects of binocular development are complete when stereoscopic acuity and all the functions that it governs reach 1' of arc.

4. Development of Eye Movements

Some aspects of the development of eye movements have already been discussed, primarily those that relate to the development of binocular function, such as vergence movements and the ability to fixate on an object. Nevertheless, it is useful to give some further details. Other aspects, such as smooth pursuit and saccadic movements, remain to be discussed.

4.1. Fixation and Refixation

Fixation in infants is short for images rich in detail. This might be expected, as the infant is interested in exploring, and an image rich in detail contains more to explore. The drift away from fixation is greater in images with detail, and so is the tendency to make a new fixation (Hainline, 1993). These processes become more sophisticated as recognition and memory develop (Bronson, 1982).

Refixation varies from infant to infant, and it does so in uninstructed adults as well (Hainline, Harris, & Krinsky, 1990). Figure 3.19 shows results from 3 infants and 3 adults, when the subjects shifted their gaze to one of four targets 7.5° from the initial fixation point. It is noticeable that the one infant who showed a performance comparable to the adults' was 14 weeks of age, and probably into the stereoptic period.

4.2. Saccades

Saccadic eye movements in infants scanning patterns can be almost as fast as in adults (400°/s), if the stimuli grab the infant's attention (Hainline, Turkel,

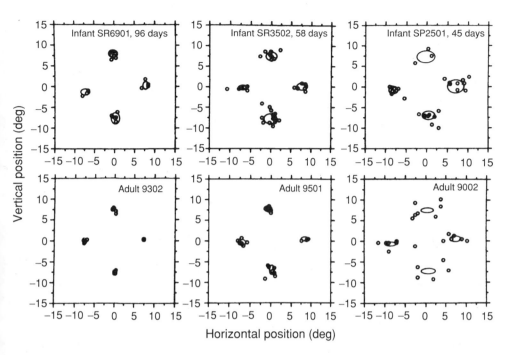

FIG. 3.19. Refixation movements in three infants and three adults. Subjects made saccades from the center to objects 7.5° away that were above, below, or to the left or right of the center. [Reprinted from Hainline, L., et al. (1990). *Infant Behavior and Development, 13*, 321–342. Copyright 1990, with permission from Elsevier.]

Abramov, Lemerise, & Harris, 1984). Saccades, when looking at textures that fill the whole screen, can be quite mature (Fig. 3.20). Saccades to forms such as squares, circles, and triangles are less mature. For less interesting stimuli, the infant may make a series of saccades rather than a single large one (Aslin & Salapatek, 1975; Roucoux, Coulee, & Roucoux, 1983). There is a linear relationship between the peak velocity and amplitude of a saccade similar to that seen in adults.

Two qualitative differences between saccades in infants and those in adults are noticeable (Hainline, 1993). Saccades in infants sometimes occur with less than 200 ms between them (see Fig. 3.20, infant LV). This almost never occurs in adults. The infant also sometimes shows an oscillatory eye movement, where the eyes saccade away from an object and then back again (see Fig. 3.20, infant BK). This is seen in adults only in pathological conditions.

Quantitatively, the accuracy of saccades in children at age 4 years is as accurate as that of saccades in adults (Fukushima, Hatta, & Fukushima, 2000). The latency decreases with age, from 305 ms at 6 years to 230 ms at 12 years. There are few, if any, measurements of saccades between 1 and 4 years of age. Thus, the mechanical aspect of saccadic eye movements matures quite early, but the control, which involves cognitive function, does not mature until close to the teenage years.

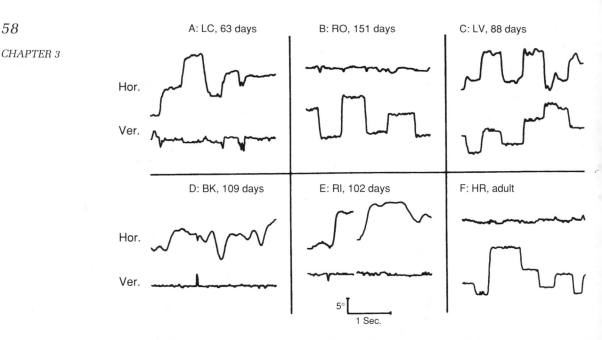

FIG. 3.20. Saccadic eye movements in 5 infants and 1 adult. [Reprinted from Hainline, L., et al. (1984). *Vision Research, 24*, 1771–1780. Copyright 1984, with permission from Elsevier.]

4.3. Smooth Pursuit

Smooth pursuit eye movements are essentially fixation on a moving target. Indeed, adults cannot make smooth pursuit eye movements unless there is a target to follow. Smooth pursuit therefore requires the ability to fixate and to detect movement.

Infants show smooth pursuit movements in response to slowly moving targets. The maximum velocity that can be followed increases with age (Roucoux et al., 1983). When this velocity is exceeded, the infant may still be able to keep up, but will use a mixture of smooth pursuit and saccades (Hainline, 1993). The results depend on the target—whether it is a large one, such as a face, or unpatterned spots, circles or bars, and whether it is repetitive, such as a stimulus with a sinusoidal movement. For a small target in a darkened room, a mixture of slow movements and saccades is seen in response to a ramp stimulus, and true following is not seen for movement at 24°/s until 102 days of age (Phillips, Finocchio, Ong, & Fuchs, 1997; Fig. 3.21). The gain of the response, the fastest velocity that can be followed, and the latency in starting an eye movement all improve between 1 and 4 months of age. There are few measurements of smooth pursuit movements published for children between a few months and several years of age, but the responses of primary school children to a sinusoidally moving stimulus are still not equal to adult responses in terms of velocity and position gain and phase (Accardo, Pensiero, Da Pozzo, & Perissutti, 1995). Presumably following a sinusoidally moving stimulus requires some anticipation that involves higher-level processes that mature late.

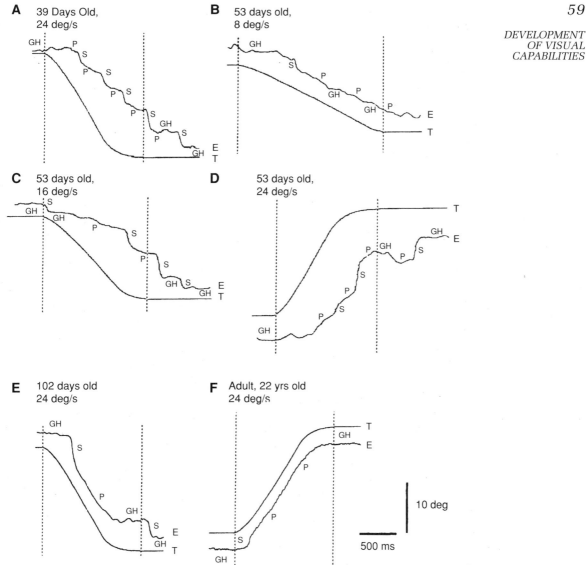

FIG. 3.21. Responses from infants at various ages and an adult to a smooth pursuit target. Abbreviations: S, saccades (defined as greater than 40°/s); P, smooth pursuit; GH, gaze holding. [Reprinted from Phillips, J. O., et al. (1997). *Vision Research, 37,* 3009–3020. Copyright 1997, with permission from Elsevier.]

4.4. Vergence and Accommodation

As discussed above, some vergence movements are seen at 1 month of age, and more pronounced movements at 2 and 3 months (Aslin, 1977). These occur in response to an object moved slowly toward or away from the infant. There is a steady improvement over the first two months (Hainline & Riddell, 1996), and a significant improvement in the number of adequate vergence movements at 4 to 5 months of age when stereopsis is rapidly developing (Mitkin & Orestova, 1988). The accuracy and peak velocity of vergence movements is adult by 4.5 years of age: only the duration remains to be improved, which happens at age 8 (Yang & Kapoula, 2004). There are no measurements in the literature that were taken between a few months and 4 years of age.

Another stimulus that is used to elicit a vergence movement in the adult is placing a base-out prism in front of one eye. The prism causes a vergence movement to keep the two eyes fixated together on the object that the adult is looking at. However, such a prism will not elicit a vergence movement in the infant. It could be that the infant notices the edge of the prism and is distracted by that because s/he has not been instructed to keep their gaze fixed on some object in the distance. However, the test pits the stereoscopic cue for depth perception against any monocular cues that may be present. Consequently, before the onset of stereopsis, the infant would not be expected to respond to this test.

Accommodation is the ability to focus on objects at different distances. It can be stimulated by blur, proximity, and vergence. Young infants tend to focus on near objects (Currie & Manny, 1997). There is considerable variability in the ability to focus on objects at other distances. Responses are poorer when blur is presented in conflict with distance. The age at which responses mature to adult levels varies considerably with the infant and the experimental situation (see table in Currie & Manny, 1997).

There is a connection between convergence (C) and accommodation (A), such that convergence can drive accommodation (AC/A) and accommodation can drive convergence (CA/C) in looking from a far object to a near one. The accommodation response to convergence stimulated by a prism is actually larger in 3 to 6 month infants than it is in adults (Bobier, Guinta, Kurtz, & Howland, 2000). For infants of all ages, the vergence response to accommodation is found to be in the normal adult range (Turner, Horwood, Houston, & Riddell, 2002). Thus, there are significant links between accommodation and vergence before binocular cues from retinal disparity enter the picture.

4.5. Optokinetic Nystagmus

Optokinetic nystagmus is elicited by a large stimulus covering a substantial amount of the visual field, and can be found in the newborn infant. The eyes follow the stimulus for a period of time, then flick back in a fast saccadelike movement. Infants can follow the stimulus better when it moves in the nasal direction than in the temporal direction (Naegele & Held, 1982). Interestingly, this direction-dependent asymmetry disappears for high-contrast stimuli around 5 months of age. Near threshold, the asymmetry may persist to 2 years of age (Lewis, Maurer, Chung, Holmes-Shannon, & Van Schaik, 2000). Optokinetic nystagmus is at least partly a subcortical phenomenon. Perhaps, after stereopsis is established at 5 months, the cortex exerts some control to make the gain of the responses in the two directions equal.

4.6. Summary

Several eye movement properties develop in synchrony with the sensory parts of the visual system. The ability to fixate improves as the fovea and acuity develop. The ability to make smooth pursuit eye movements, as opposed to saccades that keep the eyes tracking the stimulus, improves as the ability to detect the velocity of a moving stimulus improves. Vergence movements improve as depth perception becomes more acute.

On the other hand, saccadic eye movements show changes that are not related to sensory properties. These are the establishment of a 200-ms delay between saccades, the disappearance of oscillatory movements away from the object and back again, and the establishment of a single large saccade, as opposed to several smaller saccades, to small targets far away. The crucial component in the development of these properties is most likely in the brainstem, rather than in the afferent pathways.

References

Accardo, A. P., Pensiero, S., Da Pozzo, S., & Perrisutti, P. (1995). Characteristics of horizontal smooth pursuit eye movements to sinusoidal stimulation in children of primary school age. *Vision Research, 35*, 539–548.

Adams, R. J., & Courage, M. L. (2002). Using a single test to measure human contrast sensitivity from early childhood to maturity. *Vision Research, 42*, 1205–1210.

Aslin, R. N. (1977). Development of binocular fixation in human infants. *Journal of Experimental Child Psychology, 23*, 133–150.

Aslin, R. N., & Salapatek, P. (1975). Saccadic localization of visual targets by the very young human infant. *Perception and Psychophysics, 17*, 293–302.

Atkinson, J., Braddick, O. J., & Moar, K. (1977). Development of contrast sensitivity over the first 3 months of life in the human infant. *Vision Research, 17*, 1037–1044.

Banks, M. S. (1980). The development of visual accommodation during early infancy. *Child Development, 51*, 646–666.

Banks, M. S., & Bennett, P. J. (1988). Optical and photoreceptor immaturities limit the spatial and chromatic vision of human neonates. *Journal of the Optical Society of America A, 5*, 2059–2079.

Banks, M. S., & Salapatek, P. (1983). Infant visual perception. In P. H. Mussen (Ed.), *Handbook of child psychology II. Infancy and developmental psychobiology* (pp. 435–571). New York: Wiley.

Banks, M. S., Sekuler, A. B., & Anderson, S. J. (1991). Peripheral spatial vision: limits imposed by optics, photoreceptors, and receptor pooling. *Journal of the Optical Society of America A, 8*, 1775–1787.

Banks, M. S., Stephens, P. R., & Hartmann, E. E. (1985). The development of basic mechanisms of pattern vision: spatial frequency channels. *Journal of Experimental Child Psychology, 40*, 501–527.

Berns, G. S., Dayan, P., & Sejnowski, T. J. (1993). A correlational model for the development of disparity selectivity in visual cortex that depends on prenatal and postnatal phases. *Proceedings of the National Academy of Sciences of the United States of America, 90*, 8277–8281.

Birch, E. E. (1993). Stereopsis in infants and its developmental relation to visual acuity. In K. Simons (Ed.), *Early visual development, normal and abnormal* (pp. 224–236). New York: Oxford University Press.

Birch, E. E., & Hale, L. A. (1989). Operant assessment of stereoacuity. *Clinical Vision Sciences, 4*, 295–300.

Birch, E. E., & Held, R. (1983). The development of binocular summation in human infants. *Investigative Ophthalmology, 24*, 1103–1107.

Birch, E. E., & Swanson, W. H. (1992). Probability summation of acuity in the human infant. *Vision Research, 32*, 1999–2003.

Birch, E. E., Gwiazda, J., & Held, R. (1982). Stereoacuity development for crossed and uncrossed disparities in human infants. *Vision Research, 22*, 507–513.

Bobier, W. R., Guinta, A., Kurtz, S., & Howland, H. C. (2000). Prism induced accommodation in infants 3 to 6 months of age. *Vision Research, 40*, 529–537.

Braddick, O. J., Atkinson, J., Julesz, B., Kropfl, W., Bodis-Wollner, I., & Raab, E. (1980). Cortical binocularity in infants. *Nature, 288*, 363–365.

Braddick, O. J., Wattam-Bell, J., & Atkinson, J. (1986). Orientation-specific cortical responses develop in early infancy. *Nature, 320*, 617–619.

Bronson, G. W. (1982). *The scanning patterns of human infants: implications for visual learning.* Norwood, NJ: Ablex.

Brown, A. M. (1997). Vernier acuity in human infants: rapid emergence shown in a longitudinal study. *Optometry and Vision Science, 74*, 732–740.

Carkeet, A., Levi, D. M., & Manny, R. E. (1997). Development of vernier acuity in childhood. *Optometry and Vision Science, 74*, 741–750.

Ciner, E. B., Schanelklitsch, E., & Herzberg, C. (1996). Stereoacuity development—6 months to 5 years—a new tool for testing and screening. *Optometry and Vision Science, 73*, 43–48.

Currie, D. C., & Manny, R. E. (1997). The development of accommodation. *Vision Research, 37*, 1525–1533.

Daw, N. W. (1994). Mechanisms of plasticity in the visual cortex. *Investigative Ophthalmology, 35*, 4168–4179.

Dobson, V., Brown, A. M., Harvey, E. M., & Narter, D. B. (1998). Visual field extent in children 3.5–30 months of age tested with a double-arc LED perimeter. *Vision Research, 38*, 2743–2760.

Drucker, D. N., & Hendrickson, A. E. (1989). The morphological development of extrafoveal human retina. *Investigative Ophthalmology, 30*, 226.

Fiorentini, A., Pirchio, M., & Spinelli, D. N. (1983). Electrophysiological evidence for spatial frequency selective mechanisms in adults and infants. *Vision Research, 23*, 119–127.

Fox, R., Aslin, R. N., Shea, S. L., & Dumais, S. T. (1980). Stereopsis in human infants. *Science, 207*, 323–324.

Fukushima, J., Hatta, T., & Fukushima, K. (2000). Development of voluntary control of saccadic eye movements I. Age-related changes in normal children. *Brain & Development, 22*, 173–180.

Fulton, A. B., & Hansen, R. M. (1987). The relationship of retinal sensitivity and rhodopsin in human infants. *Vision Research, 27*, 697–704.

Giaschi, D. E., & Regan, D. (1997). Development of motion-defined figure-ground segregation in preschool and older children, using a letter-identification task. *Optometry and Vision Science, 74*, 761–767.

Gibson, J. J. (1950). *The perception of the visual world.* Boston: Houghton Mifflin.

Hainline, L. (1993). Conjugate eye movements of infants. In K. Simons (Ed.), *Early visual development, normal and abnormal* (pp. 47–79). New York: Oxford University Press.

Hainline, L., & Riddell, P. M. (1996). Eye alignment and convergence in young children. In F. Vital-Durand, J. Atkinson, & O. Braddock (Eds.), *Infant vision* (pp. 221–248). New York: Oxford University Press.

Hainline, L., Harris, C. M., & Krinsky, S. (1990). Variability of refixations in infants. *Infant Behaviour and Development, 13*, 321–342.

Hainline, L., Turkel, J., Abramov, I., Lemerise, E., & Harris, C. M. (1984). Characteristics of saccades in human infants. *Vision Research, 24*, 1771–1780.

Hansen, R. M., & Fulton, A. B. (1986). Pupillary changes during dark adaptation in human infants. *Investigative Ophthalmology, 27*, 1726–1729.

Held, R. (1993). Two stages in the development of binocular vision and eye alignment. In K. Simons (Ed.), *Early visual development, normal and abnormal* (pp. 250–257). New York: Oxford University Press.

Held, R., Birch, E. E., & Gwiazda, J. (1980). Stereoacuity of human infants. *Proceedings of the National Academy of Sciences of the United States of America, 77*, 5572–5574.

Hickey, T. L., & Peduzzi, J. D. (1987). Structure and development of the visual system. In P. Salapatek & L. Cohen (Eds.), *Handbook of infant perception* (pp. 1–42). Orlando: Academic Press.

Hohmann, A., & Haase, W. (1982). Development of visual line acuity in humans. *Ophthalmic Research, 14*, 107–112.

Howland, H. C. (1993). Early refractive development. In K. Simons (Ed.), *Early visual development, normal and abnormal* (pp. 5–13). New York: Oxford University Press.

Irvine, S. R. (1948). Amblyopia ex anopsia. Observations on retinal inhibition, scotoma, projection, light difference discrimination and visual acuity. *Transactions of the American Ophthalmological Society, 66*, 527–575.

Katz, B., & Sireteanu, R. (1990). The Teller acuity card test: a useful method for the clinical routine? *Clinical Vision Sciences, 5*, 307–323.

Kiorpes, L., & Bassin, S. A. (2003). Development of contour integration in macaque monkeys. *Visual Neuroscience, 20*, 567–575.

Kiorpes, L., & Movshon, J. A. (2004). Development of sensitivity to visual motion in macaque monkeys. *Visual Neuroscience, 21*, 851–859.

Kovacs, I., Kozma, P., Feher, A., & Benedek, G. (1999). Late maturation of visual spatial integration in humans. *Proceedings of the National Academy of Sciences of the United States of America, 96*, 12204–12209.

Leat, S. J., St Pierre, J., Hassan-Abadi, S., & Faubert, J. (2001). The Moving Dynamic Random Dot Stereosize test: development, age norms and comparison with the Frisby, Randot, and Stereo Smile tests. *Journal of Pediatric Ophthalmology and Strabismus, 38*, 284–294.

LeVay, S., Stryker, M. P., & Shatz, C. J. (1978). Ocular dominance columns and their development in layer IV of the cat's visual cortex: a quantitative study. *Journal of Comparative Neurology, 179*, 223–244.

LeVay, S., Wiesel, T. N., & Hubel, D. H. (1980). The development of ocular dominance columns in normal and visually deprived monkeys. *Journal of Comparative Neurology, 191*, 1–51.

Levi, D. M., Klein, S. A., & Aitsebaomo, A. P. (1985). Vernier acuity, crowding and cortical magnification. *Vision Research, 25*, 963–977.

Lewis, T. L., Maurer, D., Chung, J. Y. Y., Holmes-Shannon, R., & Van Schaik, C. S. (2000). The development of symmetrical OKN in infants: quantification based on OKN acuity for nasalward versus temporalward motion. *Vision Research, 40*, 445–453.

Mason, A. J. S., Braddick, O. J., & Wattam-Bell, J. (2003). Motion coherence thresholds in infants—different tasks identify at least two distinct motion systems. *Vision Research, 43*, 1149–1157.

Mayer, D. L., Beiser, A. S., Warner, A. F., Pratt, E. M., Raye, K. N., & Lang, J. M. (1995). Monocular acuity norms for the Teller acuity cards between ages of one month and four years. *Investigative Ophthalmology and Visual Science, 36*, 671–685.

Mitkin, A., & Orestova, E. (1988). Development of binocular vision in early ontogenesis. *Psychologische Beitrage, 30*, 65–74.

Naegele, J. R., & Held, R. (1982). The postnatal development of monocular optokinetic nystagmus in infants. *Vision Research, 22*, 341–346.

Neu, B., & Sireteanu, R. (1995). Monocular acuity in preschool children: assessment with the Teller and Keeler acuity cards in comparison to the C-test. *Strabismus, 5*, 185–201.

Norcia, A. M., & Tyler, C. W. (1985). Spatial frequency sweep VEP: visual acuity during the first year of life. *Vision Research, 25*, 1399–1408.

Norcia, A. M., Tyler, C. W., & Hamer, R. D. (1990). Development of contrast sensitivity in the human infant. *Vision Research, 30*, 1475–1486.

O'Dell, C. D., Quick, M. W., & Boothe, R. G. (1991). The development of stereoacuity in infant rhesus monkeys. *Investigative Ophthalmology, 32*, 1044.

Petrig, B., Julesz, B., Kropfl, W., Baumgartner, G., & Anliker, M. (1981). Development of stereopsis and cortical binocularity in human infants: electrophysiological evidence. *Science, 213*, 1402–1405.

Phillips, J. O., Finocchio, D. V., Ong, L., & Fuchs, A. F. (1997). Smooth pursuit in 1- to 4-month-old human infants. *Vision Research, 37*, 3009–3020.

Roucoux, A., Culee, C., & Roucoux, M. (1983). Development of fixation and pursuit eye movements in human infants. *Behavioral Brain Research, 10*, 133–139.

Salapatek, P., & Cohen, L. (1987). *Handbook of infant perception.* Orlando: Academic Press.

Salomao, S. R., & Ventura, D. F. (1995). Large sample population for visual acuities obtained with Vistech-Teller cards. *Investigative Ophthalmology and Visual Science, 36*, 657–670.

Schor, C. M. (1985). Development of stereopsis depends upon contrast sensitivity and spatial tuning. *Journal of the American Optometric Association, 56*, 628–635.

Shimojo, S., & Held, R. (1987). Vernier acuity is less than grating acuity in 2- and 3-month-olds. *Vision Research, 27*, 77–86.

Simons, K. (1983). Visual acuity norms in young children. *Survey of Ophthalmology, 28*, 84–92.

Sireteanu, R. (2000). Development of the visual system in the human infant. In A. F. Kalverboer, & A. Gramsbergen (Eds.), *Handbook of brain and behaviour in human development* (pp. 629–652). Dordrecht: Kluwer.

Skoczenski, A. M., & Norcia, A. M. (2002). Late maturation of visual hyperacuity. *Psychological Science, 13*, 537–541.

Slater, A. M., Morison, V., & Somers, M. (1988). Orientation discrimination and cortical function in the human newborn. *Perception, 17*, 597–602.

Teller, D. Y. (1977). The forced-choice preferential looking procedure: a psychophysical technique for use with human infants. *Infant Behavior and Development, 2*, 135–153.

Teller, D. Y. (1997). First glances: the vision of infants. *Investigative Ophthalmology and Visual Science, 38*, 2183–2203.

Teller, D. Y., & Bornstein, M. H. (1987). Infant color vision and color perception. In P. Salapatek & L. Cohen (Eds.), *Handbook of infant perception* (pp. 185–236). Orlando: Academic Press.

Thorn, F., Gwiazda, J., Cruz, A., Bauer, J., & Held, R. (1994). The development of eye alignment, sensory binocularity and convergence in young infants. *Investigative Ophthalmology, 35*, 544–553.

Timney, B. N. (1981). Development of binocular depth perception in kittens. *Investigative Ophthalmology, 21*, 493–496.

Turner, J. E., Horwood, A. M., Houston, S. M., & Riddell, P. M. (2002). Development of the AC/A ratio over the first year of life. *Vision Research, 42*, 2521–2532.

Walk, R. D., & Gibson, E. J. (1961). A comparative and analytical study of visual depth perception. *Psychological Monographs, 75*, 1–44.

Wattam-Bell, J. (1991). Development of motion-specific cortical responses in infancy. *Vision Research, 31*, 287–297.

Wattam-Bell, J. (1996). The development of visual motion processing. In F. Vital-Durand, J. Atkinson, & O. Braddock (Eds.), *Infant vision* (pp. 79–94). Oxford: Oxford University Press.

Weiss, M. J., & Zelazo, P. R. (1991). *Newborn attention.* Norwood, NJ: Ablex.

Wilson, H. R. (1988). Development of spatiotemporal mechanisms in the human infant. *Vision Research, 28*, 611–628.

Yang, Q., & Kapoula, Z. (2004). Saccade-vergence dynamics and interaction in children and in adults. *Experimental Brain Research, 156*, 212–223.

Yonas, A., & Granrud, C. E. (1985). The development of sensitivity to kinetic, binocular and pictorial depth information in human infants. In D. Ingle, D. Lee, & R. M. Jeannerod (Eds.), *Brain mechanisms and spatial vision* (pp. 113–145). Martinus Nijhoff Press, Amsterdam.

Yuodelis, C., & Hendrickson, A. E. (1986). A qualitative and quantitative analysis of the human fovea during development. *Vision Research, 26*, 847–855.

4

Anatomical Development
of the Visual System

The development of the nervous system is complex and amazing. The nervous system consists of nearly one hundred billion neurons, and each has its own individual job to do. Cells in the various parts of the nervous system are generated over the same period, and their projections grow out simultaneously but in different directions. To find their way to the right nucleus and, finally, to the right cells in the nucleus, these billions of projections must somehow cross many other fibers along the way, in many cases traversing a long distance.

An orderly sequence of steps is involved. The cells must first be generated, then migrate to their appropriate, often distant, destination. They form dendrites to receive their inputs and axons to transmit their outputs, sometimes while the cell bodies are still migrating. The axons find their way to the correct target structure and form an orderly pattern within that nucleus. The brain produces more cells than are used in the mature organism and many cells that project to an inappropriate nucleus may be lost. Connections are made between a cell and its target; the connections are then refined by a process of pruning of the dendrites, a retraction of axonal terminals, a sprouting of new terminals, and by a maturation of the synapses.

The initial steps are under chemical or molecular control, as suggested by Sperry in his celebrated chemoaffinity hypothesis, which was based on many observations made by early embryologists (Sperry, 1963). Molecular cues guide fibers toward the appropriate target and keep them away from inappropriate ones by mechanisms of attraction and repulsion. These mechanisms govern development before the synaptic connections are made, and before there is sensory input or motor output. Later steps are influenced by electrical activity between cells in the system. Activity governs the refinement of the strength and distribution of connections to make them conform to the correct quantitative analysis of sensory signals and control of movement. Consequently we can define two periods in the development of the nervous system: the first, in which genetic factors provide the molecular instructions, and the second, in which local environmental factors control the refinement of connections. During the second period, the system is said to be mutable or plastic, and studies discuss experience-dependent plasticity in the nervous system as a whole, and, for the visual system, sensory-dependent plasticity.

This whole process of development and plasticity has been most thoroughly studied in the visual system. We will concentrate on the mammalian visual system because that is where correlations can best be made between the anatomy, the physiology, and the psychophysical properties described in Chapter 3, and the similarity to human vision is most obvious. Considerable work has also been done on the development of connections between the retina and tectum of amphibians. Some of that work will be discussed later on, when we cover topographic projections.

Cells in the three main sensory region of the mammalian visual system—the retina, lateral geniculate nucleus, and visual cortex—are generated during overlapping periods of time. For example, cells in the retina are generated in the macaque monkey between embryonic day 30 and embryonic day 120 (E30–E120), in the lateral geniculate nucleus between E36 and E43, and in the cortex between E40 and E90 (Rakic, 1992). The comparatively long period of cell generation in the retina occurs because there is a gradient of cell generation, with the central part near the fovea being generated first and the peripheral parts later (LaVail, Rapaport, & Rakic, 1991). Thus, development in the various structures comprising the afferent pathways in the visual system occurs in parallel rather than sequentially.

1. Development of the Retina and the Projections within It

Within the retina, ganglion cells, horizontal cells, amacrine cells, and cones develop in parallel, followed by rods, bipolar cells, and Muller glial cells (Marquardt & Gruss, 2002). We are concerned primarily with the central nervous system, that is, with the development of ganglion cells and the projections of their axons to lateral geniculate nucleus and superior colliculus and then to the visual cortex. Thus, discussion of development within the retina will be brief.

In the cat, at birth ganglion cells ramify in both a and b sublaminae of the inner plexiform layer and have ON–OFF responses. Over the next two weeks, the dendritic arborizations of most ganglion cells segregate so that they are found in either the a sublamina or the b sublamina (Maslim & Stone, 1988) and the responses become either OFF or ON. This segregation does not occur if the retina is bathed in 2-amino-4-phosphonobutyric acid, which blocks all electrical responses in these immature retinas (Bodnarenko & Chalupa, 1993). The segregation also does not occur if the animals are reared in the dark (Tian & Copenhagen, 2003). Other properties of ganglion cells have not been found to be changed by these manipulations. The changes in ON and OFF responses that do occur will clearly be reflected in the responses of cells in the lateral geniculate nucleus and visual cortex.

The axons of these ganglion cells must find their way over the surface of the retina to the optic nerve head, where they exit the retina on their way to the chiasm. The first ganglion cells to be generated are located in central retina, close to the optic nerve head. A ring of chondroitin sulfate directs them towards the optic nerve head (Brittis, Canning, & Silver, 1992). Ganglion cells that are subsequently generated in the more peripheral parts of the retina are directed centrally by this ring of chondroitin sulfate, and then fasciculate with the axons of ganglion cells previously generated through the action of an immunoglobulin molecule called L1 (Brittis, Lemmon, Rutishauser, & Silver, 1995). They are also attracted to the optic nerve head by netrin (Deiner, Kennedy, Fazeli, Serafini, Tessier-Lavigne, & Sretavan, 1997) and repelled from the edge of the optic nerve by the semaphorin guidance molecule Sema 5A (Oster, Bodeker, He, & Sretavan, 2003). Thus, a combination of attractive and repulsive factors guides the retinal ganglion cell axons across the retina and into the optic nerve.

2. Crossing in the Optic Chiasm

Animals with eyes that look forward have binocular vision. To accomplish this, axons from ganglion cells that deal with the contralateral field of view cross to the other side of the brain in the optic chiasm, and axons that deal with the ipsilateral field of view project to the same side of the brain. Thus, the left lateral geniculate nucleus and the left visual cortex get input from the left temporal retina and the right nasal retina to produce binocular input from the right visual field, and vice versa for the right lateral geniculate and right visual cortex. The percentage of retinal ganglion cell axons that project ipsilaterally is almost half in primates, with decreasing percentages in cat, ferret, and rodent. In mice, it is 5% or less depending on the strain.

The retinal ganglion cell axons are guided towards the chiasm by extracellular matrix molecules called *slits*. These are inhibitory to all retinal ganglion cell axons through a receptor on the growth cones of these axons called robo (Erskine, Williams, Brose, Kidd, Rachel, Goodman, Tessier-Lavigne, & Mason, 2000). The slits are located around the chiasm, around parts of the optic nerve on the route to the chiasm, and around the optic tract on the route away from it (Erskine et al., 2000). Double mutants in mice for slit1 and slit2 show a large additional chiasm anterior to the true chiasm, axons that project into the contralateral optic nerve towards the opposite retina, and axons that extend dorsal and lateral to the chiasm (Plump, Erskine, Sabatier, Brose, Epstein, Goodman, & Mason, 2002; see Fig. 4.1). Thus, the slits guide retinal ganglion cell axons into, through, and out of the chiasm, but do not distinguish between axons projecting ipsilaterally and those projecting contralaterally.

Axons that project ipsilaterally diverge from those that project contralaterally in a palisade of glial cells in the chiasm near the midline (Marcus, Blazeski, Godemont, & Mason, 1995). The most medial of these glia express a ligand called ephrin B2. Axons from the ventrotemporal retina in the mouse, which are due to project ipsilaterally, have a receptor EphB1, which is repelled by ephrin-B2, and the axons therefore do not cross the midline (Williams, Mann, Erskine, Sakurai, Wei, Rossi, Gale, Holt, Mason, &

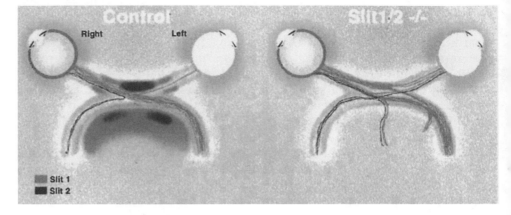

FIG. 4.1. Slits surround the optic chiasm and optic pathways nearby. In their absence, some fibers have aberrant pathways. [Reprinted from Plump, A. S., et al. (2002). *Neuron, 33*, 219–232. Copyright 2002, with permission from Elsevier.]

Henkemeyer, 2003). The expression of ephrin B varies with species according to the percentage of ipsilaterally projecting axons in those species and is also expressed at the appropriate time in development (Nakagawa, Brennan, Johnson, Shewan, Harris, & Holt, 2000). There is also a transcription factor—the zinc finger protein zic2—that is expressed in the ventrotemporal retina correlated with the degree of binocularity in various species, and whose absence results in failure of the ipsilateral projection (Herrera, Brown, Aruga, Rachel, Dolen, Mikoshiba, Brown, & Mason, 2003). Another transcription factor, Isl2, is found only in contralaterally projecting retinal ganglion cells (Pak, Hindges, Lim, Pfaff, & O'Leary, 2004). A variety of experiments suggests that it represses the ipsilateral pathfinding program involving zic2 and ephrin B2.

Other molecules are also involved in routing of retinal ganglion cell axons to their targets. Tenascin and neurocan, extracellular molecules that inhibit retinal axon growth *in vitro*, are enriched in the hypothalamus and epithalamus, which most retinal axons avoid (Tuttle, Braisted, Richards, & O'Leary, 1998). Mice deficient in netrin or its receptor DCC show unusual retinal ganglion cell axon trajectories in the hypothalamus (Deiner & Sretavan, 1999). It seems likely that a variety of molecules is involved in steering retinal ganglion cell axons away from inappropriate areas, such as the epithalamus and hypothalamus, and towards areas that they normally project, to such as the lateral geniculate nucleus and superior colliculus.

2.1. Errors at the Chiasm in Albino Animals

There are some genetic defects that affect the routing of fibers in the chiasm. For example, albino animals and humans have a band of retinal ganglion cells in the temporal retina next to the vertical meridian that project to the contralateral lateral geniculate nucleus instead of ipsilaterally (Guillery, 1974; see Fig. 4.2). This leads to two problems: first, there is a band on each side of the vertical meridian in the field of view that is handled by both

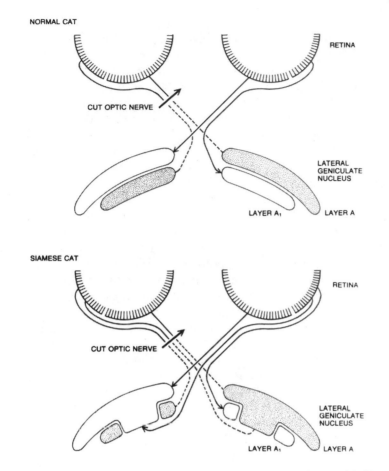

FIG. 4.2. Misrouting of connections in Siamese cats. In normal cats, the nasal half of the retina crosses to the contralateral lateral geniculate nucleus and the temporal half of the retina projects to the ipsilateral lateral geniculate nucleus (top). In Siamese cats, and other albino animals, some of the temporal half of the retina projects abnormally to the contralateral lateral geniculate (bottom). Consequently the dividing line between projections that go to one side of the brain as opposed to the other is displaced to the temporal side of the fovea. Projections are observed by cutting the optic nerve on one side, and looking at the degeneration. [From Guillery, R. W. (1974). Visual pathways in albinos. *Scientific American, 230*, 26, 97–104. Copyright 1974 by Scientific American, Inc. All rights reserved.]

the left and right hemispheres, with a consequent duplication, and second, because ganglion cells within this band from the left eye project to one hemisphere while the corresponding ganglion cells from the other eye project to the other hemisphere, there is a lack of binocular coordination. Thus, it is rather surprising that some albinos have stereoscopic vision (Apkarian & Reites, 1989; Guo, Reinecke, Fendick, & Calhoun, 1989). The hypothesis is that connections through the corpus callosum in these people make up for the deficits in the chiasm.

Studies in cats show two ways in which the system deals with the duplication owing to albinism. In one, cells in the lateral geniculate fed by the aberrant projection from the retina project to the usual place in the cortex, but the input from this projection to the cortex is suppressed (Guillery, 1974). Cats with this pattern of projection are called *Midwestern*, because they were first found by investigators working in Wisconsin. Because the projection is suppressed, they cannot see in the contralateral field of view when one eye is closed. The other way that the brain compensates is that a new part of the cortex is created for the aberrant projection from the temporal retina, so that each cortex contains a map of the central part of the field of view with topographic specificity. Cats with this pattern of projection are called *Boston*, because they were first described by investigators working in that city.

Studies with fMRI suggest that humans show neither the Boston nor the Midwestern pattern (Hoffmann, Tolhurst, Moore, & Morland, 2003). The input from the temporal retina is not substantially suppressed, and the topography is not rearranged. This is true for both striate and extrastriate visual cortex. This corresponds to the Midwestern pattern without the suppression and the authors call it the true albino pattern. Similar results were found in four albino humans. There are numerous different types of human albinos, and whether this result is true for all of them remains to be seen. However, an asymmetry in the visual evoked potential between one hemisphere and the other is found in most human albinos when only one eye is stimulated (Creel, Witkop, & King, 1974; Guo et al., 1989).

Abnormal projections at the chiasm are found in albinos who lack pigment in the skin (oculocutaneous albinos) and in albinos who lack pigment in the eye (ocular albinos) but have pigment in the skin. A variety of experiments show the melanin in the pigment epithelium in the retina is the important factor, not the defect in the chiasm (LaVail, Nixon, & Sidman, 1978; Marcus, Wang, & Mason, 1996). This clearly leads to the conclusion that lack of pigment in the retina affects guidance factors expressed by the retinal ganglion cells, such as Eph B1 and zic 2, which determine which retinal ganglion cell axons cross in the chiasm and which do not. How this might occur is a question whose answer is not yet known.

3. Development of the Lateral Geniculate Nucleus

The lateral geniculate nucleus is a layered structure; it has three main layers in the cat (the upper two are shown in Fig. 4.2), and six in the primate (see Fig. 2.8). Initially the layers are not noticeable and the endings from each eye ramify through the whole width of the structure (Rakic 1976; Sretavan & Shatz, 1986). The layers form during development as the right-eye nerve endings retract from some layers and the left-eye nerve endings retract from others (Fig. 4.3). This process does not occur in the absence of electrical activity (Shatz & Stryker, 1988), and neither does the segregation into the separate ON and OFF pathways discussed in Chapter 2. That is, although single cells in the lateral geniculate of normal kittens respond either at the onset or the offset of a stimulus, single cells in the lateral geniculate of kittens that have been reared without electrical input from the retina respond to both onset and offset (Dubin, Stark, & Archer, 1986). In the ferret there is an additional

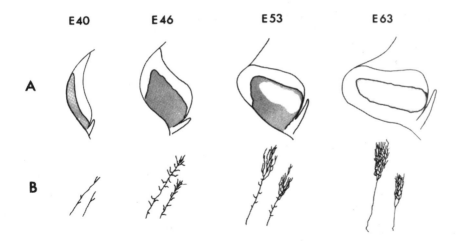

FIG. 4.3. Formation of eye-specific layers in the cat lateral geniculate nucleus. (A) Boundaries of the layers. Shading represents areas where endings from the two eyes overlap. (B) Terminals of representative axons from the retina. [Reprinted with permission from Sretavan, D. W., & Shatz, C. J. (1986). *Journal of Neuroscience, 6*, 234–251. Copyright 1986 by the Society for Neuroscience.]

sublamination into ON and OFF sublaminae, and this sublamination also does not occur in the absence of electrical input from the retina (Cramer & Sur, 1997). Interestingly, axons from ganglion cells in the M pathway in the macaque find their way to the correct two layers (the bottom two) at the start, and so do axons from ganglion cells in the P pathway (the top four layers), even though the eye-specific layers have not yet formed (Meissirel, Wikler, Chalupa, & Rakic, 1997). Thus, a mixture of molecular and activity-dependent cues are involved in the formation of the lateral geniculate layers.

The formation of the laminae in the lateral geniculate nucleus occurs prenatally in cat and macaque, and postnatally before the eyes open in the ferret. At this time the photoreceptors have not yet developed. The question therefore arises: where does the activity come from, and how does it lead to segregation of left eye input from right eye input, and of ON input from OFF input?

The fundamental mechanism is based on the Hebb (1949) hypothesis, which can be stated colloquially as cells that fire together wire together. If neighboring left eye cells fire at the same time, they will innervate neighboring lateral geniculate cells, and similarly for right eye cells. If left eye cells and right eye cells fire at different times, they will innervate different lateral geniculate cells.

It turns out that there is a mechanism in the retina to do just this. Around the time that laminae in the lateral geniculate nucleus are segregating, there are waves of ganglion cell firing in the retina that move across the retina in various directions (Meister, Wong, Baylor, & Shatz, 1991). The waves in the left retina proceed independently of the waves in the right retina. Because the waves move across the retina, neighboring ganglion cells fire together, while distant ganglion cells do not. Synchronization of these waves is believed to occur through the cholinergic amacrine cells that supply a common input to a number of ganglion cells within an area (Feller, Wellis, Stellwagen, Werblin, & Shatz, 1996). Consequently, retinogeniculate segregation is abolished in mice lacking the α2 subunit of the acetylcholine receptor (Rossi, Pizzorusso, Porciatti, Marubio, Maffei, & Changeux, 2001), which lack correlated activity between neighboring ganglion cells (McLaughlin, Torborg, Feller, & O'Leary, 2003).

4. Topography of Projections

There are topographic projections from the retina to the lateral geniculate nucleus and to the superior colliculus, and also from the lateral geniculate nucleus to the visual cortex. The formation of these maps has been studied most carefully in the superior colliculus and in its homolog in lower vertebrates, the optic tectum. This is a two-dimensional projection, with the temporal–nasal axis in the retina mapping onto the anterior–posterior axis of the superior colliculus, and the dorsal–ventral axis of the retina mapping to the lateral–medial axis of the superior colliculus. There are interesting differences between projections in frog and fish, where both retina and tectum grow during life so that the connections have to move, and in mouse and rat, where this does not happen. We will concentrate on results from mammals, primarily rodents.

The retinal ganglion cell axons enter the superior colliculus from its anterior end (for review, see McLaughlin, Hindges, & O'Leary, 2003). They do not grow initially to the correct location in the superior colliculus—they pass to each side of it and beyond it. Then, through a process of refinement of the endings, they turn towards the correct location, and the terminals that have gone beyond the correct location retract (Fig. 4.4).

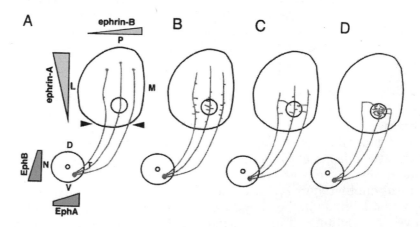

FIG. 4.4. Summary of retinocollicular topographic map development. Axon terminals initially overshoot (A) then retract to their correct location (D). A dorso–ventral gradient of EphB in the retina maps to a lateromedial gradient of ephrin-B in the superior colliculus, and a nasotemporal gradient of EphA in the retina maps to an anteroposterior gradient of ephrin-A in the superior colliculus. [Reprinted from Hindges, R., et al. (2002). *Neuron, 35,* 475–487. Copyright 2002, with permission from Elsevier.]

Mapping along both axes can be influenced by gradients of the receptor tyrosine kinase molecules, the Eph molecules, and their ligands, the ephrins (Fig. 4.4). There are two classes: ephrin-As, which are anchored to the membrane by a glycosophosphatidyl inositol linkage and bind EphA receptors; and ephrin-Bs, which have a transmembrane domain and bind EphB receptors. EphBs are expressed in a gradient from ventral to dorsal in the retina, and ephrin-Bs in a gradient from medial to lateral in the superior colliculus. Double mutants of EphB2 and EphB3 show errors in mapping along the mediolateral axis (Hindges, McLaughlin, Genoud, Henkemeyer, & O'Leary, 2002). EphAs are expressed in a gradient from temporal to nasal in the retina and ephrin-As in a gradient from posterior to anterior in the superior colliculus. The situation is not quite as clean for ephrin-As as for ephrin-Bs, because double mutants for ephrin-A2 and ephrin-A5 showed abnormalities in mapping along the anteroposterior axis, and, to a lesser extent, along the mediolateral axis (Feldheim, Kim, Bergemann, Frisen, Barabcid, & Flanagan, 2000). The fundamental mechanism depends on the response of the axon endings to the gradient, which is attractive at low concentrations and repulsive at high concentrations (Hansen, Dallal, & Flanagan, 2004).

Most work on topographic projections has been done on the superior colliculus rather than the lateral geniculate nucleus. In the lateral geniculate nucleus, an interesting problem arises. There are layers for the left eye and layers for the right eye, and they are laid out in the nucleus on top of each other in a map that goes from the vertical midline to the periphery. Are there two gradients in the retinas, from center to temporal edge in one eye, and from center to nasal edge in the other eye, mapping on to a single gradient in the lateral geniculate nucleus? Or is there a single gradient in the retina from the temporal to the nasal edge that maps to two opposing gradients in the lateral geniculate, one for left eye layers and the other for right eye layers? The first solution seems to be the correct one, with two gradients of EphAs in the retina and one gradient of ephrinAs in the lateral geniculate nucleus (Huberman, Murray, Feldhein, & Chapman, 2003). Presumably the existence of the double gradient in the retina is not noticed in species where the ipsilateral projection is 5% or less.

Ephrins are involved in turning the ipsilateral projection away at the chiasm as well as mapping projections to the lateral geniculate nucleus and the superior colliculus. As described in the next section, they are also involved in the delineation of areas in the cortex. Furthermore, ephrin-A2 and ephrin-A5 define a distinct border between the visual and auditory thalamus (Lyckman, Jhaveri, Feldheim, Vanderhaeghen, Flanagan, & Sur, 2001). This raises a question: What governs the expression of the ephrins so that they are in the right place at the right time for these multiple functions? There are various transcription factors that are responsible (e.g., Vax2 mutants exhibit flattened gradients of Eph A5, EphB2, EphB3, ephrin-B1, and ephrinB-2; Mui, Hindges, O'Leary, Lemke, & Bertuzzi, 2003), and a recent summary can be found in McLaughlin, Hindges, et al. (2003). Unfortunately, the evidence is too complicated for a brief review.

While gradients of ephrins and other molecules guide retinal axons to the appropriate place in the superior colliculus, activity also plays a role.

Treatment of the superior colliculus with antagonists to the *N*-methyl-D-aspartate glutamate receptor in rats produces arborizations of retinal ganglion cell terminals that are more spread out than in controls (Simon, Prusky, O'Leary, & Constantine-Paton, 1992). Moreover, mice that are mutant for the 2 subunit of the acetylcholine receptor, which do not show the retinal waves described above and do not have correlated activity between neighboring ganglion cells between P0 and P8, also have more widely spread ganglion cell terminals (McLaughlin, Torborg, et al., 2003). Apparently the ephrins are sufficient to guide ganglion cell terminals to approximately the correct location, but the final refinement of the map is under the control of activity, with correlated activity between neighboring ganglion cells leading to terminations in neighboring locations in the superior colliculus.

5. Development of Visual Cortex and Projections to It

The location of the visual cortex is affected by molecular factors. Three in particular are the homeodomain transcription factor *Emx2,* the secreted signaling molecule FGF8, and the paired-box containing transcription factor *Pax6. Emx2* is expressed in a low anterior to high posterior gradient, and a low lateral to high medial gradient. *Pax 6* has the reverse gradient—low medial and posterior to high lateral and anterior. FGF8 is expressed close to the anterior pole of the neocortex. Overexpression of *Emx2* leads to an expansion of the visual cortex (Hamasaki, Leingartner, Ringstedt, & O'Leary, 2004), whereas augmenting the endogenous anterior FGF8 signal shifts area boundaries posteriorly (Fukuchi-Shimogori & Grove, 2001). In *Emx2* mutants, the visual cortex contracts and is moved posteriorly whereas in *Pax6* mutants it is moved anteriorly, although this evidence is not quite as convincing because the animals die at birth (Bishop, Goudreau, & O'Leary, 2000). There are other transcription factors expressed in gradients across the cortex, but how they interact with each other remains to be seen (see O'Leary & Nakagawa, 2002).

Although the gradients of these molecules affect the position of the sensory and motor areas of the cortex, they do not specifically mark the boundaries between these areas. The visual cortex is marked more particularly by ephrins. This is most noticeable in macaque monkeys, where there is a sharp line between the striate and extrastriate cortex delineated by ephrin expression. EphA6 and EphA7 are found in the future visual cortex at E65, before afferents reach the cortical plate (Donoghue & Rakic, 1999). EphA3 is also found in visual cortex at this stage, but only in the extrastriate cortex. At E115, after the afferents have reached the cortex, ephrin A5 and EphA7 are found in striate cortex with a particularly sharp boundary (Sestan, Rakic, & Donoghue, 2001). Different Ephs and ephrins are also found in the thalamus with distinct distributions (Sestan et al., 2001). Unfortunately, experiments with mutants are not possible with macaque monkeys, so we do not yet know how particular Ephs in the thalamus may lead to particular projections in the cortex. Nevertheless, it is clear that cortical areas are marked before afferents from the thalamus reach them, in addition to the gradients that determine the general location of the areas.

An interesting question is: How do gradients of molecules create sharp boundaries between areas of cortex? In theory, this is possible if two opposing gradients of molecules such as *Emx2* and *Pax6* interact to affect other molecules localized within the same cells. In practice, the mechanism is not known. It seems likely that more molecules will be found to mark particular areas of cortex, probably more clearly than the ephrins, before the mechanism is worked out.

5.1. Development of Geniculocortical Projections

Projections from the lateral geniculate to the visual cortex and from the visual cortex to the lateral geniculate grow out at the same time and meet each other halfway (see Lopez-Bendito & Molnar, 2003). The two sets of projections may act as a scaffold for each other on the rest of the way to their terminations, a concept that is known as the *handshake hypothesis*. Projections from the lateral geniculate to the visual cortex may affect the structure of the visual cortex, for example, if a bilateral enucleation is performed in the macaque monkey, then a novel cytoarchitectonic area is found near area 17 that differs from both area 17 and area 18 (Rakic, Suner, & Williams, 1991). Various molecular factors can affect the route of the projections. As one example, both sets of projections are aberrant in *Emx2* mutants (Lopez-Bendito & Molnar, 2003). Activity also has an effect on projections from the lateral geniculate to the visual cortex at a fairly early stage of development; intracranial infusion of tetrodotoxin leads to significant projections within the subplate below cortical areas that are normally bypassed (Catalano & Shatz, 1998). In summary, both molecular influences and activity affect the course of these projections.

5.2. Formation of Layers in the Cortex

Cells destined for the visual cortex are generated in a pattern that has important consequences for the organization of the cortex. Cortical neurons are generated from stem cells located in a layer in the deepest part of the cortex called the *ventricular zone*. The young neurons migrate away from the ventricular zone to form the cortical layers (Fig. 4.5). The first cells to be generated are temporary and eventually die. Some migrate to layer I, and some to the white matter below what will become layer VI (Marin-Padilla, 1971; Rakic, 1977; Luskin & Shatz, 1985; Kostovic & Rakic, 1990). Those in layer I are known as Cajal–Retzius cells, and those below layer VI as subplate cells. The cortex itself is generated after these transitory cells in an inside-out fashion. As illustrated in Figure 4.1, the innermost layer, layer VI, is generated first, followed by layer V, then layer IV, then layer III, and finally the outermost layer, which is layer II (Rakic, 1974; Luskin & Shatz, 1985). Because the cells are generated in the ventricular zone, below layer VI, the consequence is that cells migrate past the lower layers as they move to their final position. The

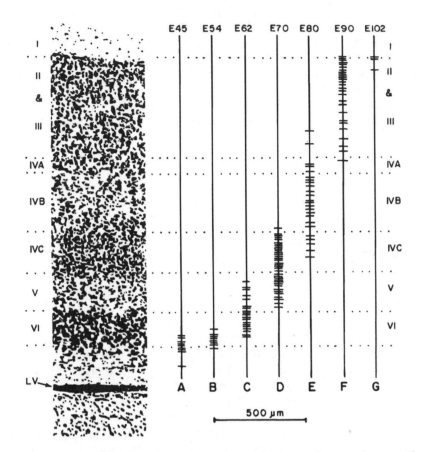

FIG. 4.5. Birthdates of neurons destined for various layers in the monkey visual cortex. The layers are shown at the left. On the right are depicted the cortical layers that will eventually be populated by neurons generated at various times in embryonic development. Each line represents a single neuron that was labeled with ^{3}H thymidine at the age shown, with its position determined 2 to 5 months after birth. Neurons ending up in white matter (WM) are the remnant of the subplate neurons. [Modified with permission from Rakic, P. (1974). *Science, 183*, 425–427. Copyright 1974 AAAS.]

whole process is a slow one. In the cat the process starts halfway through gestation at E30, and the cells for layer II do not reach their final position until 2 weeks after birth (Shatz & Luskin, 1986; see Fig. 4.6).

As the cells move through the layers, they are closely apposed to glial cells, called *radial glia*, which guide the young neurons away from the ventricular zone (Rakic, 1972; see Fig. 4.7). The young neurons develop into mature cells, the majority of whose axons and dendrites are lined up radially within the cortex. Indeed, observation of this organization by Lorente de No (1938) led him to propose that the cortex is arranged in a columnar fashion, long before the physiological evidence mentioned earlier came along. It seems likely that the radial migration of cells during development has something to do with the columnar organization of cortex, although the exact mechanism for this has not yet been worked out.

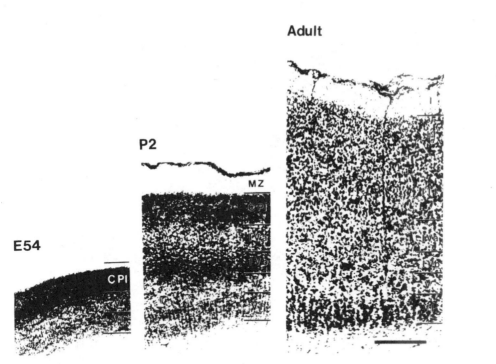

FIG. 4.6. Genesis of the visual cortex in the cat. At E54 layers V and VI are formed; 2 days after birth, at P2, layer IV is formed but layers II and III are not. Abbreviations: MZ, marginal zone; CPI, cortical plate. [Reprinted with permission from Springer, Payne B. R., et al. (1988). *Cerebral cortex* (pp. 309–389).]

5.3. Role of the Subplate Neurons

Cells in the subplate below the cortex have a significant role in the pathfinding of the afferent fibers. Axons from the lateral geniculate nucleus grow toward the cortex in the subplate (Rakic, 1976; Shatz & Luskin, 1986). When the axons reach the correct general location, they stop in the subplate for a period that was named the waiting period by Rakic (1977). This wait may last several weeks in the slowly developing primate brain. At this stage, axons from the geniculate make connections with the subplate cells. The subplate cells have axons that contact cells in layer IV; consequently, the subplate cells can be stimulated monosynaptically from the lateral geniculate nucleus, while layer IV is stimulated polysynaptically (Friauf, McConnell, & Shatz, 1990). In the cat, the connection to layer IV is polysynaptic at birth; the geniculate fibers grow into layer IV after birth (Shatz & Luskin, 1986), and the connections to layer IV become monosynaptic at some time before postnatal day 21 (Friauf & Shatz, 1991; see Fig. 4.8). If the subplate cells are deleted, the lateral geniculate fibers go past their correct location, and end up somewhere else (Ghosh, Antonini, McConnell, & Shatz, 1990; see Fig. 4.9). Thus, the subplate cells probably contain the molecular cues that govern the correct localization of the afferent fibers. This may be their prime function, because many of them die soon after the lateral geniculate fibers make contact with them (Chun & Shatz, 1989; Kostovic & Rakic, 1990).

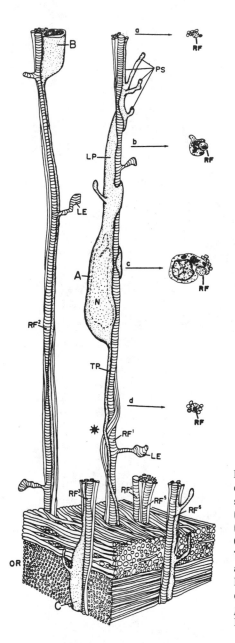

FIG. 4.7. Neurons (A, B, C) migrating through the cortex from the ventricular zone below toward the surface above in close apposition to radial glia cells (RF). Neuron A is shown with its leading process (LP), pseudopodia (PS), and trailing process (TP). Cross-sections at four levels are shown on the right. The neurons are in close contact with the radial glia at all levels. Abbreviation: OR, optic radiation. [From Rakic, P. (1972). Mode of cell migration to the superficial layers of fetal monkey neocortex. *Journal of Comparative Neurology, 145*, 61–83. Copyright © 1972. Reprinted by permission of John Wiley & Sons, Inc.]

5.4. Tangential Projections

The cells that migrate radially through the cortex along radial glia are the pyramidal cells that use glutamate as a transmitter and project out of the cortex, or to other layers within the cortex. Cells using GABA as a transmitter take a different route. They are generated in the ganglionic eminences and move tangentially through the cortex to reach their final location (Anderson, Eisenstat, Shi, & Rubenstein, 1997; Lavdas, Grigoriou, Pachnis, & Parnavelas, 1999). The glutamatergic neurons receive afferents and send out efferents

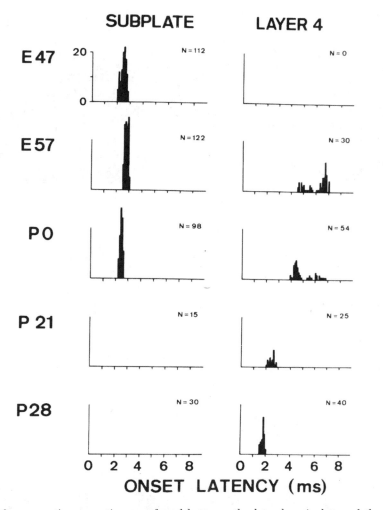

FIG. 4.8. Monosynaptic connections are found between the lateral geniculate and the subplate before birth, and between the lateral geniculate and layer IV after birth, in the cat. The figure shows the latency in the subplate and layer IV from stimulation of the lateral geniculate at various ages. A latency of around 2 ms represents monosynaptic input; around 4 ms it is disynaptic or more. The connection to layer IV becomes monosynaptic between P0 and P21. [Used with permission from Friauf, E., & Shatz, C. J. (1991). *Journal of Neurophysiology, 66*, 2059–2071.]

with a topographic organization. The GABAergic neurons are local circuit neurons, responsible for refining receptive field properties; thus, their position is not important in the way that the position of the glutamatergic neurons is important, and a different mode of migration makes sense.

5.5. Development of Connections to and from Layers in the Visual Cortex

The organization of the layers within the visual cortex is also controlled by molecular cues. Afferents come in to layer IV, efferents project back to the

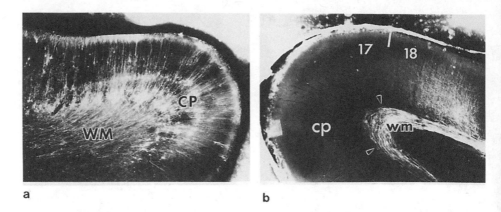

FIG. 4.9. Lateral geniculate axons do not innervate the cortex if the subplate is missing. (a) Lateral geniculate axons innervating the cortex at P2. (b) Lateral geniculate axons bypassing the cortex at P5 after lesions of the subplate. [Reprinted with permission from Ghosh, A., et al. (1990). *Nature, 347,* 179–181. Copyright 1990 MacMillan Magazines Limited.]

lateral geniculate from layer VI, and efferents to the superior colliculus come from layer V. This specificity is retained when slices of cortex and lateral geniculate or superior colliculus are placed in a culture dish (Yamamoto, Kurotani, & Toyama, 1989; Blakemore & Molnar, 1990; Novak & Bolz, 1993; see Fig. 4.10). A slice of the lateral geniculate nucleus can be placed above the pial surface of the cortex, rather than below the white matter, and the fibers from it will still grow into layer IV. This strongly suggests that there are molecular cues that attract the afferent fibers. Our old friends the ephrins are again involved—ephrin A5 is expressed in layer IV, and a knockout of ephrinA5 reduces the thalamic terminals in that layer; in contrast, overexpression of

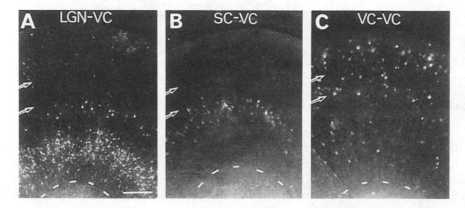

FIG. 4.10. Cells in the visual cortex establish appropriate connections when slices of visual cortex are put into coculture with slices of areas to which the visual cortex normally connects. A label is put into the target, and transported retrogradely back to the cell of origin. When the visual cortex is cocultured with the lateral geniculate (LGN-VC), cells in layer VI are labeled (A); when cocultured with superior colliculus (SC-VC), cells in layer V are labeled (B); with visual cortex (VC-VC), cells in layer II are labeled (C). Arrows mark layer IV. [Reprinted from Toyama, K., et al. (1993). *Progress in Neurobiology, 41,* 543–563. Copyright 1992, with permission from Elsevier.]

ephrin A5 increases the terminals (Mann, Peuckert, Dehner, Zhou, & Bolz, 2002).

There is a mutant mouse, called *reeler*, where the organization of the layers is disturbed (Caviness, 1976). The polymorphic cells of layer VI are found just below the pia. Pyramidal cells are found in an inverted location, with the large ones that are normally in layer V above the small ones that are normally in layers II and III. In spite of being in the wrong layer, the cells make the correct connections and have the correct receptive field properties (Lemmon and Pearlman, 1981). This also shows that there is some factor intrinsic to the cells in layer V, and another factor intrinsic to the cells in layers II and III that enables them to recognize their targets, independent of whether they are located in a normal or abnormal position in the cortex.

Connections within the cortex from one layer to another also have some specificity from the time they are made. In the primate, developing spiny neurons specifically target superficial and deep layers without forming branches in layer IVC, and layer VI pyramidal neurons that target layer IVC never form branches in layer V. Some transient branches are found—some IVC neurons may branch in 4B, and there are some transient projections to the subplate (Callaway, 1998). Some of these branches are eliminated under the influence of activity (Butler, Dantzker, Shah, & Callaway, 2001). Thus, activity-dependent cues play a role in some cases as well as molecular cues.

6. Development of Clusters of Cells with Similar Properties

As described in Chapter 2, cells in the visual cortex with similar receptive field properties cluster together. There are clusters for cells driven by the left eye and for cells driven by the right known as *ocular dominance columns*. Cells specific for a particular orientation are found together in orientation columns, arranged around focal points known as blobs. In the blobs, there is a high concentration of cells specific for color, without much specificity for orientation. Both activity and molecular cues affect the development of these columns.

6.1. Formation of Ocular Dominance Columns

Ocular dominance columns are found early in development: before birth in the macaque (Rakic, 1976; Horton & Hocking, 1996), a few days after eye opening in the cat (Crair, Horton, Antonini, & Stryker, 2001), and 2 weeks before eye opening in the ferret (Crowley & Katz, 2000). Clearly, visual experience is not required. The stage at which the columns form is earlier than the stage at which they can be affected by monocular deprivation (Crowley & Katz, 2000). Whether activity that is not dependent on vision is required or whether molecular cues drive the formation of the columns is an unresolved question. Later development of the columns can be affected by the abolition of activity with tetrodotoxin (Stryker & Harris, 1986). Crowley & Katz (2000) have suggested that the initial development may depend on molecular cues for the temporal retina versus the nasal retina. However, there is at the moment no experiment proving that molecular cues are required, and no putative molecules have been found (Katz & Crowley, 2002).

6.2. Formation of Blobs and Pinwheels

The cytochrome oxidase blobs that are found in primary visual cortex (area 17) are there before birth in the macaque (Horton & Hocking, 1996) and by 2 weeks of age, soon after the eyes open, in the cat (Murphy, Duffy, Jones, & Mitchell, 2001). They increase in density and the spacing increases as the cortex gets larger, but their initial formation does not depend on visual input because they develop in dark-reared cats in the same fashion as they do in normal cats (Murphy et al., 2001). The pinwheels of orientation selectivity that radiate from the blobs develop around the same period of time, with the development of the difference in input from the contralateral eye and ipsilateral eye. The contralateral eye input develops sharply between 7 and 14 days in the cat, and the ipsilateral eye input develops sharply between 14 and 21 days with some further maturation until 28 days (Crair, Gillespie, & Stryker, 1998). The development of pinwheels also takes place in the absence of patterned visual input until 21 days of age; the pinwheels then degenerate. This contrasts with the cytochrome oxidase blobs, which remain in the absence of any visual input.

6.3. Development of Lateral Connections

Within the adult visual cortex, lateral connections are made between columns that deal with like features: left eye columns to left eye columns, horizontal orientation columns to horizontal orientation columns, and so on. These connections also are initially spread out (Luhmann, Millan, & Singer, 1986; Callaway & Katz, 1990). The process of refining the connections also depends on electrical activity, as shown by experiments where stimulation of the retina is prevented by suturing both eyes shut, in which case the refinement of columnar connections is abolished (Callaway & Katz, 1991).

7. Other Events during Differentiation

There are several events that take place in the nervous system after the young neurons have found their way to their final location and have sent processes out to make connections. One is cell loss through the death of some cells. A second is the pruning or elimination of axon terminals, and in some cases the growth of new ones. A third is the differentiation of the dendrites. A fourth is the formation and loss of synapses. Each of these occurs during the development of the visual system.

The best-documented cell loss occurs among ganglion cells in the retina and in the lateral geniculate nucleus. Major cell loss occurs in the retina between E80 and E120 in the macaque monkey (Rakic & Riley, 1983a) and between E39 and E53 in the cat (Ng & Stone, 1982; Williams, Bastiani, Lia, & Chalupa, 1986). This loss is under genetic control, and is not affected by

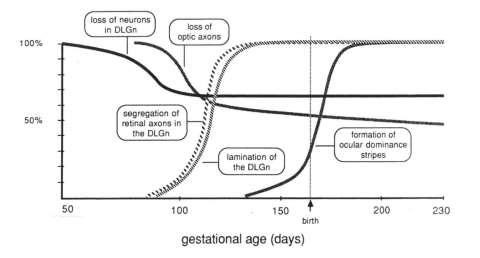

FIG. 4.11. Events in the development of the monkey visual system. DLGn refers to dorsal lateral geniculate nucleus. [From Williams, R. W., & Rakic, P. (1988). Elimination of neurons from the rhesus monkey's lateral geniculate nucleus during development. *Journal of Comparative Neurology, 272,* 424–436. Copyright © 1988. Reprinted by permission of John Wiley & Sons, Inc.]

electrical activity (Friedman & Shatz, 1990). In motor systems, the purpose of cell loss is well established; it matches the number of motoneurons to the number of muscles. In the visual system the purpose is not as clear. The loss of cells in the macaque retina occurs while the lamination of the lateral geniculate nucleus is taking place (Fig. 4.11). It can be reduced by taking out one eye, suggesting a relationship between the cell loss and the elimination of endings from one layer in the lateral geniculate nucleus (Rakic & Riley, 1983b). However, cell loss in the lateral geniculate nucleus starts at E48, before the retinal fibers arrive at the lateral geniculate, before lamination of the lateral geniculate occurs, and before cortical connections are made (Williams & Rakic, 1988). The matching of afferents and target, therefore, does not seem to be the purpose of this loss.

The pruning of axon terminals takes place all over the visual system during development. This is the mechanism whereby ocular dominance columns form in the cortex and eye-specific layers form in the lateral geniculate nucleus. The terminals of retinal ganglion cells in the lateral geniculate initially have side branches in all the layers (Fig. 4.9). The side branches in the wrong layers eventually retract (Sretavan & Shatz, 1986). Similarly, the terminals of lateral geniculate cells in layer IV of the visual cortex grow widely spread out terminals, then some side branches are lost, so that in the adult there are patches of side branches alternating with bare spaces along the axons (LeVay & Stryker, 1979). These alternating areas are the basis for the ocular dominance columns in the mature visual system. Likewise, projections to area 18 in the adult cat originate from clusters of cells in area 17. These cells of origin are distributed in bands of uniform density in newborn kittens. The formation of clusters occurs during weeks 2 and 3 by a process of axonal retraction, and possibly by cell death in the deep laminae (Price & Blakemore, 1985).

The right visual cortex, which deals with the left field of view, and the left visual cortex, which deals with the right field of view, are connected through the corpus callosum. The callosum therefore primarily handles the vertical meridian that separates the two halves of the field of view. Callosal projections are also widespread early in development, and later retract. In the cat, a wide area of the field of view is connected across the midline to start with, the area then becomes confined to the vertical meridian (Innocenti, 1981), although the initially widely spread out endings do not reach through the cortex to their normal location. In the primate, callosal fibers join the secondary visual cortex, but not the primary visual cortex. However, the same process of retraction takes place, as well as some elimination of axons (Dehay, Kennedy, Bullier, & Berland, 1988; LaMantia & Rakic, 1990).

Normally the cells that project from the retina to the lateral geniculate are different from those that project to the superior colliculus. X cells, also known as ß cells, which are responsible for fine acuity, project to the lateral geniculate nucleus but not the superior colliculus in the adult cat. However, at E38 to E43, some of these cells also project to the superior colliculus (Ramoa, Campbell, & Shatz, 1989). The projections that are not functional in the adult are eliminated by a process that must include the elimination of axons to the superior colliculus because it occurs after the period of cell death is over.

There is also sculpting of the efferent connections of the cortex. Layer V cells in the adult project to the superior colliculus. During development they also project to the spinal cord, which is a natural target for layer V cells from the motor cortex. There is some molecular specificity because they do not project to the cerebellum or many other parts of the brain that they pass along the way. At the same time there is a target specificity that occurs by pruning after the initial projections are made. The cells in the visual cortex eventually lose their projections to the spinal cord (Stanfield & O'Leary, 1985).

The dendrites of cells, like the axons, develop by a process of ramification and retraction. There are three stages in the development of dendrites after their initial growth (Lund, Boothe, & Lund, 1977). First, the dendrites grow hairlike processes while the axons are still ramifying. Then, all cells grow a dense set of spines on the dendrites, including those cells that do not have spines in the adult. Then the spines retract, until the adult stage is reached (Fig. 4.12). These stages may occur at different times in different cells, but the same general sequence occurs in all neurons (Meyer & Ferres-Torres, 1984).

Synapses are also produced in greater numbers than found in the adult, as one might expect from the general overproduction of cells, axons, and dendrites. The first cortical synapses are found in layer I and the subplate, and those on cell bodies, of course, disappear as the cells disappear (Molliver, Kostovic, & Van der Loos, 1973). In the cat there is a rapid increase of synapses between P8 and P37 (Cragg, 1975). Only 1% of synapses are present at birth. The number peaks at 4 to 8 weeks of age, then declines, in all layers (Winfield, 1983). There may be a considerable turnover of synapses during the peak of the period of rearrangements, at 4 to 6 weeks of age, but there is no marker that can be used to detect this accurately at the present time. A similar situation occurs in the macaque (Bourgeois & Rakic, 1993).

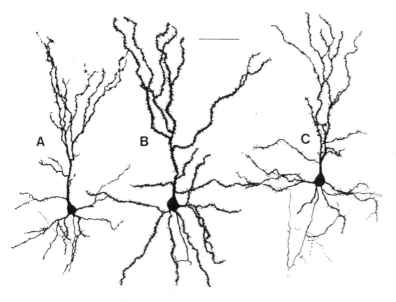

FIG. 4.12. Maturation of pyramidal cells from layer II of macaque visual cortex. Individual cells were stained using the Golgi technique. Typical cells are shown for three ages: A, at birth; B, 8 weeks postnatal; C, adult. [From Lund, J. S., et al. (1977). Development of neurons in the visual cortex (area 17) of the monkey (Macacca nemestrina): a Golgi study from fetal day 127 to postnatal maturity. *Journal of Comparative Neurology, 176*, 149–187. Copyright © 1977. Reprinted by permission of John Wiley & Sons, Inc.]

It seems likely that all these processes, except cell loss, are involved in sensory-dependent plasticity because of the time at which they occur. The pruning of axon terminals and differentiation of dendrites are both postnatal events, occurring after the eyes open and while physiological changes happen. The number of synapses peaks at the time that the system is most susceptible to sensory-dependent effects. We will discuss how these processes are involved after giving the details of sensory-dependent plasticity.

8. Summary

The initial events in the development of the visual system, which occur before the connections are formed, are under genetic and molecular control. These include the generation and migration of cells, the projection of their axons to their targets, the formation of topographic projections, the general organization of the terminals within the targets, the crossing of fibers in the chiasm, the position of areas within the cerebral cortex, and the formation of cytochrome oxidase blobs in the cortex. Most of this takes place before birth. Later events, occurring after the connections are formed, and in most cases after the eyes open, are under the control of electrical activity. This includes the refinement of maps within a nucleus, the refinement of columns within the cortex, and the formation of layers within the lateral geniculate nucleus. Some development is affected by both molecular cues and electrical activity. This includes the specificity of layers within the cortex, including the specificity of afferent connections, efferent connections, and connections within the cortex, also the formation of pinwheels around the cytochrome oxidase blobs. Given the complexity of the system, it is amazing that the various cues work together to produce the final result.

References

Anderson, S. A., Eisenstat, D. D., Shi, L., & Rubenstein, J. L. R. (1997). Interneuron migration from basal forebrain to neocortex: dependence on *Dlx* genes. *Science, 278*, 474–478.

Apkarian, P., & Reites, D. (1989). Global stereopsis in human albinos. *Vision Research, 29*, 1359–1370.

Bishop, K. M., Goudreau, G., & O'Leary, D. M. (2000). Regulation of area identity in the mammalian neocortex by *Emx2* and *Pax6. Science, 288*, 344–349.

Blakemore, C., & Molnar, Z. (1990). Factors involved in the establishment of specific interconnections between thalamus and cerebral cortex. *Cold Spring Harbor Symposia on Quantitative Biology, 55*, 491–504.

Bodnarenko, S. R., & Chalupa, L. M. (1993). Stratification of ON and OFF ganglion cell dendrites depends on glutamate-mediated afferent activity in the developing retina. *Nature, 364*, 144–146.

Bourgeois, J. P., & Rakic, P. (1993). Changes of synaptic density in the primary visual cortex of the macaque monkey from fetal to adult stage. *Journal of Neuroscience, 13*, 2801–2820.

Brittis, P. A., Canning, D. R., & Silver, J. (1992). Chondroitin sulfate as a regulator of neuronal patterning in the retina. *Science, 255*, 733–736.

Brittis, P. A., Lemmon, V., Rutishauser, U., & Silver, J. (1995). Unique changes of ganglion cell growth cone behavior following cell adhesion molecule perturbations: a time-lapse study of the living retina. *Molecular and Cellular Neurobiology, 6*, 433–449.

Butler, A. K., Dantzker, J. L., Shah, R. B., & Callaway, E. M. (2001). Development of visual cortical axons: layer-specific effects of extrinsic influences and activity blockade. *Journal of Comparative Neurology, 430*, 321–331.

Callaway, E. M. (1998). Local circuits in primary visual cortex of the macaque monkey. *Annual Review of Neuroscience, 21*, 47–74.

Callaway, E. M., & Katz, L. C. (1990). Emergence and refinement of clustered horizontal connections in cat striate cortex. *Journal of Neuroscience, 10*, 1134–1153.

Callaway, E. M., & Katz, L. C. (1991). Effects of binocular deprivation on the development of clustered horizontal connections in cat striate cortex. *Proceedings of the National Academy of Sciences of the United States of America, 88*, 745–749.

Catalano, S. M., & Shatz, C. J. (1998). Activity-dependent cortical target selection by thalamic axons. *Science, 281*, 559–562.

Caviness, V. S. (1976). Patterns of cell and fiber distribution in the neocortex of the reeler mutant mouse. *Journal of Comparative Neurology, 170*, 435–448.

Chun, J. M., & Shatz, C. J. (1989). Interstitial cells of the adult neocortical white matter are the remnant of the early generated subplate neuron population. *Journal of Comparative Neurology, 282*, 555–569.

Cragg, B. G. (1975). The development of synapses in the visual system of the cat. *Journal of Comparative Neurology, 160*, 147–166.

Crair, M. C., Gillespie, D. C., & Stryker, M. P. (1998). The role of visual experience in the development of columns in cat visual cortex. *Science, 279*, 566–570.

Crair, M. C., Horton, J. C., Antonini, A., & Stryker, M. P. (2001). Emergence of ocular dominance columns in cat visual cortex by 2 weeks of age. *Journal of Comparative Neurology, 430*, 235–249.

Cramer, K. S., & Sur, M. (1997). Blockade of afferent impulse activity disrupts on/off sublamination in the ferret lateral geniculate nucleus. *Developmental Brain Research, 98*, 287–290.

Creel, D., Witkop, C. J., & King, R. A. (1974). Asymmetric visually evoked potentials in human albinos: evidence for visual system anomalies. *Investigative Ophthalmology, 13*, 430–440.

Crowley, J. C., & Katz, L. C. (2000). Early development of ocular dominance columns. *Science, 290*, 1321–1325.

Dehay, C., Kennedy, H., Bullier, J., & Berland, M. (1988). Absence of interhemispheric connections of area 17 during development in the monkey. *Nature, 331*, 348–350.

Deiner, M. S., & Sretavan, D. W. (1999). Altered midline axon pathways and ectopic neurons in the developing hypothalamus of netrin-1- and DCC-deficient mice. *Journal of Neuroscience, 19*, 9900–9912.

Deiner, M. S., Kennedy, T. E., Fazeli, A., Serafini, T., Tessier-Lavigne, M., & Sretavan, D. W. (1997). Netrin-1 and DCC mediate axon guidance locally at the optic disc: loss of function leads to optic nerve hypoplasia. *Neuron, 19*, 575–589.

Donoghue, M. J., & Rakic, P. (1999). Molecular evidence for the early specification of presumptive functional domains in the embryonic primate cerebral cortex. *Journal of Neuroscience, 19*, 5967–5979.

Dubin, M. W., Stark, L. A., & Archer, S. M. (1986). A role for action-potential activity in the development of neuronal connections in the kitten retinogeniculate pathway. *Journal of Neuroscience, 6*, 1021–1036.

Erskine, L., Williams, S. E., Brose, K., Kidd, K., Rachel, R. A., Goodman, C. S., Tessier-Lavigne, M., & Mason, C. A. (2000). Retinal ganglion cell axon guidance in the mouse optic chiasm: expression and function of robos and slits. *Journal of Neuroscience, 20*, 4975–4982.

Feldheim, D. A., Kim, Y. I., Bergemann, A. D., Frisen, J., Barbacid, M., & Flanagan, J. G. (2000). Genetic analysis of ephrin-A2 and ephrin-A5 shows their requirement in multiple aspects of retinocollicular mapping. *Neuron, 25*, 563–574.

Feller, M. B., Wellis, D. P., Stellwagen, D., Werblin, F. S., & Shatz, C. J. (1996). Requirement for cholinergic synaptic transmission in the propagation of spontaneous retinal waves. *Science, 272*, 1182–1187.

Friauf, E., & Shatz, C. J. (1991). Changing patterns of synaptic input to subplate and cortical plate during development of visual cortex. *Journal of Neurophysiology, 66*, 2059–2071.

Friauf, E., McConnell, S. K., & Shatz, C. J. (1990). Functional synaptic circuits in the subplate during fetal and early postnatal development of cat visual cortex. *Journal of Neuroscience, 10*, 2601–2613.

Friedman, S., & Shatz, C. J. (1990). The effects of prenatal intracranial infusion of tetrodotoxin on naturally occurring retinal ganglion cell death and optic nerve ultrastructure. *European Journal of Neuroscience, 2*, 243–253.

Fukuchi-Shimogori, T., & Grove, E. A. (2001). Neocortex patterning by the secreted signaling molecule FGF8. *Science, 294*, 1071–1074.

Ghosh, A., Antonini, A., McConnell, S. K., & Shatz, C. J. (1990). Requirement for subplate neurons in the formation of thalamocortical connections. *Nature, 347*, 179–181.

Guillery, R. W. (1974). Visual pathways in albinos. *Scientific American, 230(5)*, 44–54.

Guo, S., Reinecke, R. D., Fendick, M., & Calhoun, J. H. (1989). Visual pathway abnormalities in albinism and infantile nystagmus: VECPs and stereoacuity measurements. *Journal of Pediatric Ophthalmology and Strabismus, 26*, 97–104.

Hamasaki, T., Leingärtner, A., Ringstedt, T., & O'Leary, D. M. (2004). EMX2 regulates sizes and positioning of the primary sensory and motor areas in neocortex by direct specification of cortical progenitors. *Neuron, 43*, 359–372.

Hansen, M. J., Dallal, G. E., & Flanagan, J. G. (2004). Retinal axon response to Ephrin-As shows a graded, concentration-dependent transition from growth promotion to inhibition. *Neuron, 42*, 717–730.

Hebb, D. O. (1949). *The organization of behaviour*. New York: Wiley.

Herrera, E., Brown, L., Arruga, J., Rachel, R. A., Dolen, G., Mikoshiba, K., Brown, S., & Mason, C. A. (2003). Zic2 patterns binocular vision by specifying the uncrossed retinal projection. *Cell, 114*, 545–557.

Hindges, R., McLaughlin, T., Genoud, N., Henkemeyer, M., & O'Leary, D. M. (2002). EphB forward signaling controls directional branch extension and arborization required for dorsal-ventral retinotopic mapping. *Neuron, 35*, 475–487.

Hoffmann, M. B., Tolhurst, D. J., Moore, A. T., & Morland, A. B. (2003). Organization of the visual cortex in human albinism. *Journal of Neuroscience, 23*, 8921–8930.

Horton, J. C., & Hocking, D. R. (1996). An adult-like pattern of ocular dominance columns in striate cortex of newborn monkeys prior to visual experience. *Journal of Neuroscience, 16*, 1791–1807.

Huberman, A. G., Murray, K. D., Feldheim, D. A., & Chapman, B. (2003). Ephrins mediate formation of eye-specific layers in the lateral geniculate nucleus. In *Abstract viewer/itinerary planner* (Program N. 567.21). Washington, DC: Society for Neuroscience.

Innocenti, G. M. (1981). Growth and reshaping of axons in the establishment of visual callosal connections. *Science, 212*, 824–827.

Katz, L. C., & Crowley, J. C. (2002). Development of cortical circuits: lessons from ocular dominance columns. *Nature Neuroscience Reviews, 3*, 34–42.

Kostovic, I., & Rakic, P. (1990). Developmental history of the transient subplate zone in the visual and somatosensory cortex of the macaque monkey and human brain. *Journal of Comparative Neurology, 297*, 441–470.

LaMantia, A. S., & Rakic, P. (1990). Axon overproduction and elimination in the corpus callosum of the developing rhesus monkey. *Journal of Neuroscience, 10*, 2156–2175.

LaVail, J. H., Nixon, R. A., & Sidman, R. L. (1978). Genetic control of retinal ganglion cell projections. *Journal of Comparative Neurology, 182*, 399–422.

LaVail, M. M., Rapaport, D. H., & Rakic, P. (1991). Cytogenesis in the monkey retina. *Journal of Comparative Neurology, 309*, 86–114.

Lavdas, A. A., Grigoriou, M., Pachnis, V., & Parnavelas, J. G. (1999). The medial ganglionic eminence gives rise to a population of early neurons in the developing cerebral cortex. *Journal of Neuroscience,19*, 7881–7888.

Lemmon, V., & Pearlman, A. L. (1981). Does laminar position determine the receptive field properties of cortical neurons? A study of corticotectal cells in area 17 of the normal mouse and the reeler mutant. *Journal of Neuroscience, 1*, 83–93.

LeVay, S., & Stryker, M. P. (1979). The development of ocular dominance columns in the cat. *Society for Neuroscience Symposia, 4*, 83–98.

Lopez-Bendito, G., & Molnar, Z. (2003). Thalamocortical development: how are we going to get there? *Nature Neuroscience Reviews, 4*, 276–289.

Lorente, d. N. (1938). Cerebral cortex: Architectonics, intracortical connections. In J. F. Fulton (Ed.), *Physiology of the nervous system* (pp. 288–313). New York: Oxford University Press.

Luhmann, H. J., Millan, L. M., & Singer, W. (1986). Development of horizontal intrinsic connections in cat striate cortex. *Experimental Brain Research, 63*, 443–448.

Lund, J. S., Boothe, R. G., & Lund, R. D. (1977). Development of neurons in the visual cortex (area 17) of the monkey (Macaca nemestrina): a Golgi study from fetal day 127 to postnatal maturity. *Journal of Comparative Neurology, 176*, 149–187.

Luskin, M. B., & Shatz, C. J. (1985). Neurogenesis of the cat's primary visual cortex. *Journal of Comparative Neurology, 242*, 611–631.

Lyckman, A. W., Jhaveri, S., Feldheim, D. A., Vanderhaeghen, P., Flanagan, J. G., & Sur, M. (2001). Enhanced plasticity of retinothalamic projections in an ephrin A2/A5 double mutant. *Journal of Neuroscience, 21*, 7684–7690.

Mann, F., Peuckert, C., Dehner, F., Zhou, R., & Bolz, J. (2002). Ephrins regulate the formation of terminal axonal arbors during the development of thalamocortical projections. *Development, 129*, 3945–3955.

Marcus, R. C., Blazeski, R., Godemont, P., & Mason, C. A. (1995). Retinal axon divergence in the optic chiasm: uncrossed axons diverge from crossed axons within a midline glial specialization. *Journal of Neuroscience, 15*, 3716–3729.

Marcus, R. C., Wang, L.-C., & Mason, C. A. (1996). Retinal axon divergence in the optic chiasm: midline cells are unaffected by the albino mutation. *Development, 122*, 859–868.

Marin-Padilla, M. (1971). Early prenatal ontogenesis of the cerebral cortex (neocortex) of the cat (Felix domestica). A Golgi study. I. The primordial neocortical organization. *Zeitschrift fur Anatomie und Entwicklungsgeschichte, 134*, 117–145.

Marquardt, T., & Gruss, P. (2002). Generating neuronal diversity in the retina: one for nearly all. *Trends in Neurosciences, 25*, 32–38.

Maslim, J., & Stone, J. (1988). Time course of stratification of the dendritic fields of ganglion cells in the retina of the cat. *Developmental Brain Research, 44*, 87–93.

McLaughlin, T., Hindges, R., & O'Leary, D. M. (2003). Regulation of axial patterning of the retina and its topographic mapping in the brain. *Current Opinion in Neurobiology, 13*, 57–69.

McLaughlin, T., Torborg, C. L., Feller, M. B., & O'Leary, D. J. (2003). Retinotopic map refinement requires spontaneous retinal waves during a brief critical period of development. *Neuron, 40*, 1147–1160.

Meisserel, C., Wikler, K. C., Chalupa, L. M., & Rakic, P. (1997). Early divergence of magnocellular and parvocellular functional subsystems in the embryonic primate visual system. *Proceedings of the National Academy of Sciences of the United States of America, 94*, 5900–5905.

Meister, M., Wong, R. L., Baylor, D. A., & Shatz, C. J. (1991). Synchronous bursts of action potentials in ganglion cells of the developing mammalian retina. *Science, 252*, 939–943.

Meyer, G., & Ferres-Torres, R. (1984). Postnatal maturation of nonpyramidal neurons in the visual cortex of the cat. *Journal of Comparative Neurology, 228*, 226–244.

Molliver, M. E., Kostovic, I., & Van der Loos, H. V. (1973). The development of synapses in cerebral cortex of the human fetus. *Brain Research, 50*, 403–407.

Mui, S. H., Hindges, R., O'Leary, D. M., Lemke, G., & Bertuzzi, S. (2002). The homeodomain protein Vax2 patterns the dorsoventral and nasotemporal axes of the eye. *Development, 129*, 797–804.

Murphy, K. M., Duffy, K. R., Jones, D. G., & Mitchell, D. M. (2001). Development of cytochrome oxidase blobs in visual cortex of normal and visually deprived cats. *Cerebral Cortex, 11*, 122–135.

Nakagawa, S., Brennan, C., Johnson, K. G., Shewan, D., Harris, W. A., & Holt, C. E. (2000). Ephrin-B regulates the ipsilateral routing of retinal axons at the optic chiasm. *Neuron, 25*, 599–610.

Ng, A. Y., & Stone, J. (1982). The optic nerve of the cat: appearance and loss of axons during normal development. *Developmental Brain Research, 5*, 263–271.

Novak, N., & Bolz, J. (1993). Formation of specific efferent connections in organotypic slice cultures from rat visual cortex cocultured with lateral geniculate nucleus and superior colliculus. *European Journal of Neuroscience, 5*, 15–24.

O'Leary, D. M., & Nakagawa, Y. (2002). Patterning centers, regulatory genes and extrinsic mechanisms controlling arealization of the neocortex. *Current Opinion in Neurobiology, 12*, 14–25.

Oster, S. F., Bodeker, M. O., He, F., & Sretavan, D. W. (2003). Invariant Sema5A inhibition serves as an ensheathing function during optic nerve development. *Development, 130*, 775-784.

Oster, S. F., Deiner, M. S., Birgbauer, E., & Sretavan, D. W. (2004). Ganglion cell axon pathfinding in the retina and optic nerve. *Seminars in Cell and Developmental Biology, 15*, 125–136.

Pak, W., Hindges, R., Lim, Y.-S., Pfaff, S. L., & O'Leary, D. M. (2004). Magnitude of binocular vision controlled by islet-2 repression of a genetic program that specifies laterality of retinal axon pathfinding. *Cell, 119*, 567–578.

Payne, B. R., Pearson, H. E., & Cornwell, P. (1988). Development of visual and auditory cortical connections in the cat. In A. Peters & E. G. Jones (Eds.), *Cerebral Cortex* (pp. 309–389). New York: Plenum.

Plump, A. S., Erskine, L., Sabatier, C., Brose, K., Epstein, C. J., Goodman, C. S., & Mason, Tessier-Lavigne, C. A. (2002). Slit 1 and Slit 2 cooperate to prevent premature crossing of retinal axons in the mouse visual system. *Neuron, 33*, 219–232.

Price, D. J., & Blakemore, C. (1985). Regressive events in the postnatal development of association projections in the visual cortex. *Nature, 316*, 721–724.

Rakic, P. (1972). Mode of cell migration to the superficial layers of fetal monkey neocortex. *Journal of Comparative Neurology, 145*, 61–83.

Rakic, P. (1974). Neurons in rhesus monkey cortex: systematic relation between time of origin and eventual disposition. *Science, 183*, 425–427.

Rakic, P. (1976). Prenatal genesis of connections subserving ocular dominance in the rhesus monkey. *Nature, 261*, 467–471.

Rakic, P. (1977). Prenatal development of the visual system in rhesus monkey. *Philosophical Proceedings of the Royal Society of London. Series B. Biological sciences, 278*, 245–260.

Rakic, P. (1992). An overview development of the primate visual system: from photoreceptors to cortical modules. In R. Lent (Ed.), *The visual system from genesis to maturity* (pp. 1–17). Boston: Birkhauser.

Rakic, P., & Riley, K. P. (1983a). Overproduction and elimination of retinal axons in the fetal rhesus monkey. *Science, 219*, 1441–1444.

Rakic, P., & Riley, K. P. (1983b). Regulation of axon number in primate optic nerve by prenatal binocular competition. *Nature, 305*, 135–137.

Rakic, P., Suner, I., & Williams, R. W. (1991). A novel cytoarchitectonic area induced experimentally within the primate visual cortex. *Proceedings of the National Academy of Sciences of the United States of America, 88*, 2082–2087.

Ramoa, A. S., Campbell, G., & Shatz, C. J. (1989). Retinal ganglion β cells project transiently to the superior colliculus during development. *Proceedings of the National Academy of Sciences of the United States of America, 86*, 2061–2065.

Rossi, F. M., Pizzorusso, T., Porciatti, V., Marubio, L. M., Maffei, L., & Changeux, J. P. (2001). Requirement of the nicotinic acetylcholine receptor beta-2 for the anatomical and functional development of the visual system. *Proceedings of the National Academy of Sciences of the United States of America, 98*, 6453–6458.

Sestan, N., Rakic, P., & Donoghue, M. J. (2001). Independent parcellation of the embryonic visual cortex and thalamus revealed by combinatorial Eph/ephrin gene expression. *Current Biology, 11*, 39–43.

Shatz, C. J., & Luskin, M. B. (1986). The relationship between the geniculocortical afferents and their cortical target cells during development of the cat's primary visual cortex. *Journal of Neuroscience, 6*, 3655–3668.

Shatz, C. J., & Stryker, M. P. (1988). Prenatal tetrodotoxin infusion blocks segregation of retinogeniculate afferents. *Science, 242*, 87–89.

Simon, D. K., Prusky, G. T., O'Leary, D. M., & Constantine-Paton, M. (1992). N-methyl-D-aspartate receptor antagonists disrupt the formation of a mammalian neural map. *Proceedings of the National Academy of Sciences of the United States of America, 89*, 10593–10597.

Sperry, R. W. (1963). Chemoaffinity in the orderly growth of nerve fiber patterns and connections. *Proceedings of the National Academy of Sciences of the United States of America, 50*, 703–710.

Sretavan, D. W., & Shatz, C. J. (1986). Prenatal development of retinal ganglion cell axons: segregation into eye-specific layers within the cat's lateral geniculate nucleus. *Journal of Neuroscience, 6*, 234–251.

Stanfield, B. B., & O'Leary, D. M. (1985). The transient corticospinal projection from the occipital cortex during the postnatal development of the rat. *Journal of Comparative Neurology, 238*, 236–248.

Stryker, M. P., & Harris, W. A. (1986). Binocular impulse blockade prevents the formation of ocular dominance columns in cat visual cortex. *Journal of Neuroscience, 6*, 2117–2133.

Tian, N., & Copenhagen, D. R. (2003). Visual stimulation is required for refinement of ON and OFF pathways in postnatal retina. *Neuron, 39*, 85–96.

Toyama, K., Komatsu, Y., Yamamoto, N., & Kurotani, T. (1993). In vitro studies of visual cortical development and plasticity. *Progress in Neurobiology, 41*, 543–563.

Tuttle, R., Braisted, J. E., Richards, L. J., & O'Leary, D. M. (1998). Retinal axon guidance by region-specific cues in diencephalon. *Development, 125*, 791–801.

Williams, R. W., & Rakic, P. (1988). Elimination of neurons from the rhesus monkey's lateral geniculate nucleus during development. *Journal of Comparative Neurology, 272*, 424–436.

Williams, R. W., Bastiani, M. J., Lia, B., & Chalupa, L. M. (1986). Growth cones, dying axons and developmental fluctuations in the fiber population of the cat's optic nerve. *Journal of Comparative Neurology, 246*, 32–69.

Williams, S. E., Mann, F., Erskine, L., Sakurai, T., Wei, S., Rossi, D. J., Gale, N. W., Holt, C. E., Mason, C. A., & Henkemeyer, M. (2003). Ephrin-B2 and EphB1 mediate retinal axon divergence at the optic chiasm. *Neuron, 39*, 919–935.

Winfield, D. A. (1983). The postnatal development of synapses in the different laminae of the visual cortex in the normal kitten and in kittens with eyelid suture. *Developmental Brain Research, 9*, 155–169.

Yamamoto, N., Kurotani, T., & Toyama, K. (1989). Neural connections between the lateral geniculate nucleus and visual cortex in vitro. *Science, 245*, 192–194.

5

Development of Receptive Field Properties

The physiological properties of most cells in the visual system continue to develop for some time after birth. The connections of many cells are not completely formed when the eyes open, and the visual performance of all higher mammals is initially uncertain and groping. Only with use can one analyze the visual image fully and respond to it. There is clearly a learning process going on. The key questions are: Which properties develop? Where in the visual system does the development occur? And when does it happen?

Most work on the development of receptive field properties has been done in cat and ferret. These are the animals of choice for correlating receptive field properties with anatomical changes. Unfortunately, they are hard to work with in behavioral experiments. Monkeys give more precise results in behavioral studies but there are not many studies on the development of receptive field properties in monkeys. Consequently, this chapter will emphasize the cat and ferret but give evidence from the monkey wherever possible.

The initial experiments on the development of receptive field properties were prompted by the nature–nurture controversy that was discussed in Chapter 1. At first, authors took somewhat extreme positions. Hubel and Wiesel (1963) were surprised that cells in young kittens respond to the orientation of a bar when it is moved through the receptive field of the cell, that cells with similar orientation sensitivity are located near each other, and that the binocular convergence of input from the two eyes onto single cells in kittens is like adult binocularity. For them, the crucial feature distinguishing cortical cells from lateral geniculate cells was orientation sensitivity, so they emphasized that "much of the richness of visual physiology in the cortex of the adult cat is present in very young kittens without visual experience." They were surprised because vision, as measured by behavior, is poor in kittens at the time of eye-opening. Avoidance of objects is not seen until 14 days, and pursuit, following movements, and visual placing appear at 20 to 25 days (Windle, 1930). Pettigrew (1974), on the other hand, reported that the selectivity of cells for disparity improves substantially over the first few weeks. He consequently emphasized the development of receptive field properties after birth. From their different points of view, they were both correct. The properties and location of cells in the visual cortex do have an organization at birth, and these properties are refined by visual experience.

Most studies of receptive field properties in the developing visual system are done in anesthetized, paralyzed animals. This ensures that the eyes will not move, and that a stimulus can be repeated several times to give a reliable response. A single cell in the visual system is isolated with a microelectrode, then stimuli are projected onto a tangent screen in front of the animal. Because the response of the cell can vary with the length, width, orientation, direction, and velocity of movement, color, spatial frequency, and disparity of the object, and because there may be interactions between these properties such as movement and depth, several experiments may be required before the properties are fully understood. Three major papers explored the properties of ganglion cells in the cat retina between 1950 and 1974, each one providing a new classification. Since 1968, three major papers have explored the properties of cells in primary visual cortex of the macaque, with numerous details added in the years since they were published. It seems likely that we now understand the retina, that some new discoveries will be made in primary visual cortex, and that many more experiments will need to be done on the cells in higher visual areas before their properties are fully understood. Consequently, this chapter will not discuss levels of the visual system higher than primary visual cortex.

All authors who have studied the receptive fields of cells in the visual cortex in young kittens have noted that the cells are not very responsive. The cells habituate, so that stimuli need to be presented several seconds apart to give the best response, and even then the response is substantially less than in the adult. Close attention needs to be paid to the condition of the animal by monitoring heart rate, blood pressure, and expired CO_2, as a deterioration of these can reduce the specificity of the response even further. However, the susceptibility of young animals to the effects of anesthetic does not account for the lack of specific receptive fields found in well-monitored animals, because cells with receptive fields that are specific for the orientation and direction of movement of the stimulus are found near cells that are not specific for these properties in the same animal under the same conditions.

An important consideration in studying the response of cells in the cat visual system is that the optics are not clear when the eyes open. There is a hyaloid membrane on the posterior surface of the lens (Thorn, Gollender, & Erickson, 1976). This blurs the image on the retina distinctly at 16 days of age, and slightly at 30 days (Bonds & Freeman, 1978). However, for many tasks the effect is not significant because of the nature of the optical distortions involved. This consideration does not apply to the macaque, where the optical media are clear at birth.

Finally, it is important to emphasize that it is impossible, in a single experiment, to characterize all aspects of the receptive field of a particular cell, and to obtain a substantial sample of cells. This is particularly true when working with young animals. Scientists have tended to concentrate on one aspect of the receptive field of the cell and study it thoroughly. Conclusions have therefore been modified as scientists attack the same general problem with new and modified stimuli.

1. Development in the Retina and Lateral Geniculate Nucleus

From the anatomical point of view, the retina, lateral geniculate nucleus, and visual cortex develop in parallel. So, clearly, the maturation of properties of cells in the cortex will depend on the maturation of the properties of cells at lower levels of the system.

An interesting comparison can be made in the monkey between its behavioral response and the responses of cells at various levels of the system by using the contrast sensitivity curve. Contrast sensitivity develops in the monkey over the first year of life (Boothe, Kiorpes, Williams, & Teller, 1988). Acuity improves, contrast sensitivity improves at all spatial frequencies, and the peak of the curve moves to higher spatial frequency, as it does in the human (Fig. 5.1).

The theoretical limit of spatial resolution imposed by the spacing of the photoreceptors has been calculated by Jacobs and Blakemore (1988) for the monkey. It is called the *Nyquist limit*, and it increases from 8 to 10 cycles/degree at 1 week of age to 40 to 50 cycles/degree in the adult (Fig. 5.2) for the same reasons discussed in Chapter 3 for humans: the photoreceptors move closer together and the eyeball gets larger. Grating acuity for the most selective neurons in the lateral geniculate is worse than the Nyquist limit at 1 week of age by a factor of 2 (Blakemore & Vital-Durand, 1986), and gets close to the Nyquist limit at around 1 year of age. Cortical neurons are a little worse than lateral geniculate neurons between 10 weeks and 1 year of age.

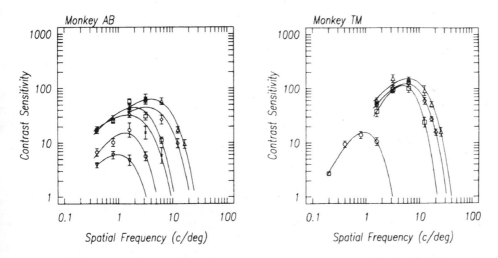

FIG. 5.1. Development of the spatial contrast sensitivity curve for two monkeys. Points for monkey AB taken at 10 (∇), 11 (○), 14 (X), 15 (□), 25 (◇), and 38 (△) weeks, Points for monkey TM taken at 5 (○), 12 (□), 20 (◇), and 32 (△) weeks. [Reprinted from Boothe, R. G., et al. (1988), *Vision Research, 28*, 387–396. Copyright 1988, with permission from Elsevier.]

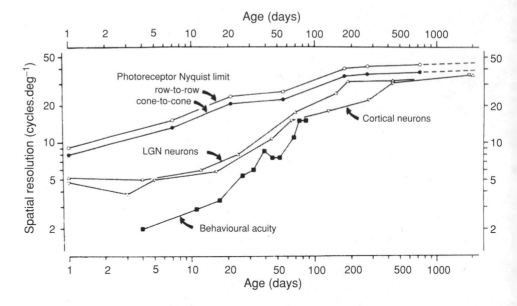

FIG. 5.2. Development of acuity in the monkey, measured in behavioral experiments, compared with the capabilities of neurons in the lateral geniculate nucleus and cortex and the theoretical limit of acuity based on the spacing of photoreceptors. [Reprinted from Jacobs, D. S., & Blakemore, C. (1988). *Vision Research, 28*, 947–958. Copyright 1988, with permission from Elsevier.]

Acuity measured by behavioral tests is worse than the performance of the lateral geniculate and cortical neurons by a factor of 2 at 1 week of age, and catches up around 12 weeks of age. Kiorpes and Movshon (2004) have performed a similar analysis and come to rather different conclusions; they find that changes in the photoreceptors are confined to the first 4 weeks, whereas the bulk of the change measured behaviorally takes place after 4 weeks. In any case, something degrades the performance between the photoreceptors and the lateral geniculate neurons, and something degrades it further between the cortex and behavior, until the performances at all levels of the system converge at around 1 year of age.

A clue as to what some of these degrading factors might be can be obtained from the cat, where the relationship between the anatomy and physiology of the cells involved is more clearly understood. The fine-detail cells in the retina of the cat are called X cells when studied physiologically, and ß cells when studied anatomically (Boycott & Wassle, 1974). The best spatial frequency for an individual cell is related to the size of the center of its receptive field and varies with the cell's distance from the center of the retina (Cleland, Harding, & Tulunay-Keesey, 1979; see Fig. 5.3). During the first 2 weeks of life, there are no cells with very small receptive centers measured physiologically, and this corresponds with the poor acuity (Tootle, 1993). However, anatomically, the size of ß cells in young kittens is small, smaller than in the adult (Rusoff & Dubin, 1978). Consequently, the physiological size of the receptive field exceeds the anatomical size of the cell at this age, presumably due to some convergence of lateral excitatory connections within the retina.

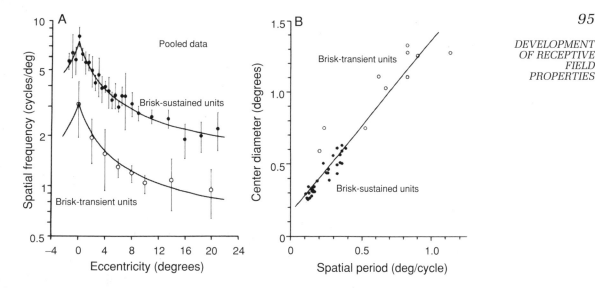

FIG. 5.3. (A) Highest spatial frequency that can be detected, measured with a drifting grating for individual ganglion cells. Results plotted for X (brisk-sustained) cells and Y (brisk-transient) cells as a function of distance from the center of the retina (eccentricity). (B) The highest detectable spatial frequency is linearly related to the diameter of the center of the receptive field, measured with a bar moved slowly across the receptive field. [Reprinted with permission from Cleland, B. G., et al. (1979). *Science, 205*, 1015–1017. Copyright 1979 AAAS.]

The terminal axons of the ß cells in the lateral geniculate nucleus contract between 3 and 12 weeks of age (Sur, Weller, & Sherman, 1984). Correspondingly, the spatial resolution of the X cells in the lateral geniculate develops between 3 and 16 weeks of age, in parallel with behavioral measurements and measurements of the visually evoked response from the cortex (Ikeda and Tremain, 1978). Lateral inhibition, which produces the surround of the receptive field of retinal cells, matures over the first 4 to 5 weeks (Rusoff & Dubin, 1977; Hamasaki & Flynn, 1977). This occurs in parallel with the development of the center of the receptive field (Tootle, 1993). The additional lateral inhibition that occurs in the lateral geniculate nucleus is immature at 4 weeks of age (Tootle and Friedlander, 1986) and matures after that. As lateral inhibition at both these levels develops, contrast sensitivity at frequencies that are low compared with contrast sensitivity at the peak of the contrast sensitivity curve (low frequency fall-off) increases correspondingly.

Y cells are primarily responsible for the detection of movement. Their temporal resolution, measured in the lateral geniculate, improves substantially between 2 and 8 weeks of age, and a little more after that (Wilson, Tessin, & Sherman, 1982). It is difficult to distinguish Y cells from X cells in 3-week-old kittens (Rusoff & Dubin, 1977; Daniels, Pettigrew, & Norman, 1978). However, their morphological counterparts, the α and ß cells, can be distinguished from each other at this age by anatomical criteria (Tootle, 1993). Thus, the distinction between X and Y cells is conferred by synaptic mechanisms that develop after the anatomy is established. The spatial resolution of Y cells in the lateral geniculate gets worse with age (Tootle and Friedlander, 1989), probably because the terminal arbors in the lateral geniculate nucleus of α cells from the retina expand between 3 and 12 weeks of age (Sur et al., 1984).

The conclusion is that the development of acuity and the low frequency fall-off in the contrast sensitivity curve depend on processing beyond the photoreceptors as well as on the development of the photoreceptors, just as predicted for the human (Banks & Bennett, 1988). Changes in the physiological properties of cells in the retina, as well as in the size of their terminal arborizations in the lateral geniculate, contribute to changes in acuity. Changes in lateral inhibitory mechanisms in both the retina and lateral geniculate contribute to low frequency fall-off. There are also additional factors in the cortex, suggested by the comparison studied by Jacobs and Blakemore (1988), but these have not been specifically identified.

2. Development in the Visual Cortex

The properties of cortical cells in the cat that depend particularly on the retina and lateral geniculate, such as spatial and temporal resolution, develop in parallel with the retina and lateral geniculate. This shows up as an increase in spatial frequency selectivity (Derrington & Fuchs, 1981) and a decrease in the size of the center of the receptive field (Braastad & Heggelund, 1985). In addition, the sensitivity to contrast for a stimulus of the optimal spatial frequency improves dramatically. A contrast of no more than 50% can be detected at 2 weeks of age, while a contrast of 1% can be detected at 8 weeks of age (Derrington & Fuchs, 1981).

The proportion of cortical cells that respond to visual stimuli also increases with age, as it does in the retina and lateral geniculate. However, more unresponsive cells are found in layers II, III, and V in young animals than in the other layers (Albus & Wolf, 1984). This difference occurs partly because layers II and III are the last to develop anatomically, and partly because layers IV and VI are the ones that receive direct input from the lateral geniculate nucleus and are therefore the first to get visual input.

The distinguishing physiological features of the visual cortex, as opposed to the lateral geniculate, are selectivity for direction of movement and for orientation, convergence of ON and OFF inputs onto a single cell, convergence of left and right eye inputs onto a single cell, and selectivity for the disparity of the stimulus for binocular cells. One might expect that these would develop with a different time course from the retina and lateral geniculate because of the complexity of the stimulus features encoded, but in fact they develop pretty much in parallel.

Some cells specific for the direction of movement of a stimulus are found in the youngest animals recorded from (Hubel & Wiesel, 1963; Pettigrew, 1974; Blakemore & Van Sluyters, 1975; see Fig. 5.4). When one considers specificity for the *orientation* of the stimulus, the situation becomes complicated by the definition of exactly what is meant. For cells that respond to stationary stimuli, the situation is clear: one flashes a stimulus on the receptive field in various different orientations, and tests whether the response to one orientation (the preferred orientation) is greater than the response to other orientations. Unfortunately, this test cannot always be applied in young animals because

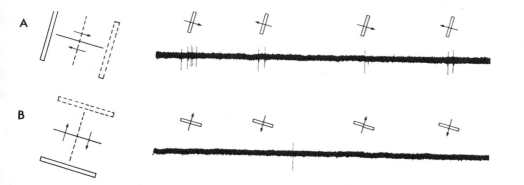

FIG. 5.4. A cell responding to direction of movement from the cortex of an 8-day-old kitten with no previous visual experience. A bar of light, 1° by 5°, was moved across the receptive field of the cell at 5°/s. On the left is shown the bar in relation to the center of the receptive field, which was in the middle. On the right is shown the train of action potentials, with the movement of the stimulus shown above. The cell responded to a bar moving from 4 o'clock to 10 o'clock and back, but not to a bar moving from 7 o'clock to 1 o'clock and back. [Used with permission from Hubel, D. H., & Wiesel, T. N. (1963). *Journal of Neurophysiology, 26,* 994–1002.]

the rather unresponsive cells that are found often respond fairly clearly to moving stimuli, but not at all clearly to stationary stimuli (Hubel & Wiesel, 1963; Albus & Wolf, 1984).

When the cell does not respond clearly to stationary stimuli, scientists have measured how the response changes as the stimulus is moved in directions away from the preferred direction. The quantitative measurement of response as a function of the angle of the direction of movement is known as a *direction tuning curve* (see Fig. 5.5). A direction tuning curve can be

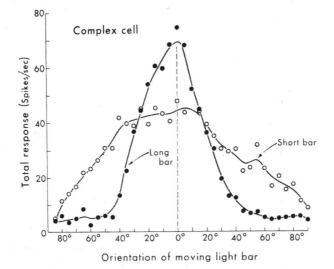

FIG. 5.5. Orientation tuning curves produced in a complex cell by light bars of different lengths. The tuning sharpens as the bar is lengthened from 1° (short) to 4° (long). [Used with permission from Henry G. L., et al. (1974). *Journal of Neurophysiology, 37,* 1394–1409.]

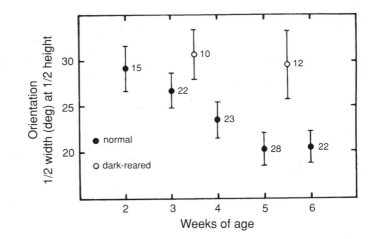

FIG. 5.6. Development of orientation specificity in the visual cortex of the cat. To obtain an orientation tuning curve (for an example of such a curve, see Fig. 5.5), responses to movement of a stimulus through the receptive field at various orientations are recorded and the angle at which the response falls to half of the peak response is noted. The graph above represents how far this angle is from that giving the peak response, and the points were calculated by taking half the angle (1/2 width) between the two orientations where the response falls to half the peak (1/2 height). Orientation specificity falls from 30° at 2 weeks of age to 20° at 5 to 6 weeks of age. Note that orientation specificity remains immature if the animal is reared in the dark. [Reprinted with permission from Bonds, A. B. (1979). *Developmental neurobiology of vision* (pp. 31–41).]

measured for the movement of a spot and also for the movement of a bar. If the curve is narrower for bars than for spots, this implies that the cell is more specific for the bar than for the spot; thus, the cell is said to be specific for the orientation of the stimulus, as well as for the direction of movement. There is no doubt that the direction tuning curve gets narrower between 2 and 5 weeks of age (Bonds, 1979; see Fig. 5.6). A less time-consuming measurement is to compare the response to the preferred orientation and direction of movement with the response to movement perpendicular to it over a sample of cells. The number of cells in which there is little or no response for movement of a bar perpendicular to the preferred orientation (orientation selective cells) increases substantially with age (Blakemore & Van Sluyters, 1975; see Fig. 5.7).

The picture is complicated in the cat by the cloudiness of the optics at early ages. This factor does not counter the point that orientation selectivity exists soon after eye opening. However, it may complicate the measurement of the increase in orientation selectivity with age. In the ferret, the optics of the eye are clear from the time of eye opening, and maturation of orientation selectivity can be more clearly measured (Chapman & Stryker, 1993).

While the selectivity of individual cells for orientation improves with age, the general organization for orientation is established at birth (Fig. 5.8). Cells responding to similar orientations are located near each other in both the cat (Hubel & Wiesel, 1963) and the monkey (Wiesel & Hubel, 1974).

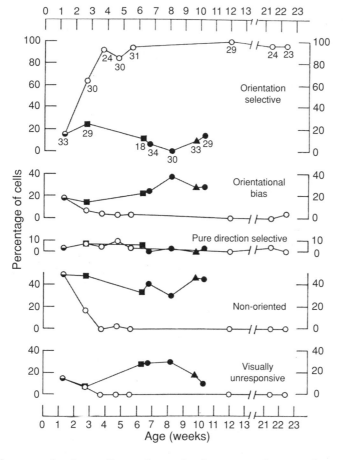

FIG. 5.7. Development of various cell types in cat visual cortex as a function of age. *Open symbols* give data from normal cats, and *closed symbols* from binocularly deprived cats. Note the large increase in orientation selective cells between 1 and 4 weeks of age, and the decrease in nonoriented and visually unresponsive cells. Note also that binocular deprivation maintains the cortex in the immature state. Orientation selective cells give little or no response for movement of a bar oriented perpendicular to the preferred orientation. Orientation bias cells give a response that is significantly larger for the preferred orientation than for the perpendicular one. [Reprinted with permission from Blakemore, C., & Van Sluyters, R. C. (1975). *Journal of Physiology, 248*, 663–716. Copyright 1975 Blackwell Publishing Ltd.]

The maturation of orientation selectivity can also be seen using the 2-deoxyglucose technique. 2-Deoxyglucose is taken up by active cells but not metabolized, and consequently can be used as a marker of cellular activity. To test orientation selectivity, the animal is stimulated with moving stripes of a particular orientation, then its cortex is assayed for ^{3}H-2-deoxyglucose taken up by the cells. In the adult, there are patches of cells demonstrating orientation columns. Before 21 days of age, patchiness is only found in layer IV (Thompson, Kossut, & Blakemore, 1983). Between 21 and 35 days of age, the patches mature. As the orientation tuning demonstrated by physiological techniques becomes tighter, the orientation columns demonstrated by anatomical techniques become sharper.

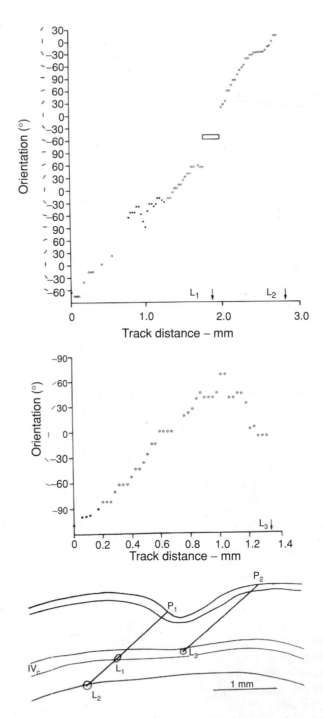

FIG. 5.8. Data from two penetrations of the visual cortex of a rhesus monkey with no prior visual experience at 17 days of age. There is a regular progression of orientations as the electrode is advanced at an oblique angle. Reconstruction of the tracks shown at bottom. [From Wiesel, T.N., & Hubel, D.H. (1974). Ordered arrangement of orientation columns in monkeys lacking visual experience. *Journal of Comparative Neurology, 158,* 307–318. Copyright © 1974. Reprinted by permission of John Wiley & Sons, Inc.]

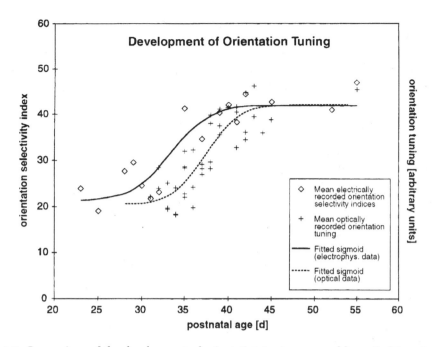

FIG. 5.9. Comparison of the development of orientation tuning assessed by optical imaging and electrophysiology. From Chapman, B., et al. (1999). Development of orientation preference in the mammalian visual cortex. *Journal of Neurobiology, 41,* 18–24. Copyright © 1999. Reprinted by permission of John Wiley and Sons, Inc.]

Another technique is optical imaging. In the ferret, where orientation selectivity is not formed at birth, because the animal is born earlier in its development than is the cat, orientation selectivity, as measured by optical imaging, lags orientation selectivity as measured in single unit recordings by about 4 days (Chapman, Godecke, & Bonhoeffer, 1999; Fig. 5.9). In the cat, the outlines of an orientation map can be seen at P14 when stimulating the contralateral eye, but not when stimulating the ipsilateral eye (Crair, Gillespie, & Stryker, 1998). The sharpness of the map then increases until 4 to 5 weeks of age. Interestingly, the map is lost if one eye is closed in young animals, and if the closed eye is then reopened and the open eye closed (reverse suture), the map in the newly opened eye is the same as that in the originally open eye (Kim & Bonhoeffer, 1994). Presumably, orientation selectivity depends on intracortical connections that form independent of the afferent input. This point is supported by the fact that intracortical connections develop in parallel with the development of orientation selectivity (Nelson & Katz, 1995).

An interesting study in the ferret compares the development of orientation selectivity in the ferret with the development of other receptive field properties, such as segregation of ON and OFF responses, whether the receptive field is circular or elongated, and whether the response is dominated by ON or OFF modalities (McKay & Thompson, 2004). Orientation selectivity improves between weeks 4 and 8 as cells become more ON–OFF than ON or OFF, the ON and OFF subfields segregate, and the receptive fields become more elongated. It seems clear that adultlike orientation tuning reflects qualitative changes in the receptive field structure. This should be contrasted with studies in the macaque, which show that orientation tuning, direction selectivity, and surround suppression do not change between birth and the adult (Kiorpes & Movshon, 2004). Presumably the difference arises because the macaque is born at a much later stage of development.

One might expect from the anatomy that binocular convergence would change substantially after birth. As described in Chapter 3, the endings in layer IV of the cortex coming from the lateral geniculate overlap at 3 weeks of age and segregate into eye-specific bands over the next few weeks (LeVay, Stryker, & Shatz, 1978). Consequently, long penetrations in layer IV of 10 to 17 day animals show a lot of binocular cells, while similar recordings in adult animals jump from cells driven largely by one eye to cells driven largely by the other. However, there is substantial convergence from the two eyes onto cells in other layers in adult animals, so that this effect is not very noticeable in ocular dominance histograms that include a sample of cells from all layers (Hubel & Wiesel, 1963; Albus & Wolf, 1984; Stryker & Harris, 1986).

One of the first studies on development in the visual cortex dealt with disparity selectivity in the cat (Pettigrew, 1974). This was an excellent choice of subject, given the observation that stereoscopic depth perception, which depends on disparity, develops late after birth. Pettigrew found a substantial improvement in disparity selectivity with age, using bars of light as the stimulus (Fig. 5.10). Experiments with gratings (Freeman & Ohzawa, 1992) suggest that the improvement may be largely due to the increase in spatial frequency selectivity of the cells. In the macaque, cells sensitive to disparity are found soon after birth, several weeks before the onset of stereopsis (Chino, Smith, Hatta, & Cheng, 1997). Their spatial frequency response and response amplitude develop over the first 4 postnatal weeks. However, we do not know anything about the development of cells excited by positive and negative disparity, cells responding to objects nearer than the fixation point compared with cells responding to objects further away, and cells inhibited by a specific disparity. This is unfortunate, given that behavioral observations show that stereoscopic vision has a rapid onset that is more clearly defined than most other properties in the visual system.

The bulk of these studies have been carried out on primary visual cortex (area 17) in the cat. The three main areas that area 17 projects to in the cat are areas 18, 19, and the lateral suprasylvian gyrus. Studies on cells in area 18 (Blakemore & Price, 1987; Milleret, Gary-Bobo, & Buisseret, 1988) and the lateral suprasylvian gyrus (Price, Zumbroich, & Blakemore, 1988) give results that are not remarkably different from those in area 17.

3. Development in the Absence of Light and Activity

Early in the history of this field, the nature–nurture controversy prompted the question: What happens to the receptive field properties of cells in the visual cortex in the absence of light? Do they mature, do they remain immature, or do they degenerate?

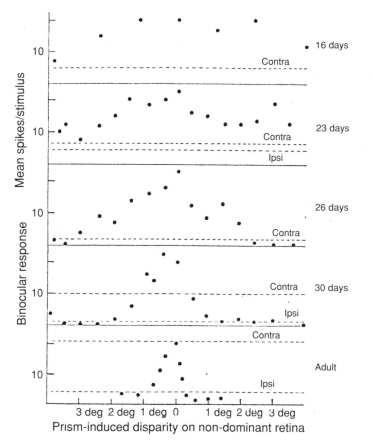

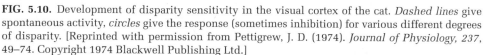

FIG. 5.10. Development of disparity sensitivity in the visual cortex of the cat. *Dashed lines* give spontaneous activity, *circles* give the response (sometimes inhibition) for various different degrees of disparity. [Reprinted with permission from Pettigrew, J. D. (1974). *Journal of Physiology, 237,* 49–74. Copyright 1974 Blackwell Publishing Ltd.]

The initial experiments were done with animals reared in the light with the eyelids of both eyes sutured shut, an experimental condition known as binocular deprivation (Wiesel & Hubel, 1965; Pettigrew, 1974; Singer & Tretter, 1976). Receptive fields were found to be immature, that is, not very specific for the orientation or direction of movement of the stimulus (Fig. 5.7). However, light does reach the retina through closed eyelids and cells in the visual cortex of such animals can detect the direction of movement of a stimulus (Spear, Tong, & Langsetmo, 1978), so binocular lid suture does not involve total deprivation.

To avoid all stimulation of the visual system, a better procedure is to rear animals in total darkness. In this case, the receptive fields of most cells are also immature and not very specific for orientation and direction of movement (Blakemore & Van Sluyters, 1975; Buisseret & Imbert, 1976; Cynader, Berman, & Hein, 1976; Bonds, 1979; see Fig. 5.6). Sensitivity to the contrast of the stimulus remains low and the preferred spatial frequency improves up to 3 weeks of age, but not after that (Derrington, 1984). The cells that do retain some specificity for orientation tend to be monocularly driven (Blakemore & Van Sluyters, 1975; Leventhal & Hirsch, 1980).

Few laboratories have made a direct comparison between the effects of dark rearing and binocular deprivation. The ocular dominance histogram from dark-reared animals is normal, while the histogram from binocularly deprived animals contains more monocular cells (Mower, Berry, Burchfiel, & Duffy, 1981). The retinas of binocularly deprived animals can detect movement of bright objects (see above) but their eyes are not aligned (Sherman, 1972). Consequently, the stimulation of cells through the two eyes is not concordant, as in strabismus (see Chapter 7), and this probably accounts for the lack of binocular cells. In addition, binocularly deprived animals have many cells that can not be driven by any visual stimulus, and dark-reared animals have many cells that can be driven by all orientations and directions of movement (Mower et al., 1981). Imaging the cortex in ferret shows that there are orientation columns in dark-reared animals, but almost none in lid-sutured animals (White, Coppola, & Fitzpatrick, 2001). Thus, while there are differences between the two procedures due to the fact that there is some visual stimulation in binocular deprivation and none in dark-rearing, the final result from both procedures is a cortex with few physiologically normal cells.

One can compare the receptive fields of cells in dark-reared animals with those of normal animals of the same age. There is some improvement in the specificity of the receptive fields up to 3 to 5 weeks of age (Buisseret & Imbert, 1976; Derrington, 1984), followed by a loss of specificity after that. This probably accounts for the point that orientation selectivity, after binocular deprivation until 4 weeks of age, looks normal (Sherk & Stryker, 1976). The orientation map also develops up to 2 to 3 weeks of age and then degenerates (Crair et al., 1998; Fig. 5.11). Therefore, the answer to the nature–nurture question, as so often happens in biology, is not either/or, but both. There is maturation of receptive field properties up to 3 to 5 weeks of age in visually inexperienced animals, some degeneration after that, and the final result is that the receptive fields are immature.

Experiments on dark-reared animals are complicated by an important point that has not yet been analyzed. Rearing in the dark leads to disruption of the day–night cycle and disturbances in the levels of circulating hormones, particularly melatonin and the adrenal hormones (Evered & Clark, 1985). Morphological effects, such as a reduction in the thickness of the cortex, are found in all parts of cortex in dark-reared animals. Are the results found in the visual cortex in dark-reared animals due to changes in the activity in the afferent fibers, or to more general hormonal changes? Unfortunately, with one or two exceptions (Aoki & Siekevitz, 1985; Daw, 1986) nobody has studied this question by comparing effects on the visual system with effects on other systems. It seems likely that there are both direct and indirect effects.

What are the mechanisms that cause the receptive fields of cells in dark-reared animals to lose their orientation and directional selectivity? There are few anatomical differences between light- and dark-reared animals. The number of cells under 1 mm^2 of cortical surface remains normal. There is a delay in the development of the number of synapses, but the effect is not large (Winfield, 1983). The cortex is thinner, and this reflects a decrease in the amount of neuropil, but which element of neuropil is not yet clear (Takacs,

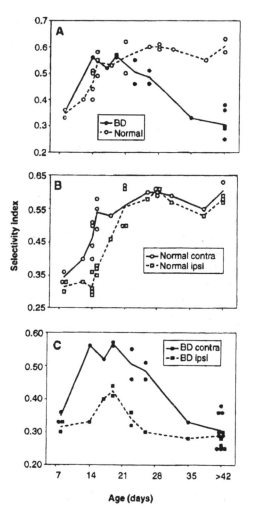

FIG. 5.11. Development of orientation selectivity and elimination of contralateral bias. (A) Comparison of orientation selectivity as a function of age for the contralateral eye of cats reared under normal and binocularly deprived (BD) conditions. (B and C) Development of orientation selectivity for contralateral and ipsilateral eyes of normal and BD cats. [[Reprinted with permission from Crair, M. C., et al. (1998). *Science, 279*, 566–570. Copyright 1998 AAAS.]

Saillour, Imbert, Bogner, & Hamori, 1992). On the positive side, there is a decrease in the extent of the basal dendrites in pyramidal cells at the border of layers II and IV in dark-reared animals (Reid & Daw, 1995).

Some people predict that there should be a difference in the physiology of the inhibitory GABA system because the orientation and direction specificity of cells is at least partly due to inhibitory mechanisms in the adult (Sillito, 1984). There may be a reduction or a delay in the development of the number of symmetric synapses, which are the inhibitory synapses (Winfield, 1983; Gabbott & Stewart, 1987). However, the percentage of cells that contain GABA and the parameters of binding to GABA receptors are the same in normal and dark-reared animals (Mower, Rustad, & White, 1988). Moreover, GABA mechanisms can clearly be shown to be present in dark-reared animals (Tanaka, Freeman, & Ramoa, 1987; Tsumoto & Freeman, 1987). Consequently, no clear mechanism has yet been found to account for the physiological and functional changes found in dark-reared animals.

A more drastic form of deprivation than either rearing in the dark or binocular lid suture is to abolish all activity with the sodium channel blocker tetrodotoxin. As described in Chapter 4, this prevents the formation of ocular dominance columns. It also prevents the development of orientation selectivity (Chapman & Stryker, 1993). Interestingly, the drug 2-amino-4-phosphononbutyrate (APB), which blocks activity in the ON pathways, also prevents the development of orientation selectivity (Chapman & Godecke, 2000). Thus, patterns of neuronal activity carried in the separate ON- and OFF-center visual pathways are necessary for the development of orientation selectivity.

4. Summary

The summary of all this work is that some elements of the organization of the visual system are present at birth, that there is very substantial development over the first 4 weeks of age in parallel with the large increase in the number of synapses during this period, and that there is a further refinement of visual properties over the next 3 months or so. These ages apply to the cat and are different in the primate, but the same general sequence of events occurs in both.

The elements of a system of orientation columns are there at birth, but the selectivity of individual cells within this system of columns develops after birth. Some cells are definitely responsive to direction of movement at birth. On the other hand, the input from the two eyes to the cortex initially overlaps, and only segregates into eye-specific columns after birth. Sensitivity to disparity develops over the same period as segregation of ocular dominance. Acuity improves as the size of the center of the receptive fields of the sustained cells gets smaller and the eyeball gets larger. Movement sensitivity improves as the temporal properties of the Y cell system improves.

The development of physiological properties, therefore, tallies with the development of psychophysical properties. In both cases, most properties, with the exception of stereopsis, exist at birth, but substantial refinement and tuning occurs postnatally.

References

Albus, K., & Wolf, W. (1984). Early postnatal development of neuronal function in the kitten's visual cortex: a laminar analysis. *Journal of Physiology, 348*, 153–185.

Aoki, C., & Siekevitz, P. (1985). Ontogenetic changes in the cyclic adenosine 3',5'-monophosphate stimulable phosphorylation of cat visual cortex proteins, particularly of microtubule-associated protein 2 (MAP 2): effects of normal and dark rearing and of the exposure to light. *Journal of Neuroscience, 5*, 2465–2483.

Banks, M. S., & Bennett, P. J. (1988). Optical and photoreceptor immaturities limit the spatial and chromatic vision of human neonates. *Journal of the Optical Society of America A, 5*, 2059–2079.

Blakemore, C., & Price, D. J. (1987). The organization and post-natal development of area 18 of the cat's visual cortex. *Journal of Physiology, 384*, 263–292.

Blakemore, C., & Van Sluyters, R. C. (1975). Innate and environmental factors in the development of the kitten's visual cortex. *Journal of Physiology, 248,* 663–716.

Blakemore, C., & Vital-Durand, F. (1986). Organization and post-natal development of the monkey's lateral geniculate nucleus. *Journal of Physiology, 380,* 453–491.

Bonds, A. B. (1979). Development of orientation tuning in the visual cortex of kittens. In R. D. Freeman (Ed.), *Developmental neurobiology of vision* (pp. 31–41). New York: Plenum.

Bonds, A. B., & Freeman, R. D. (1978). Development of optical quality in the kitten eye. *Vision Research, 18,* 391–398.

Boothe, R. G., Kiorpes, L., Williams, R. A., & Teller, D. Y. (1988). Operant measurements of spatial contrast sensitivity in infant macaque monkeys during normal development. *Vision Research, 28,* 387–396.

Boycott, B. B., & Wassle, H. (1974). The morphological type of ganglion cells of the domestic cat's retina. *Journal of Physiology, 240,* 397–419.

Braastad, B. O., & Heggelund, P. (1985). Development of spatial receptive field organization and orientation selectivity in kitten striate cortex. *Journal of Neurophysiology, 53,* 1158–1178.

Buisseret, P., & Imbert, M. (1976). Visual cortical cells: their developmental properties in normal and dark-reared kittens. *Journal of Physiology, 255,* 511–525.

Chapman, B. & Godecke, I. (2000) Cortical cell orientation selectivity fails to develop in the absence of ON-center retinal ganglion cell activity. *Journal of Neuroscience 20,* 1922–1930.

Chapman, B., & Stryker, M. P. (1993). Development of orientation selectivity in ferret visual cortex and effects of deprivation. *Journal of Neuroscience, 13,* 5251–5262.

Chapman, B., Godecke, I., & Bonhoeffer, T. (1999). Development of orientation preference in the mammalian visual cortex. *Journal of Neurobiology, 41,* 18–24.

Chino, Y. M., Smith, E. L., Hatta, S., & Cheng, H. (1997). Postnatal development of binocular disparity sensitivity in neurons of the primate visual cortex. *Journal of Neuroscience, 17,* 296–307.

Cleland, B. G., Harding, T. H., & Tulunay-Keesey, U. (1979). Visual resolution and receptive field size: examination of two kinds of cat retinal ganglion cell. *Science, 205,* 1015–1017.

Crair, M. C., Gillespie, D. C., & Stryker, M. P. (1998). The role of visual experience in the development of columns in cat visual cortex. *Science, 279,* 566–570.

Cynader, M. S., Berman, N. J., & Hein, A. (1976). Recovery of function in cat visual cortex following prolonged deprivation. *Experimental Brain Research, 25,* 139–156.

Daniels, J. D., Pettigrew, J. D., & Norman, J. L. (1978). Development of single-neuron responses in kitten's lateral geniculate nucleus. *Journal of Neurophysiology, 41,* 1373–1393.

Daw, N. W. (1986). Effect of dark rearing on development of myelination in cat visual cortex. *Society for Neuroscience Abstracts, 12,* 785.

Derrington, A. M., & Fuchs, A. F. (1981). The development of spatial-frequency selectivity in kitten striate cortex. *Journal of Physiology, 316,* 1–10.

Derrington, A. M. (1984). Development of spatial frequency selectivity in striate cortex of vision-deprived cats. *Experimental Brain Research, 55,* 431–437.

Evered, D., & Clark, S. (1985). *Photoperiodism, melatonin and the pineal.* London: Pitman.

Freeman, R. D., & Ohzawa, I. (1992). Development of binocular vision in the kitten's striate cortex. *Journal of Neuroscience, 12,* 4721–4736.

Gabbott, P. A., & Stewart, M. G. (1987). Quantitative morphological effects of dark rearing and light exposure on the synaptic connectivity of layer 4 in the rat visual cortex (area 17). *Experimental Brain Research, 68,* 103–114.

Hamasaki, D. I., & Flynn, J. T. (1977). Physiological properties of retinal ganglion cells of 3-week-old kittens. *Vision Research, 17,* 275–284.

Henry, G. L., Dreher, B., & Bishop, P. O. (1974). Orientation specificity of cells in cat striate cortex. *Journal of Neurophysiology, 37,* 1394–1409.

Hubel, D. H., & Wiesel, T. N. (1963). Receptive fields of cells in striate cortex of very young, visually inexperienced kittens. *Journal of Neurophysiology, 26,* 994–1002.

Ikeda, H., & Tremain, K. E. (1978). The development of spatial resolving power of lateral geniculate neurones in kitten. *Experimental Brain Research, 31,* 193–206.

Jacobs, D. S., & Blakemore, C. (1988). Factors limiting the postnatal development of visual acuity in the monkey. *Vision Research, 28,* 947–958.

Kim, D.-S., & Bonhoeffer, T. (1994). Reverse occlusion leads to a precise restoration of orientation preference maps in visual cortex. *Nature, 370,* 370–372.

Kiorpes, L., & Movshon, J. A. (2004). Neural limitations on visual development in primates. In L. M. Chalupa & J. S. Werner (Eds.), *The visual neurosciences* (pp. 158–173). Cambridge, MA: MIT Press.

LeVay, S., Stryker, M. P., & Shatz, C. J. (1978). Ocular dominance columns and their development in layer IV of the cat's visual cortex: a quantitative study. *Journal of Comparative Neurology, 179,* 223–244.

Leventhal, A. G., & Hirsch, H. B. (1980). Receptive field properties of different classes of neurons in visual cortex of normal and dark-reared cats. *Journal of Neurophysiology, 43,* 1111–1132.

McKay, S. M., Smyth, D., Akerman, C. J., & Thompson, I. D. (2001). Changing receptive fields and response properties underlie development of orientation tuning in ferret primary visual cortex. *Society for Neuroscience Abstracts, 27,* 475.13.

Milleret, C., Gary-Bobo, E., & Buisseret, P. (1988). Comparative development of cell properties in cortical area 18 of normal and dark-reared kittens. *Experimental Brain Research, 71,* 8–20.

Mower, G. D., Berry, D., Burchfiel, J. L., & Duffy, F. H. (1981). Comparison of the effects of dark rearing and binocular suture on development and plasticity of cat visual cortex. *Brain Research, 220,* 255–267.

Mower, G. D., Rustad, R., & White, W. F. (1988). Quantitative comparisons of Gamma-Aminobutyric acid neurons and receptors in the visual cortex of normal and dark-reared cats. *Journal of Comparative Neurology, 272,* 293–302.

Nelson, D. A., & Katz, L. C. (1995). Emergence of functional circuits in ferret visual cortex visualized by optical imaging. *Neuron, 15,* 23–34.

Pettigrew, J. D. (1974). The effect of visual experience on the development of stimulus specificity by kitten cortical neurones. *Journal of Physiology, 237,* 49–74.

Price, D. J., Zumbroich, T. J., & Blakemore, C. (1988). Development of stimulus selectivity and functional organisation in the suprasylvian visual cortex of the cat. *Transactions of the Royal Society of London. Series B. Biological sciences, 233,* 123–163.

Reid, S. M., & Daw, N. W. (1995). Dark-rearing changes microtubule-associated protein 2 (MAP 2) dendrites but not subplate neurons in cat visual cortex. *Journal of Comparative Neurology, 359,* 38–47.

Rusoff, A. C., & Dubin, M. W. (1977). Development of receptive field properties of retinal ganglion cells in kittens. *Journal of Neurophysiology, 40,* 1188–1198.

Rusoff, A. C., & Dubin, M. W. (1978). Kitten ganglion cells: dendritic field size at 3 weeks of age and correlation with receptive field size. *Investigative Ophthalmology, 17,* 819–821.

Sherk, H., & Stryker, M. P. (1976). Quantitative study of cortical orientation selectivity in visually inexperienced kitten. *Journal of Neurophysiology, 39,* 63–70.

Sherman, S. M. (1972). Development of interocular alignment in cats. *Brain Research, 37,* 187–203.

Sillito, A. M. (1984). Functional considerations of the operation of GABAergic inhibitory processes in the visual cortex. In E. G. Jones & A. Peters (Eds.), *Cerebral cortex.* (pp. 91–117). New York: Plenum.

Singer, W., & Tretter, F. (1976). Receptive field properties and neuronal connectivity in striate and parastriate cortex of contour-deprived cats. *Journal of Neurophysiology, 39,* 613–630.

Spear, P. D., Tong, L., & Langsetmo, A. (1978). Striate cortex neurons of binocularly deprived kittens respond to visual stimuli through the closed eyelids. *Brain Research, 155,* 141–146.

Stryker, M. P., & Harris, W. A. (1986). Binocular impulse blockade prevents the formation of ocular dominance columns in cat visual cortex. *Journal of Neuroscience, 6,* 2117–2133.

Sur, M., Weller, R. E., & Sherman, S. M. (1984). Development of X- and Y-cell retinogeniculate terminations in kittens. *Nature, 310,* 246–249.

Takacs, J., Saillour, P., Imbert, M., Bogner, M., & Hamori, J. (1992). Effect of dark rearing on the volume of visual cortex (areas 17 and 18) and the number of visual cortical cells in young kittens. *Journal of Neuroscience Research, 32,* 449–459.

Tanaka, K., Freeman, R. D., & Ramoa, A. S. (1987). Dark-reared kittens: GABA sensitivity of cells in the visual cortex. *Experimental Brain Research, 65,* 673–675.

Thompson, I. D., Kossut, M., & Blakemore, C. (1983). Development of orientation columns in cat striate cortex revealed by 2 deoxyglucose autoradiography. *Nature, 301,* 712–715.

Thorn, F., Gollender, M., & Erickson, P. (1976). The development of the kitten's visual optics. *Vision Research, 16*, 1145–1149.

Tootle, J. S. (1993). Early postnatal development of visual function in ganglion cells of the cat retina. *Journal of Neurophysiology, 69*, 1645–1660.

Tootle, J. S., & Friedlander, M. J. (1986). Postnatal development of receptive field surround inhibition in kitten dorsal lateral geniculate nucleus. *Journal of Neurophysiology, 56*, 523–541.

Tootle, J. S., & Friedlander, M. J. (1989). Postnatal development of the spatial contrast sensitivity of X- and Y-cells in the kitten retinogeniculate pathway. *Journal of Neuroscience, 9*, 1325–1340.

Tsumoto, T., & Freeman, R. D. (1987). Dark-reared cats: responsivity of cortical cells influenced pharmacologically by an inhibitory antagonist. *Experimental Brain Research, 65*, 666–672.

White, L. E., Coppola, D., & Fitzpatrick, D. (2001). The contribution of sensory experience to the maturation of orientation selectivity in ferret visual cortex. *Nature, 411*, 1049–1052.

Wiesel, T. N., & Hubel, D. H. (1965). Comparison of the effects of unilateral and bilateral eye closure on cortical unit responses in kittens. *Journal of Neurophysiology, 28*, 1029–1040.

Wiesel, T. N., & Hubel, D. H. (1974). Ordered arrangement of orientation columns in monkeys lacking visual experience. *Journal of Comparative Neurology, 158*, 307–318.

Wilson, J. R., Tessin, D. E., & Sherman, S. M. (1982). Development of the electrophysiological properties of Y-cells in the kitten's medial interlaminar nucleus. *Journal of Neuroscience, 2*, 562–571.

Windle, W. F. (1930). Normal behavioral reactions of kittens correlated with the postnatal development of nerve-fiber density in the spinal cord. *Journal of Comparative Neurology, 50*, 479–497.

Winfield, D. A. (1983). The postnatal development of synapses in the different laminae of the visual cortex in the normal kitten and in kittens with eyelid suture. *Developmental Brain Research, 9*, 155–169.

II

Amblyopia and the Effects
of Visual Deprivation

6

Modifications to the Visual Input that Lead to Nervous System Changes

Early in life, if a patient has an optical deficit that degrades the image on the retina, the visual cortex can adapt to allow the patient to cope with his or her visual problems. Unfortunately, such deficits are all too common. In the worst cases, the image on the left retina is not coordinated with the image on the right retina. In such cases, the visual cortex will receive mismatched signals, and either suppress one image or change its wiring to try to bring the signals into synchrony with each other. In this chapter, we will briefly describe the deficits found in humans. The next chapter considers animal models that describe the behavioral, anatomical, and physiological results of such deficits. Then, we will come back to the nature of the deficits found in humans and describe them in more detail in the light of the mechanisms that have been discovered. Finally, the concept of a critical period will be discussed, as well as how the critical period varies with the deficit, and how this variation can affect what treatment is used. Deficits in humans include strabismus, anisometropia, astigmatism, myopia, and cataract.

The general clinical term for the pathology resulting from optical deficits in childhood is *amblyopia*. The literal translation from Greek is blunt sight, and this is a good description. The result is not blindness, but a distortion and muddling of the connections in the cortex. How the connections get rewired depends on the nature of the optical deficit. In most cases there is a loss of acuity, but there can be other effects, and these vary with the cause of the amblyopia. How amblyopia varies from case to case is a fascinating question that will be discussed later, after its causes and the underlying anatomical and physiological mechanisms have been described.

1. Strabismus

Strabismus is a deficit in the muscular control of the eyes, so that the eyes look in different directions. One eye may look inward (esotropia) or outward (exotropia), and sometimes upward (hypertropia) or downward (hypotropia).

There are numerous causes of strabismus; some are motor defects and some sensory (Von Noorden, 1990). The causes include paralysis of an eye muscle, mechanical problems in movements of the eye, a poor image on the retina so that there is no good signal for fixation, refractive errors that disrupt the normal relationship between focusing and convergence of the eyes, and poor control of eye movements by the central nervous system.

Esotropia is the leading cause of amblyopia in children. Frequently it is associated with hyperopia, where the image in the resting condition is focused behind the retina (Atkinson, 1993). To bring the image into focus, the eye has to accommodate. The eyes tend to converge when they accommodate (Fig. 6.1). This is a useful mechanism in normal vision, designed to keep the image in focus and at the same time have it fall on corresponding parts of the two retinas when looking from a distant object to a near one. The connection between accommodation and convergence is automatic and involuntary. Thus, hyperopia automatically leads to convergence. Many children are born with hyperopia and their focus becomes normal over time through growth of the eyeball. However, some have high hyperopia that continues

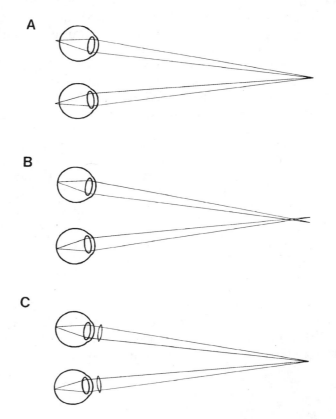

FIG. 6.1. Hyperopia leads to the eyes turning inward. (A) The image is focused behind the retina in the resting state. (B) Accommodation, which attempts to bring the image into focus, leads to the eyes turning inward because of the connection between accommodation and convergence. Therefore, the image will not be in focus for both eyes, but will fall on noncorresponding parts of the two retinas. (C) This condition can easily be corrected with spectacles.

until they are 2 to 3 years old due to an abnormally small eyeball, and these patients tend to become esotropic (Ingram, Walker, Wilson, Arnold, & Dally, 1986). The continued convergence associated with the hyperopia upsets the mechanism for binocular fusion.

There is a genetic component to strabismus, which was first noted by Hippocrates 24 centuries ago. The relationship is particularly strong for children who have relatives with strabismus and are highly hyperopic (<greater than> 3D). The risk of developing strabismus in such children is 4 to 6 times the risk in the whole population, and if one follows such children one will identify almost half the cases of strabismus in the population (Abrahamsson, Magnusson, & Sjostrand, 1999).

Esotropia may also be associated with an abnormal relationship between accommodation and convergence in people who are emmetropic. For some people, the amount of convergence associated with accommodation is excessive (this is called a high AC/A ratio). Thus, any attempt to look at a nearby object tends to make the person cross-eyed. Binocular fusion can sometimes compensate for this problem by reducing the amount of convergence needed to perceive a single image. In some cases, however, this fusion mechanism is not powerful enough to compensate, and the result is esotropia (Fawcett & Birch, 2003).

Some children are born with esotropia or develop it by 12 months of age, and such esotropia is not associated with hyperopia or a high AC/A ratio. In the case of albino children, the cause has been pinned down, but in the majority of cases it has not. Albino children tend to be esotropic due to the misrouting of fibers in the optic chiasm (Kinnear, Jay, & Witkop, 1985). The projection from the contralateral eye to the central nervous system is larger than normal (see Chapter 4), and the projection from the ipsilateral eye is smaller than normal (Creel, Witkop, & King, 1974), as first described in Siamese cats (Guillery, 1974). As a result, there are very few cells with binocular input in the visual cortex, and presumably there is therefore poor control of binocular fusion.

Our understanding of the misrouting of fibers in albinos raises the question of whether other esotropes might have a misrouting of fibers at the optic chiasm. In most cases, evidence from evoked potentials in the visual cortex suggests that the projection to the central nervous system is normal (McCormack, 1975; Hoyt & Caltrider, 1984). An exception to this is a class of infantile esotropes with a large angle of deviation and jerky movements of the eyes (nystagmus). Asymmetric visual evoked potentials (VEPs) are seen in these children, although the asymmetry does not always show an enlarged contralateral projection (Ciancia, 1994). In other cases, there could be a misrouting of fibers that does not show up with the VEP techniques that have been used. Thinking of this possibility, it is intriguing that strabismus has a genetic component, and that its incidence is higher in light-skinned Caucasians than in dark-skinned non-Caucasian people (see Simons, 1993). It is unfortunate that only VEPs have so far been used to study this question because the technique only shows gross abnormalities. There is currently no anatomical study of the projections from the eye to the central nervous system in infantile esotropes. Consequently the question remains unsettled.

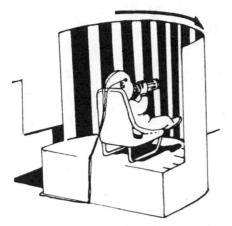

FIG. 6.2. Apparatus used to test optokinetic nystagmus in infants. The infant faces a semicircular screen on which stripes are projected continually moving in one direction. [Reprinted from Naegele, J. R., & Held, R. (1982). *Vision Research, 22,* 341–346. Copyright 1982, with permission from Elsevier.]

There are various hypotheses about the causes of esotropia in unexplained cases. One is that there may be a tendency to develop esotropia because stereopsis for crossed disparity develops before stereopsis for uncrossed disparity (Held, 1993). Crossed disparity is a cue to look at near objects, so this could lead to a tendency toward convergence between the times that crossed and uncrossed disparity develop. However, no study so far has compared the timing of onset of disparity for crossed compared with uncrossed stimuli in children who become esotropic, to see if this is a tendency that is stronger in children with esotropia than in normal children.

Another hypothesis involves the system for detection of movement. There is an interesting correlation in children with infantile esotropia between the development of the esotropia and the development of monocular optokinetic nystagmus (MOKN). Optokinetic nystagmus can be elicited by allowing a subject to view a drum that has vertical stripes on it and moves in one direction (Fig. 6.2). The eyes involuntarily follow the drum, then flick back in the reverse direction with a saccadelike eye movement, and the whole cycle is repeated indefinitely. When one eye is open, adults follow the drum equally well in both directions. Normal infants follow the drum better when it is moving in the nasal direction (Atkinson, 1979; Naegele & Held, 1982; see Fig. 6.3). The discrepancy between following in the nasal direction and following in the temporal direction continues until sometime between 3 and 6 months of age.

Adults who had infantile esotropia show the same movement asymmetry that is seen in infants (Atkinson & Braddick, 1981). This is particularly true when the esotropia appears between birth and 6 months. It happens less frequently when the age of onset is 6 to 12 months, and is comparatively rare for onset after 1 year of age (Demer & Von Noorden, 1988). Besides the asymmetry in MOKN, there is an asymmetry in the patient's ability to judge target velocity and in the initiation of smooth pursuit eye movements (Tychsen & Lisberger, 1986). Whether the eye movement abnormality leads to esotropia or esotropia leads to the eye movement abnormality is not known. However, the direction of the asymmetry in the eye movement abnormality is related to the direction of the strabismus that is common in infants: movement toward

MODIFICATIONS
TO THE VISUAL
INPUT THAT
LEAD TO
NERVOUS
SYSTEM
CHANGES

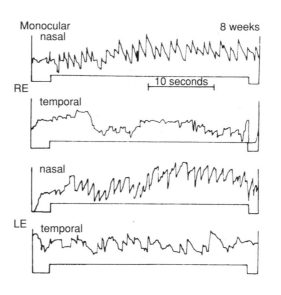

FIG. 6.3. Asymmetry of optokinetic nystagmus in a normal human infant at 8 weeks of age. Diagonal traces represent eye movements following the drum and vertical traces represent the saccadelike flick back. Each eye follows well in a temporal to nasal direction, and poorly in a nasal to temporal direction. [Reprinted from Naegele, J. R., & Held, R. (1982). *Vision Research, 22,* 341–346. Copyright 1982, with permission from Elsevier.]

the nose is perceived better and leads to a stronger eye movement response, and the eyes tend to turn inward toward the nose (Tychsen & Lisberger, 1986).

Very likely the preference for movements toward the nose is overcome as binocularity and fusion develop (Wattam-Bell, Braddick, Atkinson, & Day, 1987). This would fit with the time course of the development of various visual properties. Preference for movement toward the nose is present at birth, along with some binocular fixation. During the first 4 months, this preference gradually disappears. Then, at 4 to 6 months of age, there is a sudden onset of stereopsis and strong vergence movements. However, more detailed experiments need to be done to dissect the cause from the effect.

Sometimes the eyes move together in strabismus, and there is a constant angle of divergence between them (comitant strabismus). Sometimes one eye moves and the other tends not to (incomitant strabismus). Different strategies are used in different cases to avoid double vision (diplopia). With incomitant strabismus, the eye that does not move becomes amblyopic and the image in that eye is usually suppressed. With comitant strabismus, the result depends on the angle of deviation (Pasino & Maraini, 1964; see Fig. 6.4). For small angles of deviation, one eye will become amblyopic, and this may be enough to avoid double vision (diplopia). For large angles of deviation, suppression may be the main mechanism. For moderate angles of deviation, where the deviation is constant over a substantial period of time, the deviating eye can acquire a new point of fixation that is correlated at some level in the cortex with the projection from the fovea of the normal eye. This is called *anomalous retinal correspondence*. Strabismic patients who do not suppress the image in one eye will report an extra letter on the Snellen chart (Pugh, 1962; see Fig. 6.5).

Anomalous retinal correspondence can lead to double vision in one eye if the original projection from the new fixation point in the deviating eye is not eliminated or suppressed. In such a case, the projections from the new fixation

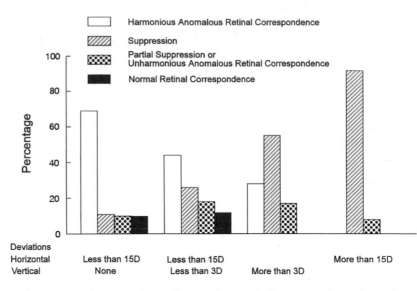

FIG. 6.4. Occurrence of suppression and anomalous retinal correspondence for various degrees of deviation. [Reprinted with permission from Pasino, L., & Maraini, G. (1964). *British Journal of Ophthalmology, 48*, 30–34. Published by BMJ Publishing Group.]

point will go to some portion of the cortex that deals with central vision and also to the part of the cortex that deals with an area outside central vision; this second set of projections is present at birth. However, the maintenance of both sets of projections is quite rare.

Exotropia is less common and less well understood than esotropia, except in cases with an obvious cause, such as paralysis of the muscle that pulls the eye outward. The general rule is that congenital esotropia is found most

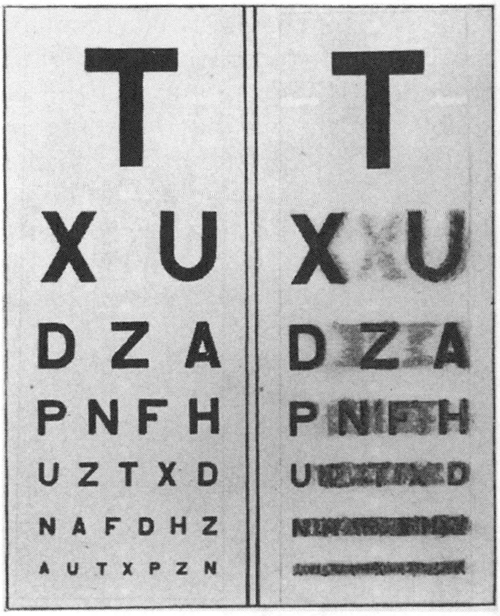

FIG. 6.5. Double vision in a strabismic patient. When asked what she saw on the Snellen chart, an extra X was described on the line of large letters, and the line of small letters was blurred. [Reprinted with permission from Pugh, M. (1962). *British Journal of Ophthalmology, 46*, 193–211. Published by BMJ Publishing Group.]

119

MODIFICATIONS
TO THE VISUAL
INPUT THAT
LEAD TO
NERVOUS
SYSTEM
CHANGES

frequently before 2 years of age, with an angle of deviation that is large and constant; accommodative esotropia is found most frequently after 2 years of age, with an angle of deviation that is smaller and more variable; and exotropia is found most frequently at older ages, and is expressed in an intermittent fashion.

In summary, there are many different types of strabismus, and a large number of factors that can contribute to them. The development of binocular fusion requires the appropriate quantitative relationship between sensory signals and vergence movements. As discussed in Chapter 3, there is a feedback relationship between increased binocularity and better vergence movements during development. Disruption of the pathway at any point can lead to a lack of binocular fusion, and to strabismus. Some contributing factors are understood (a short eyeball, excessive convergence, misrouting of fibers at the optic chiasm) and some are speculative (a tendency to prefer movement toward the nose, a development of crossed stereopsis before uncrossed stereopsis). In a large percentage of cases, exactly what has disturbed the development of binocular fusion and vergence movements is not precisely known.

2. Anisometropia

Anisometropia is a difference in focal point between the two eyes, probably because of a difference in the size of the eyeballs. It can lead to amblyopia if the difference persists until the age of 3 or later (Abrahamsson, Andersson, & Sjostrand, 1990; von Noorden, 1990). It is associated with strabismus in approximately one third of the cases. The cause and effect in this association is not clear because few patients have been followed over a substantial period of time before their amblyopia becomes apparent. In some cases, anisometropia occurs with a very small amount of strabismus (Helveston & Von Noorden, 1967). It seems likely in these cases that the anisometropia leads to a poorly defined fixation area in the unfocused eye, which in turn leads to a small angular deviation in the unfocused eye, but it could be the other way around. In other cases, anisometropia develops in the deviating eye after strabismus occurs (Lepard, 1975; see Fig. 6.6). What is known is that acuity in children with both strabismus and anisometropia is worse than acuity in children with strabismus alone or anisometropia alone (Flom & Bedell, 1985). Anisometropia leads to amblyopia, monofixation, and loss of stereopsis if one eye is more than 2 diopters myopic, or if one eye is more than 1 diopter hyperopic (see Fig. 6.7), and the extent of amblyopia is related to the size of the anisometropia (Weakley, 2001).

3. Astigmatism

Astigmatism is a cylindrical component in the refractive system of the eye, usually in the cornea, so that when lines along one axis are in focus, lines along the perpendicular axis are out of focus (Fig. 6.8). A large number of infants have astigmatism at birth that goes away over the first year of life

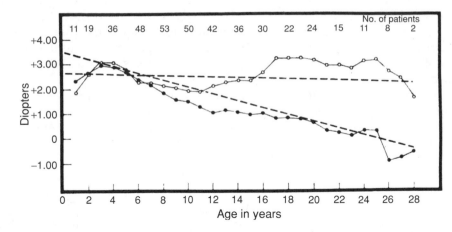

FIG. 6.6. Average refractive error of fixing eyes (*closed circles*) and amblyopic eyes (*open circles*) of 55 patients with growth and development at yearly intervals. The amblyopic eye remains hyperopic. The numbers at the top show the number of patients seen at any one age. [Published with permission from Lepard, C. W. (1975). *The American Journal of Ophthalmology, 80*, 485–490. Copyright by The Ophthalmic Publishing Company.]

(Atkinson, Braddick, & French, 1980; see Fig. 6.9). Those that still have significant astigmatism at 1 year of age do not show deficits when the optics of their eyes are corrected (Gwiazda, Mohindra, Brill, & Held, 1985). If the astigmatism persists, however, acuity for lines along the axis of astigmatism is poor compared with acuity along the axis in focus, even after correction of the optics (Mitchell, Freeman, Millodot, & Haegerstrom, 1973; see Fig. 6.10). In some cases the eyes may grow to have good optics by about 7 years of age,

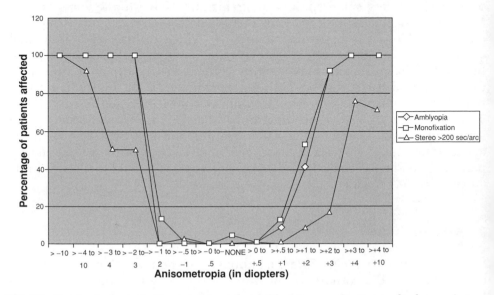

FIG. 6.7. Graph of spherical anisometropia versus amblyopia, monofixation, and subnormal stereopsis. [Reprinted with permission from Weakley, D. R. (2001). *Ophthalmology*, 108, 163–171.]

121

*MODIFICATIONS
TO THE VISUAL
INPUT THAT
LEAD TO
NERVOUS
SYSTEM
CHANGES*

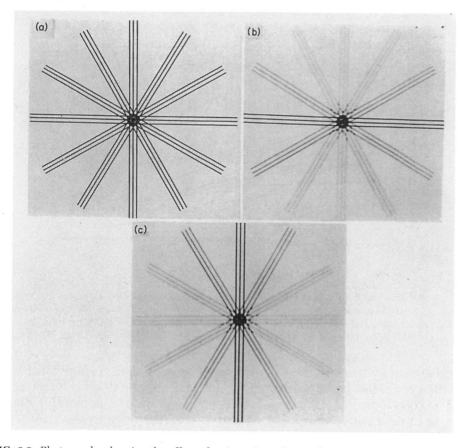

FIG. 6.8. Photographs showing the effect of astigmatic optics on the appearance of objects: (a) as seen by a normal eye; (b) as seen by an eye with astigmatism along the vertical axis; (c) as seen by an eye with astigmatism along the horizontal axis. [Reprinted from Mitchell, D. E., et al. (1973). *Vision Research, 13,* 535–558. Copyright 1973, with permission from Elsevier.]

and still have meridional amblyopia if they were astigmatic earlier (see Held, Thorn, McLellan, Grice, & Gwiazda, 2000). There is probably a genetic component to astigmatism and the consequent meridional amblyopia. Chinese are less likely to be affected than Caucasians (Held et al., 2000), while North American Indians of the Tohonu O'Odham Nation are more likely to be affected (Dobson, Miller, Harvey, & Mohan, 2003).

4. Cataract

Cataract is a clouding of the lens of the eye. Congenital cataract can be inherited or caused by a disease such as German measles in the mother. If it is confined to the center of the lens, light passing through the edge of the lens can form a partially clear image on the retina. If it covers the whole lens, then the image on the retina is diffused and blurred. The cure is to take the lens out. After this is done, the focus of the eye can be corrected for

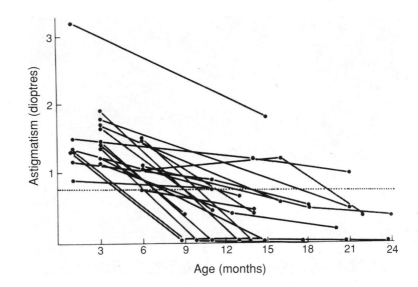

FIG. 6.9. Astigmatism in infants and its disappearance with age. The vertical axis shows the difference in refraction between the axis of astigmatism and the perpendicular axis. Each line represents results from one infant who was followed over a period of several months. [Reprinted from Atkinson, J., et al. (1980). *Vision Research, 20,* 891–893. Copyright 1980, with permission from Elsevier.]

one distance by a spectacle, an intraocular lens implant, or a contact lens, but the eye cannot accommodate. Thus, in cases of unilateral cataract, there will be some anisometropia at some distances. Moreover, depending on the type of optical correction, there will be some difference in the size of the

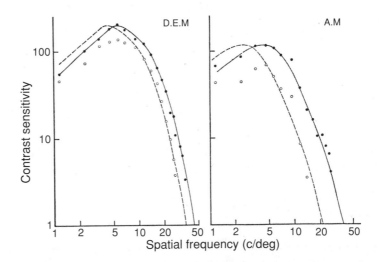

FIG. 6.10. Measurements of contrast sensitivity along the axis of normal focus and the axis of astigmatism, with corrected optics, for two meridional amblyopes. Acuity, represented by the place where the curve intersects the horizontal axis, was reduced by a factor of 1.5 in observer D.E.M. and by a factor of 2 in observer A.M. [Reprinted from Mitchell, D. E., & Wilkinson, F. E. (1974). *Journal of Physiology, 243,* 739–756. By permission of Oxford University Press.]

image on the retina between the normal and treated eye. Strabismus may also develop. Controlled experiments with monkeys show that intraocular lenses combined with a contact lens give a better result than contact lenses alone (Boothe, Louden, Aiyer, Isquierdo, Drews, & Lambert, 2000). This confirms results from humans. However, intraocular lens implants often require further operations (Lambert, 2000). For all these reasons, the neural changes that can occur as a result of cataracts are extremely hard to treat. Only the most persistent physicians, in collaboration with the most persistent parents, have been successful (Jacobson, Mohindra, & Held, 1981; Birch, Stager, & Wright, 1986; Drummond, Scott, & Keach, 1989; Maurer & Lewis, 1993).

5. Myopia

Myopia occurs when the eyeball is too long. If the eyeball is too short, it is farsighted, but one can overcome this to a certain extent by an effort of accommodation. However, one cannot relax the lens much beyond the resting level, and therefore one cannot compensate for an eyeball that is too long. Thus, infants tend to be born hyperopic so that their eyeballs can achieve the correct size by growing (see Fig. 6.6).

The growth of the eyeball is under the control of visual input (see Chapter 13). Over the first 4 to 5 years of life, the growth of the eyeball brings the image into focus on the retina in a relaxed state of accommodation for most people (Gwiazda, Bauer, Thorn,, & Held, 1996). However, the eyeball cannot shrink. Somebody who is born with an eyeball that is too long may be able to compensate for it by a slow rate of growth, but somebody whose eyeball grows to a size that is longer than adult over the first few years of life cannot reverse the process. Thus, the percentage of the population that is myopic increases with age (Curtin, 1985). Children who become myopic tend to do so between 7 and 13 years of age (Gwiazda et al., 1996).

Myopia can be brought on by near work, that is, continuous viewing of objects nearby. This point was noted by Kepler in 1611, emphasized by Tscherning in 1882, and has been consistently confirmed (see Curtin, 1985; Owens, 1991). Interestingly, the prevalence of myopia increases with education; the percentage of myopes goes up from elementary school to middle school to high school, and is highest among university students (Curtin, 1985). Perhaps myopic students tend to become readers rather than football players, but the influence of visual input on the size of the eyeball, to be discussed in Chapter 13, suggests that the reverse is also a definite factor—lots of reading can lead to myopia.

Myopia is also associated with a high AC/A ratio, from a prospective study in 6- to 18-year-old children (Gwiazda, Thorn, and Held, 2005). The significantly higher AC/A ratios in the children who became myopic were a result of significantly reduced accommodation. The findings suggest that the abnormal oculomotor factors found before the onset of myopia may have produced hyperopic retinal defocus when the child was engaged in near-viewing tasks.

Uncorrected myopia, for strong myopes, leads to a substantial reduction in contrast sensitivity at all spatial frequencies (Fiorentini & Maffei, 1976; see

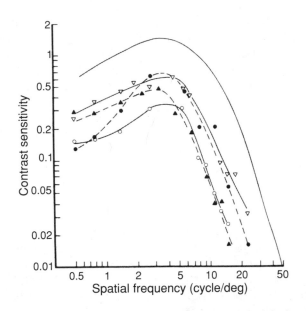

FIG. 6.11. Contrast sensitivity curves from four myopes compared with the normal curve. Top curve shows the contrast sensitivity curve from normal adults. Points and curves drawn through them show the results from the four myopes. Contrast sensitivity is degraded for them at all spatial frequencies. [Reprinted from Fiorentini, A., & Maffei, L. (1976). *Vision Research, 16,* 437–438. Copyright 1976, with permission from Elsevier.]

Fig. 6.11). Acuity is reduced, and so is sensitivity to contrast for coarser spatial frequencies. The result of myopia is like the result of severe anisometropia, which is to be expected because they are the same condition except that the problem occurs in both eyes in the myopia discussed in this section, whereas the problem occurs in one eye in anisometropia, and some anisometropes are hyperopic in their poor eye rather than myopic.

There are genetic as well as environmental effects on myopia. This is born out by parent–offspring relationships and twin studies (Feldkamper & Schaeffel, 2003). Myopia is found in connective tissue deficits such as Marfan's syndrome and Stickler's syndrome, but this represents a minority of the cases. Four loci have been identified in various families, but which genes are actually affected has not yet been resolved (Young, 2004).

6. Summary

This short discussion shows that a number of different problems can lead to disruption of the signals reaching the visual cortex. On the sensory side, there is diffusion of the image on the retina (cataract), poor focus of the image on one retina compared with the image on the other (anisometropia), poor focus along one axis (astigmatism), and excessive growth of the eyeball (myopia). On the motor side, there are a number of causes of misalignment of the two eyes and mismatch of the information from the two retinas (strabismus). As emphasized in the chapter on the development of the visual system, there is an interaction between sensory and motor systems so that deficits in one will lead to deficits in the other. In all cases there is a danger that the connections in the visual cortex will become rewired to compensate for the deficit, and that the rewiring will become permanent if the underlying deficit is not treated.

125

MODIFICATIONS
TO THE VISUAL
INPUT THAT
LEAD TO
NERVOUS
SYSTEM
CHANGES

References

Abrahamsson, M., Andersson, A. K., & Sjostrand, J. (1990). A longitudinal study of a population based sample of astigmatic children I. Refraction and amblyopia II. The changeability of anisometropia (Fabian). *Acta Ophthalmologica Copenhagen, 68*, 428–434.

Abrahamsson, M., Magnusson, G., & Sjostrand, J. (1999). Inheritance of strabismus and the gain of using heredity to determine populations at risk of developing strabismus. *Acta Ophthalmologica Scandinavica, 77*, 653–657.

Atkinson, J. (1979). Development of optokinetic nystagmus in the human infant and monkey infant. In R. D. Freeman (Ed.), *Developmental neurobiology of vision* (pp. 277–287). New York: Plenum.

Atkinson, J. (1993). Infant vision screening: prediction and prevention of strabismus and amblyopia from refractive screening in the Cambridge photorefraction program. In K. Simons (Ed.), *Early visual development, normal and abnormal* (pp. 335–348). New York: Oxford University Press.

Atkinson, J. & Braddick, O. J. (1981). Development of optokinetic nystagmus in the human infant and monkey infant. In D. F. Fisher, R. A. Monty, & J. W. Senders (Eds.), *Eye movements: cognition and perception* (pp. 53–64). Hillside, NJ: Erlbaum.

Atkinson, J., Braddick, O. J., & French, J. (1980). Infant astigmatism: its disappearance with age. *Vision Research, 20*, 891-893.

Birch, E. E., Stager, D. R., & Wright, W. W. (1986). Grating acuity development after early surgery for congenital unilateral cataract. *Archives of Ophthalmology, 104*, 1783–1787.

Boothe, R. G., Louden, T., Aiyer, A., Izquierdo, A., Drews, C., & Lambert, S. R. (2000). Visual outcome after contact lens and intraocular lens correction of neonatal monocular aphakia in monkeys. *Investigative Ophthalmology and Visual Science, 41*, 110–119.

Ciancia, A. O. (1994). On infantile esotropia with nystagmus in abduction. *Transactions of the ISA Congress, 7*, 1–16.

Creel, D., Witkop, C. J., & King, R. A. (1974). Asymmetric visually evoked potentials in human albinos: evidence for visual system anomalies. *Investigative Ophthalmology, 13*, 430–440.

Curtin, B. J. (1985). *The myopias: basic science and clinical management.* Philadelphia: Harper & Row.

Demer, J. L., & Von Noorden, G. K. (1988). Optokinetic asymmetry in esotropia. *Journal of Pediatric Ophthalmology and Strabismus, 25*, 286–292.

Dobson, V., Igartua, I., De la Rosa, E. J., & de la Villa, P. (2003). Amblyopia in astigmatic preschool children. *Vision Research, 43*, 1081–1090.

Dobson, V., Miller, J. M., Harvey, E. M., & Mohan, K. M. (2003). Amblyopia in astigmatic pre-school children. *Vision Research, 43*, 1081–1090.

Drummond, G. T., Scott, W. E., & Keach, R. V. (1989). Management of monocular congenital cataracts. *Archives of Ophthalmology, 107*, 45–51.

Fawcett, S. L., & Birch, E. E. (2003). Risk factors for abnormal binocular vision after successful realignment of accommodative esotropia. *Journal American Association of Pediatric Ophthalmology and Strabismus, 7*, 256–262.

Feldkamper, M., & Schaeffel, F. (2003). Interaction of genes and environment in myopia. In B. Wissinger, S. Kohl, & U. Langenbeck (Eds.), *Genetics in ophthalmology* (pp. 34–49). Basel: Karger.

Fiorentini, A., & Maffei, L. (1976). Spatial contrast sensitivity of myopic subjects. *Vision Research, 16*, 437–438.

Flom, M. C., & Bedell, H. E. (1985). Identifying amblyopia using associated conditions, acuity, and nonacuity features. *American Journal of Optometry and Physiological Optics, 62*, 153–160.

Guillery, R. W. (1974). Visual pathways in albinos. *Scientific American, 230 (5)*, 44–54.

Gwiazda, J., Bauer, J., Thorn, F., & Held, R. (1996). Prediction of myopia in children. In F. Vital-Durand, J. Atkinson, & O. J. Braddick (Eds.), *Infant vision* (pp. 125–134). New York: Oxford University Press.

Gwiazda, J., Mohindra, I., Brill, S., & Held, R. (1985). Infant astigmatism and meridional amblyopia. *Vision Research, 25*, 1269–1276.

Gwiazda, J., Thorn, F., & Held, R. (2005). Accommodation, accommodative convergence, and response AC/A ratios before and at the onset of myopia in children. *Optometry and Vision Science, 82*, 273–278.

Held, R. (1993). Two stages in the development of binocular vision and eye alignment. In K. Simons (Ed.), *Early visual development, normal and abnormal* (pp. 250–257). New York: Oxford University Press.

Held, R., Thorn, F., McLellan, J., Grice, K., & Gwiazda, J. (2000). Early astigmatism contributes to the oblique effect and creates its Chinese-Caucasian difference. In J. Andre, D. A. Owens, & L. O. Harvey (Eds.), *Visual perception: the influence of H.W. Leibowitz* (pp. 81–94). Washington, DC: American Psychological Association.

Helveston, E. M., & Von Noorden, G. K. (1967). Microtropia. *Archives of Ophthalmology, 78*, 272–281.

Hoyt, C. S., & Caltrider, N. (1984). Hemispheric visually-evoked responses in congenital esotropia. *Journal of Pediatric Ophthalmology and Strabismus, 21*, 19–21.

Ingram, R. M., Walker, C., Wilson, J. M., Arnold, P. E., & Dally, S. (1986). Prediction of amblyopia and squint by means of refraction at age 1 year. *British Journal of Ophthalmology, 70*, 12–15.

Jacobson, S. G., Mohindra, I., & Held, R. (1981). Development of visual acuity in infants with congenital cataracts. *British Journal of Ophthalmology, 65*, 727–735.

Kinnear, P. E., Jay, B., & Witkop, C. J. (1985). Albinism. *Survey of Ophthalmology, 30*, 75–101.

Lambert, S. R. (2000). A comparison of grating acuity, strabismus and reoperation outcomes among aphakic and pseudophakic children after unilateral cataract surgery during infancy. *Journal American Association of Pediatric Ophthalmology and Strabismus, 5*, 70–75.

Lepard, C. W. (1975). Comparative changes in the error of refraction between fixing and amblyopic eyes during growth and development. *American Journal of Ophthalmology, 80*, 485–490.

Maurer, D., & Lewis, T. L. (1993). Visual outcomes after infantile cataract. In K. Somons (Ed.), *Early visual development, normal and abnormal* (pp. 454–484). New York: Oxford University Press.

McCormack, E. L. (1975). Electrophysiological evidence for normal optic nerve projections in normally pigmented squinters. *Investigative Ophthalmology, 14*, 931–935.

Mitchell, D. E., & Wilkinson, F. E. (1974). The effect of early astigmatism on the visual resolution of gratings. *Journal of Physiology, 243*, 739–756.

Mitchell, D. E., Freeman, R. D., Millodot, M., & Haegerstrom, G. (1973). Meridional amblyopia: evidence for modification of the human visual system by early visual experience. *Vision Research, 13*, 535–558.

Naegele, J. R., & Held, R. (1982). The postnatal development of monocular optokinetic nystagmus in infants. *Vision Research, 22*, 341–346.

Owens, D. A. (1991). Near work, accommodative tonus, and myopia. In T. Grosvenor & M. C. Flom (Eds.), *Refractive anomalies* (pp. 318–344). Stoneham, MA: Butterworth-Heinemann.

Pasino, L., & Maraini, G. (1964). Importance of natural test conditions in assessing the sensory state of the squinting subject with some clinical considerations on anomalous retinal correspondence. *British Journal of Ophthalmology, 18*, 30–34.

Pugh, M. (1962). Amblyopia and the retina. *British Journal of Ophthalmology, 46*, 193–211.

Simons, K. (1993). Stereoscopic neurontropy and the origins of amblyopia and strabismus. In K. Simons (Ed.), *Early visual development, normal and abnormal* (pp. 409–453). New York: Oxford University Press.

Tychsen, L., & Lisberger, S. G. (1986). Maldevelopment of visual motion processing in humans who had strabismus with onset in infancy. *Journal of Neuroscience, 6*, 2495–2508.

Von Noorden, G. K. (1990). *Binocular vision and ocular motility*. St. Louis: Mosby.

Wattam-Bell, J., Braddick, O. J., Atkinson, J., & Day, J. (1987). Measures of infant binocularity in a group at risk for strabismus. *Clinical Vision Sciences, 1*, 327–336.

Weakley, D. R. (2001). The association between nonstrabismic anisometropia, amblyopia, and subnormal binocularity. *Ophthalmology, 108*, 163–171.

Young, T. L. (2004). Dissecting the genetics of human high myopia: a molecular biologic approach. *Transactions of the American Ophthalmological Society, 102*, 43–66.

7

Physiological and Anatomical Changes that Result from Optical and Motor Deficits

Our understanding of what happens in various forms of visual deprivation has increased enormously over the last 40 years as a result of experiments with animals. The seminal experiments were done by David Hubel and Torsten Wiesel in the early 1960s. They were awarded the Nobel Prize in 1981 for this work (Wiesel, 1982), and for their work on the organization of the visual system in normal animals. Since then this has been one of the most productive areas of research on the visual system. We now understand a number of the physiological and anatomical changes that occur and where the changes take place.

1. Monocular Deprivation

The most thorough analysis of these physiological and anatomical changes has been done with monocular deprivation in cats and monkeys. This corresponds to unilateral cataract, which is a comparatively uncommon form of deficit in humans. However, it gives the simplest and clearest results, and is therefore the most useful in pursuing the fundamental mechanisms. The eyelids of one eye are sutured shut for a period of time, resulting in light perception but allowing very little patterned image on the retina. The direction of movement of an object can be detected (Spear, Tong, & Langsetmo, 1978), but the shape and form are difficult to see.

If a cat or monkey is monocularly deprived for a period of 3 months from the time of eye opening, it becomes severely amblyopic in that eye (Wiesel & Hubel, 1963b; Dews & Wiesel, 1970). When one records cells in the visual cortex after opening both eyes for the experiment, very few cells can be activated by the eye that was sutured (Wiesel & Hubel, 1963b; Hubel, Wiesel, & LeVay, 1977; see Fig. 7.1). The animal is essentially blind in this eye because there is little input left from the sutured eye to the visual cortex.

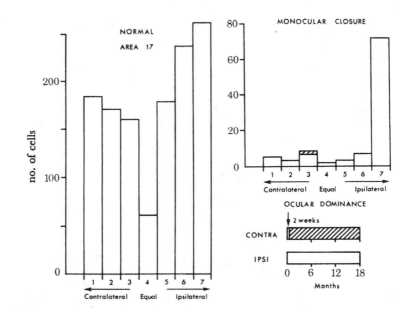

FIG. 7.1. Ocular dominance histograms in normal and monocularly deprived monkeys. For the histograms, electrophysiological recordings were taken from a sample of cells in the visual cortex. Each cell was categorized according to whether it was driven solely by the contralateral eye (group 1), solely by the ipsilateral eye (group 7), equally by both eyes (group 4), or somewhere in between (groups 2, 3, 5, and 6). The histogram on the left was created from recordings of 1256 cells in the visual cortex of juvenile and adult monkeys. The histogram on the right was obtained by recording from cells in the left hemisphere of the visual cortex of a monkey whose right eye was closed from 2 weeks to 18 months. [Reprinted with permission from Hubel, D.H., et al. (1977). Plasticity of ocular dominance columns in monkey striate cortex. *Philosophical Transaction of the Royal Society of London. Series B. Biological sciences, 278,* 377–409. Figure 1. Copyright 1977 Royal Society, London.]

In contrast, the retina in the sutured eye is normal (Wiesel & Hubel, 1963b; Sherman & Stone, 1973). The physiological properties of cells in the lateral geniculate that are driven by the sutured eye are grossly normal (Wiesel & Hubel, 1963a). However, the arbors of X (fine detail) cells in the lateral geniculate coming from the sutured eye are larger than normal, and the arbors of Y (movement) cells are smaller than normal (Sur, Humphrey, & Sherman, 1982). As a result, fewer Y cells are recorded, and the spatial contrast sensitivity of the X cells is reduced (see Sherman, 1985).

Major changes occur in the projections from the lateral geniculate nucleus to the visual cortex. These can be observed by putting radioactive amino acids into one eye; the labeled amino acids are transported from the eye to the cortex, and mark the input from that eye to layer IV of the cortex. The normal pattern of terminals from one eye is a pattern of stripes, like those on a zebra. When one eye is sutured from an early age, the stripes from the sutured eye are narrower than normal, and the stripes from the open eye are wider (Hubel, Wiesel, & LeVay, 1975; see Fig. 7.2). In other words, the terminal arborization in the cortex, coming from cells in the lateral geniculate nucleus driven by the sutured eye, is shrunken (Tieman, 1984). As a result, the cells in the lateral

129

*PHYSIOLOGICAL
AND
ANATOMICAL
CHANGES THAT
RESULT FROM
OPTICAL AND
MOTOR
DEFICITS*

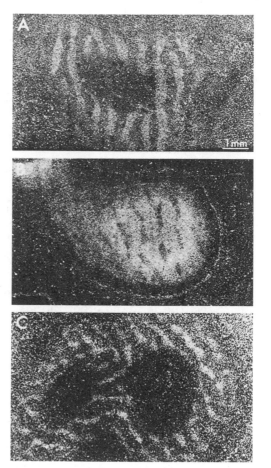

FIG. 7.2. Ocular dominance stripes in layer IV of visual cortex of monkeys. Radioactive tracer is injected into one eye and transported to the cortex to reveal the projections from that eye. White dots represent the tracer. (A) Normal monkey. (B) Monocularly deprived monkey, normal eye injected, white stripes wider. (C) Monocularly deprived monkey, deprived eye injected, white stripes narrower. [Reprinted with permission from Hubel, D.H., et al. (1975). *Cold Spring Harbor Symposia on Quantitative Biology, 40,* 581–589.]

geniculate for this eye are smaller than usual because they have a smaller terminal arbor to support (Wiesel & Hubel, 1963a).

There are further changes within the cortex. Projections from layer IV to other layers of the cortex are also altered to strengthen connections from the open eye and weaken connections from the sutured eye. This can be deduced from physiological recordings, which show substantial effects in layers II, III, V, and VI even when the effects in layer IV are quite small (Shatz & Stryker, 1978; Mower, Caplan, Christen, & Duffy, 1985; Daw, Fox, Sato, & Czepita, 1992). Indeed, there is evidence that ocular dominance changes in layers II and III precede those in layer IV (Trachtenberg, Trepel, & Stryker, 2000). Changes in the extragranular layers also show up with anatomical methods that mark the ocular dominance columns in all layers of the cortex (Tumosa, Tieman, & Tieman, 1989). The remaining cells that can be driven by the deprived eye show a lack of orientation selectivity and are centered on the pinwheels (see Chapter 2), which can be seen by stimulating the nondeprived eye (Crair, Ruthazer, Gillespie, & Stryker, 1997).

The ocular dominance changes occur in a particular sequence. At the peak of the critical period, at 4 to 6 weeks in the kitten (see Chapter 9), 2 days

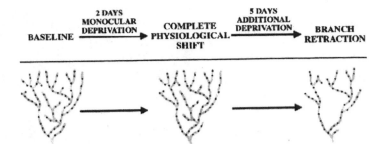

FIG. 7.3. Two days of monocular deprivation has no effect on the relative numerical synapse density or synaptic vesicle protein density in deprived and nondeprived geniculocortical afferents, despite the fact that 2 days of monocular deprivation causes a saturating ocular dominance shift. Seven days of monocular deprivation results in the coordinate retraction of deprived-eye geniculocortical axon branches and removal of deprived-eye geniculocortical presynaptic sites. [Reprinted with permission from Silver, M. A., & Stryker, M. P. (1999). *Journal of Neuroscience, 19*, 10829–10842. Copyright 1999 by the Society for Neuroscience.]

of monocular deprivation produces a saturating ocular dominance shift. At this stage, the terminal arborizations of the geniculocortical afferents have not changed. Over the first week, the terminal arborizations coming from the deprived eye shrink, and this occurs before the arborizations coming from the nondeprived eye expand (Antonini & Stryker, 1996). The synaptic density on these terminal arborizations remains the same, so the number of synapses between the deprived eye and cells in layer IV is reduced in proportion to the shrinkage of the terminal arborizations (Silver & Stryker, 1999; see Fig. 7.3). Presumably the continued existence of some synapses is what allows recovery from the effects of monocular deprivation (see below).

The effects of monocular deprivation involve competition between the inputs from the two eyes. The effects cannot be explained simply by a loss of connections from the deprived eye. This can be seen by comparing the results from monocular deprivation with those from binocular deprivation. In the case of long-term monocular deprivation from an early age, almost no cells in the visual cortex can be driven by the deprived eye. In the case of long-term binocular deprivation, up to one third of the cells can be driven by one or both eyes, and the cells have normal receptive fields (Wiesel & Hubel, 1965). Although a substantial number of cells in these animals do not have visual responses, binocular deprivation is not the sum of two monocular deprivations.

To a certain extent, the sculpting of connections that occurs as a result of monocular deprivation is a modification of the changes that occur during development. As described in Chapter 4, the projections from the lateral geniculate nucleus to the visual cortex from the two eyes overlap each other at birth. Then they segregate into eye-specific columns around the time that stereopsis develops. Consequently, the terminals from each eye retract into half the space that they previously occupied. In the case of monocular deprivation, the terminals from the deprived eye retract until they cover a small fraction of the space, and the terminals from the normal eye do not retract. Thus, very few cells in the cortex can be activated by the deprived eye because the input to the cortex from that eye is substantially reduced.

131

PHYSIOLOGICAL
AND
ANATOMICAL
CHANGES THAT
RESULT FROM
OPTICAL AND
MOTOR
DEFICITS

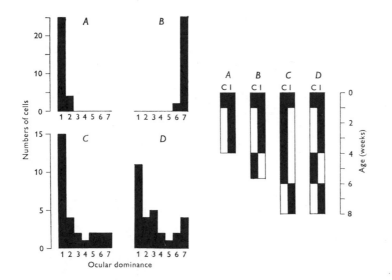

FIG. 7.4. Reversal of the effects of monocular deprivation in cats. Ocular dominance histograms from four animals whose visual experience through the contralateral (C) and ipsilateral (I) eyes is shown on the right. Filled regions indicate periods of eye closure. Closure of one eye (ipsilateral) until 4 weeks of age resulted in cells being monocularly driven by the contralateral eye (histogram A). Closure of the contralateral eye at 4 weeks for 10 days completely reversed the effect of the previous closure of the ipsilateral eye (histogram B), and closure at 6 weeks substantially reversed it (histogram C). Reopening the originally open eye at 6 weeks, after 2 weeks of reverse suture, changed the ocular dominance of some cells back again (compare B with D). [Reprinted with permission from Movshon, J. A. (1976). *Journal of Physiology, 261*, 125–174. Copyright 1976 Blackwell Publishing Ltd.]

However, the response of the cortex is more complicated than this scenario would suggest. Monocular deprivation continues to have an effect for some time after the process of segregation of afferents from the lateral geniculate to the cortex is finished. Moreover, one can close the left eye until nearly all cells are dominated by the right eye, and then open the left eye and close the right eye until nearly all cells are dominated by the left eye, a process known as *reverse suture* (Blakemore & Van Sluyters, 1974; Movshon, 1976; see Fig. 7.4). This recovery is due more to the retraction of terminals coming from the originally nondeprived eye than to the sprouting of the terminals coming from the originally deprived eye (Antonini, Gillespie, Crair, & Stryker, 1998).

Binocular recovery can occur following monocular deprivation, but not by reverse suture, which produces a shift from dominance by one eye to dominance by the other with very few cells driven binocularly. For full recovery of acuity and binocular vision, one needs monocular vision through the previously deprived eye to bring up the acuity in that eye as well as binocular vision to get the two eyes to work together and prevent vision in the previously nondeprived eye from declining. The ideal procedure, from behavioral experiments with cats, is to patch the nondeprived eye for one half to three quarters of the time, reflecting clinical experience with infants (Mitchell & MacKinnon, 2002; see Fig. 7.5). Unfortunately, even the best procedure

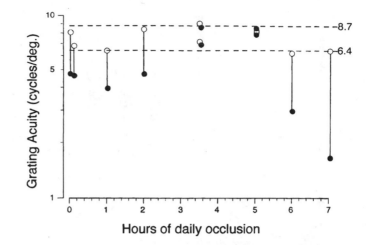

FIG. 7.5. Effects of part-time reverse occlusion on acuities of the initially deprived (*filled symbols*) and nondeprived (*open symbols*) eyes of kittens that had been monocularly deprived to 6 weeks of age. Vertical lines join data for the two eyes of the same animal. Horizontal dashed lines represent upper and lower bounds for acuities of normal cats. [Reprinted with permission from Mitchell, D. E., & MacKinnon, S. (2002). *Clinical and Experimental Optometry, 85,* 5–17.]

does not yield normal depth perception, again reflecting clinical experience with infants (Mitchell, Ptito, & Lepore, 1994; Birch, Fawcett, & Stager, 2000).

In summary, the major effects of monocular deprivation occur within the visual cortex and involve competition between left and right eye inputs. If the left eye is sutured closed, then there is a retraction of terminals in the visual cortex coming from the left eye and an expansion of terminals coming from the right eye, so that, after a period of time, cells in the visual cortex are driven almost exclusively by the right eye. As a result, in severe cases, the animal becomes almost totally blind in the left eye.

2. Orientation and Direction Deprivation

Changes in the visual cortex also occur from a variety of other forms of visual deprivation. Animals can be reared in an environment of stripes of one orientation. If the stripes are vertical, then there is an increase in the percentage of cells in the visual cortex preferring vertical orientations, and a decrease in the percentage of cells preferring horizontal orientations (Blakemore & Cooper, 1970; Hirsch & Spinelli, 1970; Sengpiel, Stawinski, & Bonhoeffer, 1999; see Fig. 7.6). The opposite occurs for animals reared in an environment of horizontal stripes.

There is an additional change if the stripes are moving in one direction or if an animal is reared in a pattern of dots moving in one direction. With a stimulus moving to the right, there is an increase in the percentage of cells preferring movement to the right and a decrease in the percentage of cells

133

*PHYSIOLOGICAL
AND
ANATOMICAL
CHANGES THAT
RESULT FROM
OPTICAL AND
MOTOR
DEFICITS*

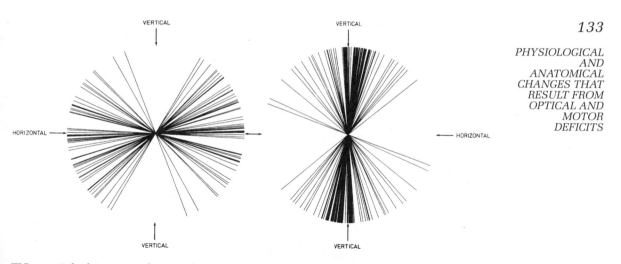

FIG. 7.6. Polar histograms showing the distributions of optimal orientations for 52 neurons from a horizontally experienced cat (left) and 72 neurons from a vertically experienced cat (right). Each line represents the preferred orientation for a single cell in the visual cortex. [Reprinted with permission from Blakemore C., & Cooper, G. F. (1970). *Nature, 228*, 477–478. Copyright 1970 MacMillan Magazines Limited.]

preferring movement to the left (Cynader, Berman, & Hein, 1975; Daw & Wyatt, 1976; see Fig. 7.7). When the stimulus moves to the left, there is an increase in the percentage of cells preferring leftward movement.

These effects on orientation and direction selectivity occur in primary visual cortex, which is the lowest level where such cells are found in higher mammals. There is a rearrangement of the synaptic connections within the visual cortex that produce selectivity for particular orientations and particular directions. Whether this involves axonal changes, dendritic changes, or just changes in synaptic efficacy is not known, because the synaptic mechanisms

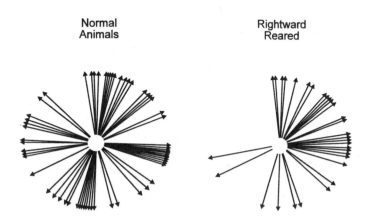

FIG. 7.7. Distribution of preferred directions of direction-selective cells in the cortex of normal animals (left) and the cortex of animals reared in an environment moving to the right (right). Each arrow represents the preferred direction of movement for a single cell. [Reprinted with permission from Daw, N. W., & Wyatt, H. J. (1976). *Journal of Physiology, 257*, 155–170. Copyright 1976 Blackwell Publishing Ltd.]

underlying orientation and direction selectivity are still controversial, but the effect on the physiological properties of the cells in the cortex is clear.

3. One Eye Out of Focus

One eye can be put out of focus by rearing an animal with a substantial concave lens over the eye that is sufficiently powerful to prevent the eye from accommodating enough to overcome it. An eye can also be put out of focus by instilling atropine into the conjunctival sac of the eye. This paralyzes accommodation and keeps the pupil dilated. Both methods give the same behavioral result as anisometropia in humans: the contrast sensitivity curve measured through the out-of-focus eye shows reduced contrast sensitivity at medium and high spatial frequencies (Eggers & Blakemore, 1978; Smith, Harwerth, & Crawford, 1985; see Fig. 7.8).

The most careful study of the physiological and anatomical results of putting one eye out of focus has been carried out in primates with atropinization of one eye. As with monocular deprivation, the main effect is seen in the visual cortex (Movshon, Eggers, Gizzi, Hendrickson, & Kiorpes, 1987). Cells driven by the atropinized eye have reduced contrast sensitivity. This effect is most prominent in the layers of the striate cortex outside layer IV, is noticeable in layer IV, and is not seen in the lateral geniculate nucleus. There is also a reduction in the percentage of binocularly driven neurons and a small shift in ocular dominance toward the normal eye.

Although physiological techniques do not show an effect of atropinization on the lateral geniculate, there are anatomical differences (Hendrickson, Movshon, Eggers, Gizzi, Boothe, & Kiorpes, 1987). Cells in the layers driven

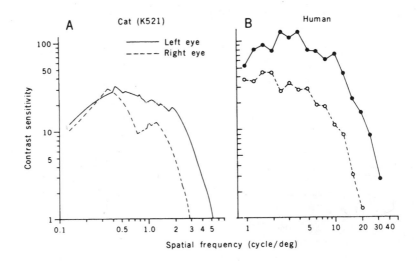

FIG. 7.8. (A) Average contrast sensitivity curve drawn from recordings of cells in the visual cortex of a cat reared with a −12 diopter lens over the right eye. (B) Contrast sensitivity curves for an anisometropic human: normal eye (•), amblyopic eye (○). [Reprinted with permission from Eggers, H. M., & Blakemore, C. (1978). *Science, 201*, 264–266. Copyright 1978 AAAS.]

135

*PHYSIOLOGICAL
AND
ANATOMICAL
CHANGES THAT
RESULT FROM
OPTICAL AND
MOTOR
DEFICITS*

by the atropinized eye are smaller. This is seen in the parvocellular layers, which deal with high spatial frequencies, and not in the magnocellular layers, which deal primarily with movement. As expected, the main effect is found in the pathway that deals with fine details. It is likely that the terminal arbors of these cells are diminished, causing the reduction in cell size, so that the anatomical change found in the lateral geniculate is a reflection of the changes in the visual cortex.

The ocular dominance columns seen from the transport of radioactive substances put into the eye do not show any deficits: the areas occupied by the out-of-focus eye and the normal eye are similar. However, staining with cytochrome oxidase shows pale bands along the boundaries of the ocular dominance columns (Horton, Hocking, & Kiorpes, 1997). This is presumably related to the loss of binocular cells found in anisometropic animals (Kiorpes, Kiper, O'Keefe, Cavanaugh, & Movshon, 1998).

Thus, results from monocular deprivation and anisometropia are very similar in the level at which they occur. The major physiological effects, which lead to the behavioral consequences of the deficit, occur in the primary visual cortex, where signals from the two eyes come together. However, the behavioral deficits are larger than the deficits seen in single cells in the striate cortex, suggesting that there are further deficits to be found at higher levels of the system (Kiorpes et al., 1998).

4. Strabismus

There are several different ways of creating experimental strabismus. Part of an eye muscle can be removed (myectomy); a tendon cut (tenotomy); an eye muscle cut and reinserted at a different position (recession); botulinum toxin infused into one eye muscle to paralyze it; or prisms can be placed over the eyes. Strabismus also occurs naturally in a population of cats (Distler and Hoffmann, 1991) and a population of monkeys (Kiorpes and Boothe, 1981), providing useful models for human strabismus. As with humans, the different causes of strabismus have different results. For example, myectomy or tenotomy produce a pattern of binocular correspondence that varies as the unaffected eye moves (incomitant strabismus), whereas recession or placing prisms over the eyes will produce a binocular mismatch with an angle of mismatch that remains comparatively constant as the eyes move (comitant strabismus).

There are four results of strabismus: amblyopia, suppression of the image in one eye, loss of binocular function, and anomalous retinal correspondence. These occur in various combinations in different cases. Loss of binocular function is due to a reduction in the number of cells in the visual cortex that can be activated by both eyes. This was first observed by Hubel and Wiesel in cats (1965; see Fig. 7.9), and has been confirmed in subsequent studies using a variety of treatments. Along with the loss of binocularity goes loss of stereoscopic depth perception (Crawford, Smith, Harwerth, & Von Noorden, 1984). The few binocular cells that can be found tend to prefer horizontal orientations (Singer, Rauschecker, & Von Grunau, 1979; Cynader, Gardner, &

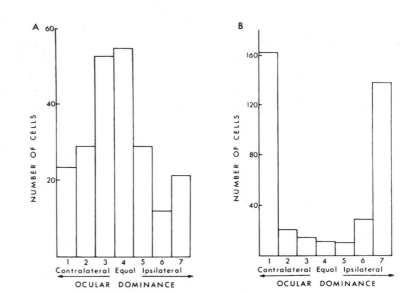

FIG. 7.9. Ocular dominance of 223 cells recorded from normal cats (A) compared to ocular dominance of 384 cells from strabismic cats (B). [Used with permission from Hubel, D. H., & Wiesel, T. N. (1965). *Journal of Neurophysiology, 28*, 1041–1059.]

Mustari, 1984; see Fig. 7.10). This occurs because the displacement that is created is usually in the horizontal direction. Consequently a single cell will be activated by a horizontal line through both eyes, but not by a vertical line.

Various physiological properties that underlie amblyopia have been found. A reduction in acuity and contrast sensitivity is observed in animals with naturally occurring strabismus (Kiorpes & Boothe, 1981) and in various forms of experimental strabismus (Von Noorden, Dowling, & Ferguson, 1970; Von Grunau & Singer, 1980). There is also a reduction in the number of cells

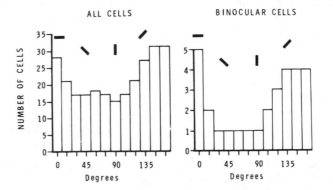

FIG. 7.10. Distribution of preferred orientations among neurons in the visual cortex of strabismic cats. 0° represents cells preferring horizontal orientations and 90° represents cells preferring vertical. [Reprinted with permission from Cynader, M. S., et al. (1984). *Experimental Brain Research, 53*, 384–399. Copyright 1984 Springer-Verlag.]

in the visual cortex that are driven by the deviating eye that is dependent on the part of the field of view that is being recorded (Kalil, Spear, & Langsetmo, 1984), although not all authors find this (Kiorpes et al., 1998). Both of these factors contribute to the amblyopia found in strabismus.

The level at which the reduction in acuity and contrast sensitivity occurs depends on the type of experimental strabismus used. With tenotomy, there is a small reduction in acuity at the retina/lateral geniculate synapse in cats (Chino, Cheng, Smith, Garraghty, Roe, & Sur, 1994), but little change in this synapse is found in primates, and the main deficit occurs in the visual cortex in both animals (Crewther & Crewther, 1990). With myectomy, there is a deficit in acuity in the lateral geniculate nucleus (Ikeda & Wright, 1976) that is much more substantial than that found after tenotomy (Crewther, Crewther, & Cleland, 1985). Both procedures produce the same effect as far as the mismatch between the image on the right and left retina is concerned. The difference presumably occurs because removing part of the eye muscle has some additional effect, perhaps caused by the loss of input from the sensory endings in the eye muscle.

Several changes are found in the primary visual cortex. Various markers are altered at the borders between the ocular dominance columns where binocular neurons are normally found, agreeing with the lack of binocular neurons in strabismic monkeys (Horton, Hocking, & Adams, 1999; Fenstemaker, Kiorpes, & Movshon, 2001). The horizontal connections have an increased tendency to connect areas dominated by the same eye (Tychsen, Wong, & Burkhalter, 2004). The layout of the orientation columns is normal—they are continuous at the boundaries between the ocular dominance columns and cross at a high angle (Lowel, Schmidt, Kim, Wolf, Hoffsummer, Singer, & Bonhoeffer, 1998)—but the orientation specificity is reduced (Schmidt, Singer, & Galuske, 2004). Visually evoked potentials are also reduced (Schmidt et al., 2004). The connections between ocular dominance columns for the normal eye are enhanced relative to other connections (Roelfsema, Konig, Engel, Sireteanu, & Singer, 1994), and there is a rapid process of anatomical changes underlying these results that occurs over 2 days (Trachtenberg & Stryker, 2001). However, many cells that appear monocular when only one eye is stimulated show binocular interactions when both eyes are stimulated, although these cells have reduced disparity tuning (Smith, Chino, Ni, Cheng, Crawford, & Harwerth, 1997).

There are also changes at levels other than primary visual cortex. Contrast sensitivity measured from single cells in area 17 of strabismic macaque monkeys does not fully account for the losses seen behaviorally in the same animals (Kiorpes et al., 1998). Cells in areas 17 and 18 of the cat do not show much bias towards the normal eye compared with the amblyopic eye, but cells in area 21a, which is on the ventral pathway, do (Schroeder, Fries, Roelfsema, Singer, & Engel, 2002). Experiments with functional magnetic resonance imaging in humans show that both V1 and areas outside V1 are affected in strabismic amblyopes (Barnes, Hess, Dumoulin, Achtman, & Pike, 2001). In the temporal cortex, there are separate areas for recognizing faces and buildings. Face-related areas show a severe disconnection from the amblyopic eye, while building-related areas remain essentially normal (Lerner, Pianka,

137

PHYSIOLOGICAL
AND
ANATOMICAL
CHANGES THAT
RESULT FROM
OPTICAL AND
MOTOR
DEFICITS

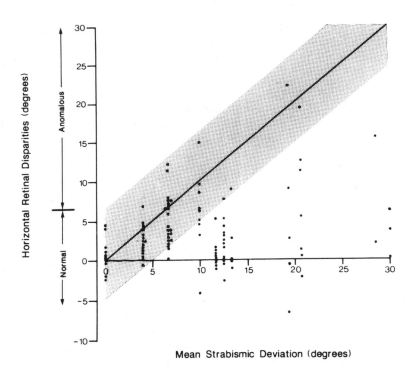

FIG. 7.11. Retinal correspondence found in binocular cells from area LS in cats with various degrees of strabismus. For cells with normal or innate correspondence, the disparity will be 0°. For cells with anomalous correspondence that produce a single image, the disparity will equal the degree of strabismic deviation (45° line). Cells with anomalous correspondence are not seen very often when the strabismic deviation is greater than 10°. [Reprinted from Grant, S., & Berman, N. J. (1991). *Visual Neuroscience, 7*, 259–281, with the permission of Cambridge University Press.]

Azmon, Leiba, Stolovitch, Loewenstein, Harel, Hendler, & Malach, 2003). However, considerable work will be required before we understand which deficits can be attributed to changes in V1 and which to changes in the numerous other areas of visual cortex.

Anomalous retinal correspondence is found primarily when the angle of strabismus is constant and moderate. Presumably axons in the cortex can affect a new location that is nearby, but not a new location that is a long distance away. In experiments on cats, anomalous retinal correspondence is seen with angles of strabismus of less than 10° (Grant & Berman, 1991; see Fig. 7.11), corresponding to experience in humans (see Wong, Lueder, Burkhalter, & Tychsen, 2000).

Cortical cells with anomalous retinal correspondence are not found in primary visual cortex (area 17). They are found in the lateral suprasylvian gyrus of the cat (LS), which contains several areas of secondary visual cortex (Grant & Berman, 1991; Sireteanu & Best, 1992), and some are also found in area 18 (Cynader et al., 1984). Cells in the primary visual cortex tend to have small receptive fields, while cells in LS tend to have large ones. Thus, in the normal animal, a point in LS will receive input from a wide area of retina, and the intracortical connections will not have to be long to generate

139

PHYSIOLOGICAL
AND
ANATOMICAL
CHANGES THAT
RESULT FROM
OPTICAL AND
MOTOR
DEFICITS

anomalous retinal correspondence. Essentially what happens with small angles of strabismus is that the cells in primary visual cortex become monocular, and the site of binocular convergence is moved to the secondary visual cortex where the compensation for the lack of correspondence in the retina takes place.

Where the images in the two eyes are not brought together through anomalous retinal correspondence because the intracortical connections are not long enough, there will be two images reaching the visual cortex that are not in register. In this case, one image will be inhibited or suppressed, or diplopia will result. The mechanism of image suppression is still not fully understood. Suppression occurs in normal people as well as in amblyopes, and the mechanisms are likely the same. Where the angle of strabismus is large, and the image in the deviating eye corresponding to the fixation point in the fixating eye falls on a peripheral part of the retina, the signals generated should cause an out-of-focus image in the deviating eye on top of an in-focus image in the fixating eye. Such images are suppressed in normal people (see Daw, 1962). Where the angle of strabismus is small, the result may be like a stereoscopic image where portions of the image behind the edge of the object being fixated fall on the retina of one eye but not the other. In some cases where the angle of strabismus is moderate, the result could be like two in-focus images with different contours falling on the two retinas, which leads to binocular rivalry in normal people—that is, suppression of one image alternating with suppression of the other.

Inhibition of the cortical response from the deviated eye by stimulation of the nondeviated eye has been documented (Singer, Von Grunau, & Rauschecker, 1980; Freeman & Tsumoto, 1983). Freeman and Tsumoto (1983) reported that the frequency and strength of the inhibition in exotropic cats was similar to that seen in normal cats, while the deviated eye was more effectively suppressed by and less able to suppress the nondeviated eye in esotropic cats (Fig. 7.12). This tallies with the clinical observation that there is a tendency for exotropes to have alternating fixation, while esotropes tend to fixate with their normal eye and become amblyopic in the deviating eye. When both eyes are stimulated with gratings, the response to the grating in the normal eye is suppressed by the grating in the deviated eye for all relative orientations of the two gratings, with a few exceptions in cells that are binocularly driven (Sengpiel, Blakemore, Kind, & Harrad, 1994). This contrasts with results in normal cats, where suppression occurs with gratings of different orientation, but stimuli of the same orientation increase the response. The difference may occur because monocularly driven cells are suppressed by stimuli of all orientations whereas binocularly driven cells are suppressed by stimuli of a different orientation, and there are more binocularly driven cells in normal cats and more monocularly driven cells in strabismic cats. Complex cells in particular show suppression when stimulated with gratings of the same orientation, no matter what the phase relationship of the gratings (Smith et al., 1997; see Fig. 7.13). Thus, there appear to be a variety of mechanisms underlying suppression in strabismic amblyopes, some of which have been studied with experiments on animals and some of which have not.

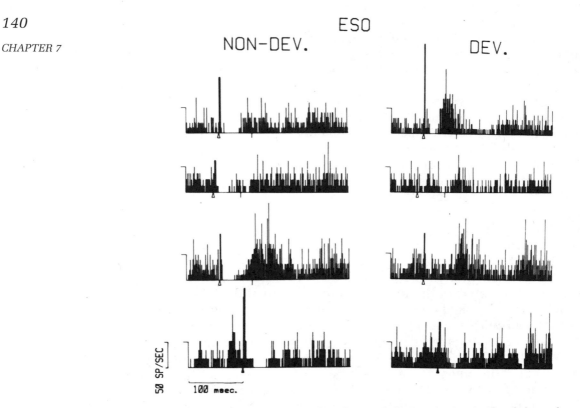

FIG. 7.12. Stronger inhibition is seen when the nondeviating eye is stimulated than when the deviating eye is stimulated. Poststimulus time histograms from four cells in the visual cortex of an esotropic cat (A–D). The optic nerve was stimulated at the times marked by triangles. [Used with permission from Freeman, R. D., & Tsumoto, T. (1983). *Journal of Neurophysiology, 49,* 238–253.]

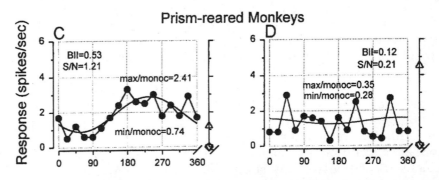

FIG. 7.13. Response of cells in strabismic monkeys to gratings stimulating the two eyes as a function of the relative phase of the gratings. Left, a simple cell; right, a complex cell. *Upward triangle* shows the response to monocular stimulation of the dominant eye. [Used with permission from Smith, E. L., et al. (1997). *Journal of Neurophysiology, 78,* 1353–1362.]

5. Summary

The general conclusion is that mammals compensate for optical deficits occurring at a young age by anatomical and physiological changes in the visual cortex. Not much compensation is found at the level of the retina or the lateral geniculate nucleus. In the case of binocular function, orientation selectivity, and direction selectivity, this is what one would expect because these are all properties of the visual cortex rather than of the retina or lateral geniculate. The mechanisms that produce acuity and contrast sensitivity changes are also often found at the cortical level, even though acuity and contrast sensitivity are properties of the retina and lateral geniculate as well.

The compensation is specific for the deficit. Monocular deprivation affects ocular dominance rather than orientation selectivity, and orientation deprivation affects orientation selectivity rather than ocular dominance. There is a rearrangement of the connections within the cortex and the columns specific for the deprived features contract, while the columns specific for the nondeprived features expand. The physiological properties of the cells change correspondingly.

There is a limit to how far compensation can occur through anatomical and physiological changes. This is not important for monocular orientation and direction deprivation because columns for left and right eyes are near each other, and so are columns for vertical and horizontal orientations and cells for rightward and leftward movement. It is, however, important for strabismus when the angle of strabismus is large. In this case, compensation occurs through some form of physiological suppression rather than through anatomical rearrangements.

References

Antonini, A., & Stryker, M. P. (1996). Plasticity of geniculocortical afferents following brief or prolonged monocular occlusion in the cat. *Journal of Comparative Neurology, 369,* 64–82.

Antonini, A., Gillespie, D. C., Crair, M. C., & Stryker, M. P. (1998). Morphology of single geniculocortical afferents and functional recovery of the visual cortex after reverse monocular deprivation in the kitten. *Journal of Neuroscience, 18,* 9896–9909.

Barnes, G. R., Hess, R. F., Dumoulin, S. O., Achtman, R. L., & Pike, G. B. (2001). The cortical deficit in humans with strabismic amblyopia. *Journal of Physiology, 533,* 281–297.

Birch, E. E., Fawcett, S., & Stager, D. R. (2000). Why does early surgical alignment improve stereoacuity outcomes in infantile esotropia? *Journal American Association of Pediatric Ophthalmology and Strabismus, 4,* 10–14.

Blakemore, C., & Cooper, G. F. (1970). Development of the brain depends on the visual environment. *Nature, 228,* 477–478.

Blakemore, C., & Van Sluyters, R. C. (1974). Reversal of the physiological effects of monocular deprivation in kittens: further evidence for a sensitive period. *Journal of Physiology, 237,* 195–216.

Chino, Y. M., Cheng, H., Smith, E. L., Garraghty, P. E., Roe, A. W., & Sur, M. (1994). Early discordant binocular vision disrupts signal transfer in the lateral geniculate nucleus. *Proceedings of the National Academy of Sciences of the United States of America, 91,* 6938–6942.

Crair, M. C., Ruthazer, E. S., Gillespie, D. C., & Stryker, M. P. (1997). Relationship between the ocular dominance and orientation maps in visual cortex of monocularly deprived cats. *Neuron, 19,* 307–318.

Crawford, M. J., Smith, E. L., Harwerth, R. S., & Von Noorden, G. K. (1984). Stereoblind monkeys have few binocular neurons. *Investigative Ophthalmology, 25*, 779–781.

Crewther, S. G., & Crewther, D. P. (1990). Neural site of strabismic amblyopia in cats: X-cell acuities in the LGN. *Experimental Brain Research, 72*, 503–509.

Crewther, S. G., Crewther, D. P., & Cleland, B. G. (1985). Convergent strabismic amblyopia in cats. *Experimental Brain Research, 60*, 1–9.

Cynader, M. S., Berman, N. J., & Hein, A. (1975). Cats raised in a one-directional world: effects on receptive fields in visual cortex and superior colliculus. *Experimental Brain Research, 22*, 267–280.

Cynader, M. S., Gardner, J. P., & Mustari, M. J. (1984). Effects of neonatally induced strabismus on binocular responses in cat area 18. *Experimental Brain Research, 53*, 384–399.

Daw, N. W. (1962). Why after-images are not seen in normal circumstances. *Nature, 196*, 1143–1145.

Daw, N. W., & Wyatt, H. J. (1976). Kittens reared in a unidirectional environment: evidence for a critical period. *Journal of Physiology, 257*, 155–170.

Daw, N. W., Fox, K. D., Sato, H., & Czepita, D. (1992). Critical period for monocular deprivation in the cat visual cortex. *Journal of Neurophysiology, 67*, 197–202.

Dews, P. D., & Wiesel, T. N. (1970). Consequences of monocular deprivation on visual behaviour in kittens. *Journal of Physiology, 206*, 437–455.

Distler, C., & Hoffmann, K. P. (1991). Depth perception and cortical physiology in normal and innate microstrabismic cats. *Visual Neuroscience, 6*, 25–41.

Eggers, H. M., & Blakemore, C. (1978). Physiological basis of anisometropic amblyopia. *Science, 201*, 264–266.

Fenstemaker, S. B., Kiorpes, L., & Movshon, J. A. (2001). Effects of experimental strabismus on the architecture of macaque monkey striate cortex. *Journal of Comparative Neurology, 438*, 300–317.

Freeman, R. D., & Tsumoto, T. (1983). An electrophysiological comparison of convergent and divergent strabismus in the cat: electrical and visual activation of single cortical cells. *Journal of Neurophysiology, 49*, 238–253.

Grant, S., & Berman, N. J. (1991). Mechanism of anomalous retinal correspondence: maintenance of binocularity with alteration of receptive-field position in the lateral suprasylvian (LS) visual area of strabismic cats. *Visual Neuroscience, 7*, 259–281.

Hendrickson, A. E., Movshon, J. A., Eggers, H. M., Gizzi, M. S., Boothe, R. G., & Kiorpes, L. (1987). Effects of early unilateral blur on the macaque's visual system II anatomical observations. *Journal of Neuroscience, 7*, 1327–1339.

Hirsch, H. B., & Spinelli, D. N. (1970). Visual experience modifies distribution of horizontally and vertically oriented receptive fields in cats. *Science, 168*, 869–871.

Horton, J. C., Hocking, D. R., & Adams, D. L. (1999). Metabolic mapping of suppression scotomas in striate cortex of macaques with experimental strabismus. *Journal of Neuroscience, 19*, 7111–7129.

Horton, J. C., Hocking, D. R., & Kiorpes, L. (1997). Pattern of ocular dominance columns and cytochrome oxidase activity in a macaque monkey with naturally occurring anisometropic amblyopia. *Visual Neuroscience, 14*, 681–689.

Hubel, D. H., & Wiesel, T. N. (1965). Binocular interaction in striate cortex of kittens reared with artificial squint. *Journal of Neurophysiology, 28*, 1041–1059.

Hubel, D. H., Wiesel, T. N., & LeVay, S. (1975). Functional architecture of area 17 in normal and monocularly deprived macaque monkeys. *Cold Spring Harbor Symposia on Quantitative Biology, 40*, 581–589.

Hubel, D. H., Wiesel, T. N., & LeVay, S. (1977). Plasticity of ocular dominance columns in monkey striate cortex. *Philosophical Transaction of the Royal Society of London. Series B. Biological sciences, 278*, 377–409.

Ikeda, H., & Wright, M. J. (1976). Properties of LGN cells in kittens reared with convergent squint: a neurophysiological demonstration of amblyopia. *Experimental Brain Research, 25*, 63–77.

Kalil, R. E., Spear, P. D., & Langsetmo, A. (1984). Response properties of striate cortex neurons in cats raised with divergent or convergent strabismus. *Journal of Neurophysiology, 52*, 514–537.

Kiorpes, L., & Boothe, R. G. (1981). Naturally occurring strabismus in monkeys (Macaca nemestrina). *Investigative Ophthalmology, 20*, 257–263.

Kiorpes, L., Kiper, D. C., O'Keefe, L. P., Cavanaugh, J. R., & Movshon, J. A. (1998). Neuronal correlates of amblyopia in the visual cortex of macaque monkeys with experimental strabismus and anisometropia. *Journal of Neuroscience, 18*, 6411–6424.

143

PHYSIOLOGICAL
AND
ANATOMICAL
CHANGES THAT
RESULT FROM
OPTICAL AND
MOTOR
DEFICITS

Lerner, Y., Pianka, P., Azmon, B., Leiba, H., Stolovitch, C., Loewenstein, A., Harel, M., Hendler, T., & Malach, R. (2003). Area-specific amblyopic occipitotemporal object effects in human representations. *Neuron, 40*, 1023–1029.

Lowel, S., Schmidt, K. E., Kim, D.-S., Wolf, W., Hoffsummer, F., Singer, W., & Bonhoeffer, T. (1998). The layout of orientation and ocular dominance domains in area 17 of strabismic cats. *European Journal of Neuroscience, 10*, 2629–2643.

Mitchell, D. E., & MacKinnon, S. (2002). The present and potential impact of research on animal models for clinical treatment of stimulus deprivation amblyopia. *Clinical and Experimental Optometry, 85*, 5–17.

Mitchell, D. M., Ptito, M., & Lepore, F. (1994). Depth perception in monocularly deprived cats following part-time reverse occlusion. *European Journal of Neuroscience, 6*, 967–972.

Movshon, J. A. (1976). Reversal of the physiological effects of monocular deprivation in the kitten's visual cortex. *Journal of Physiology, 261*, 125–174.

Movshon, J. A., Eggers, H. M., Gizzi, M. S., Hendrickson, A. E., & Kiorpes, L. (1987). Effects of early unilateral blur on the macaque's visual system III. Physiological observations. *Journal of Neuroscience, 7*, 1340–1351.

Mower, G. D., Caplan, C. J., Christen, W. G., & Duffy, F. H. (1985). Dark rearing prolongs physiological but not anatomical plasticity of the cat visual cortex. *Journal of Comparative Neurology, 235*, 448–466.

Roelfsema, P. R., Konig, P., Engel, A. K., Sireteanu, R., & Singer, W. (1994). Reduced synchronization in the visual cortex of cats with strabismic amblyopia. *European Journal of Neuroscience, 6*, 1645–1655.

Schmidt, K. E., Singer, W., & Galuske, R. W. (2004). Processing deficits in primary visual cortex of amblyopic cats. *Journal of Neurophysiology, 91*, 1661–1671.

Schroder, J. H., Fries, P., Roelfsema, P. R., Singer, W., & Engel, A. K. (2002). Ocular dominance in extrastriate cortex of strabismic amblyopic cats. *Vision Research, 42*, 29–39.

Sengpiel, F., Blakemore, C., Kind, P. C., & Harrad, R. (1994). Interocular suppression in the visual cortex of strabismic cats. *Journal of Neuroscience, 14*, 6855–6871.

Sengpiel, F., Stawinski, P., & Bonhoeffer, T. (1999). Influence of experience on orientation maps in cat visual cortex. *Nature Neuroscience, 2*, 727–732.

Shatz, C. J., & Stryker, M. P. (1978). Ocular dominance in layer IV of the cat's visual cortex and the effects of monocular deprivation. *Journal of Physiology, 281*, 267–283.

Sherman, S. M. (1985). Development of retinal projections to the cat's lateral geniculate nucleus. *Trends in Neurosciences, 8*, 350–355.

Sherman, S. M., & Stone, J. (1973). Physiological normality of the retina in visually deprived cats. *Brain Research, 60*, 224–230.

Silver, M. A., & Stryker, M. P. (1999). Synaptic density in geniculocortical afferents remains constant after monocular deprivation in cat. *Journal of Neuroscience, 19*, 10829–10842.

Singer, W., Rauschecker, J. P., & Von Grunau, M. W. (1979). Squint affects striate cortex cells encoding horizontal image movements. *Brain Research, 170*, 182–186.

Singer, W., Von Grunau, M. W., & Rauschecker, J. P. (1980). Functional amblyopia in kittens with unilateral exotropia I. Electrophysiological assessment. *Experimental Brain Research, 40*, 294–304.

Sireteanu, R., & Best, J. (1992). Squint-induced modification of visual receptive fields in the lateral suprasylvian cortex of the cat: binocular interaction, vertical effect and anomalous correspondence. *European Journal of Neuroscience, 4*, 235–242.

Smith, E. L., Chino, Y. M., Ni, J., Cheng, H., Crawford, M. J., & Harwerth, R. S. (1997). Residual binocular interactions in the striate cortex of monkeys reared with abnormal binocular vision. *Journal of Neurophysiology, 78*, 1353–1362.

Smith, E. L., Harwerth, R. S., & Crawford, M. J. (1985). Spatial contrast sensitivity deficits in monkeys produced by optically induced anisometropia. *Investigative Ophthalmology, 26*, 330–342.

Spear, P. D., Tong, L., & Langsetmo, A. (1978). Striate cortex neurons of binocularly deprived kittens respond to visual stimuli through the closed eyelids. *Brain Research, 155*, 141–146.

Sur, M., Humphrey, A. H., & Sherman, S. M. (1982). Monocular deprivation affects X- and Y-cell terminations in cats. *Nature, 300*, 183–185.

Tieman, S. B. (1984). Effects of monocular deprivation on geniculocortical synapses in the cat. *Journal of Comparative Neurology, 222*, 166–176.

Trachtenberg, J. L., & Stryker, M. P. (2001). Rapid anatomical plasticity of horizontal connections in the developing visual cortex. *Journal of Neuroscience, 21*, 3476–3482.

Trachtenberg, J. L., Trepel, C., & Stryker, M. P. (2000). Rapid extragranular plasticity in the absence of thalamocortical plasticity in the developing primary visual cortex. *Science, 287,* 2029–2031.

Tumosa, N., Tieman, S. B., & Tieman, D. G. (1989). Binocular competition affects the pattern and intensity of ocular activation columns in the visual cortex of cats. *Visual Neuroscience, 2,* 391–407.

Tychsen, L., Wong, A. M. F., & Burkhalter, A. (2004). Paucity of horizontal connections for binocular vision in V1 of naturally strabismic macaques: cytochrome oxidase compartment specificity. *Journal of Comparative Neurology, 474,* 261–275.

Von Grunau, M. W., & Singer, W. (1980). Functional amblyopia in kittens with unilateral exotropia II. Correspondence between behavioural and electrophysiological assessment. *Experimental Brain Research, 40,* 305–310.

Von Noorden, G. K., Dowling, J. E., & Ferguson, D. C. (1970). Experimental amblyopia in monkeys. *Archives of Ophthalmology, 84,* 206–214.

Wiesel, T. N. (1982). Postnatal development of the visual cortex and the influence of environment. *Nature, 299,* 583–591.

Wiesel, T. N., & Hubel, D. H. (1963a). Effects of visual deprivation on morphology and physiology of cells in the cat's lateral geniculate body. *Journal of Neurophysiology, 26,* 978–993.

Wiesel, T. N., & Hubel, D. H. (1963b). Single cell responses in striate cortex of kittens deprived of vision in one eye. *Journal of Neurophysiology, 26,* 1003–1017.

Wiesel, T. N., & Hubel, D. H. (1965). Comparison of the effects of unilateral and bilateral eye closure on cortical unit responses in kittens. *Journal of Neurophysiology, 28,* 1029–1040.

Wong, A. M. F., Lueder, G. T., Burkhalter, A., & Tychsen, L. (2000). Anomalous retinal correspondence: neuroanatomic mechanism in strabismic monkeys and clinical findings in strabismic children. *Journal American Association of Pediatric Ophthalmology and Strabismus, 4,* 168–174.

8

What Is Amblyopia?

In the last chapter we looked at deficits in animals and at the physiological and anatomical changes that accompany them. In this chapter, we will consider visual deficits in humans that are collectively known as amblyopia. Amblyopia was originally defined as poor vision, or blunt sight. The aspect of the deficit that is most commonly assessed is acuity, which is usually done in the ophthalmologist's office with a Snellen chart. However, the deficit as a whole is much more complicated. There may be a loss of connections or a distortion or rearrangement of connections within the visual cortex. What happens varies with the deficit because the compensation in the central nervous system is specific to the optical or motor problem that causes the amblyopia. In some cases, as we shall see, there can even be a distortion of vision without any loss of acuity. Thus, the term *amblyopia* covers a variety of different forms of poor vision. As far as is currently possible, this chapter will describe these variations.

Amblyopia has been studied almost entirely by psychophysical means. However, some of the most interesting observations have come from asking patients what they see. One can make psychophysical measurements, such as contrast sensitivity, in animals, and tally the results with anatomical and physiological measurements. Unfortunately, one cannot ask animals what they see. Thus, the anatomical and physiological mechanisms that underlie details of the various forms of amblyopia are, in many cases, speculative. The animal studies, described in the last chapter, suggest a number of explanations for amblyopia. However, the experiments to prove these suggestions have not been done.

1. Amblyopia from Anisometropia

The easiest situation to describe and understand is anisometropia. In cases where there is no strabismus, the two eyes look in approximately the same direction. Most of the time the image in one eye is out of focus, and, therefore, the image on the retina is degraded. As a result, the connections between the retina and the cortex do not form as precise a topographic map as they do in a normal person. We do not yet know if the normal topographic map forms and then degenerates, or if there is a normal process of refinement of the topographic map over the first few years of life that does not occur when the image on the retina is out of focus. In any case, the image is poor and vision is poor over most of the field of view of one eye.

Acuity, as measured by gratings, is diminished in the amblyopic eye, as is contrast sensitivity. The contrast sensitivity curve tends to show substantial losses at high spatial frequencies and not much loss at low spatial frequencies (Bradley & Freeman, 1981). Acuity can be measured with gratings or with letters, and the results correspond with each other (Levi & Klein, 1982). Vernier acuity is also reduced. The fraction by which acuity is reduced varies from patient to patient, but for a particular patient, vernier, grating, and Snellen acuity are all reduced by the same fraction (Levi & Klein, 1982; see Fig. 8.1).

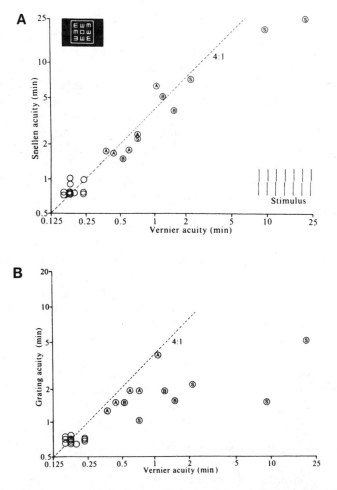

FIG. 8.1. Relationship between (A) Snellen acuity and vernier acuity, and (B) grating acuity and vernier acuity for anisometropic amblyopes (A), strabismic amblyopes (S), amblyopes that are both anisometropic and strabismic (B), and normal people (O). For anisometropic amblyopes, grating acuity, vernier acuity. and letter (Snellen) acuity are linearly related. [Reprinted with permission from Levi, D.M., & Klein, S. (1982). *Nature, 298*, 268–270. Copyright 1982 MacMillan Magazines Limited.]

The acuity loss is also found in the peripheral part of the binocular field of view, and the same amount of loss is seen in both the nasal and temporal parts of the field (Sireteanu & Fronius, 1981). This suggests that the grain of the whole system is degraded by an amount that depends on the extent of the anisometropia.

Interestingly, monocularly driven acuity is spared. In the far periphery of the temporal field, there is a region that is driven by one eye only because the nose blocks the view from the other eye. In this area, anisometropic amblyopes do not show deficits (Hess & Pointer, 1985; see Fig. 8.2). Consequently, the deficits seen in the binocular part of the field of view must be due to binocular interactions. Presumably, the good eye competes with the blurred eye and takes over space in the cortex from the blurred eye, just as it does in monocular deprivation. This tallies with the small shift in ocular dominance found in animal models.

Spatial localization is degraded in anisometropic amblyopes in proportion to their contrast sensitivity loss (Hess & Holliday, 1992). To test this, one

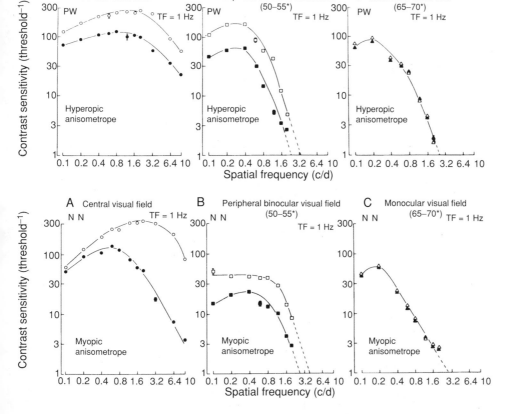

FIG. 8.2. Contrast sensitivity in the binocular and monocular parts of the field of view for two hyperopic anisometropes. *Filled symbols* show contrast sensitivity in the amblyopic eye, and *open symbols* show contrast sensitivity in the normal eye. [Reprinted from Hess, R. F., & Pointer, J. S. (1985). *Vision Research, 25,* 1577–1594. Copyright 1985, with permission from Elsevier.]

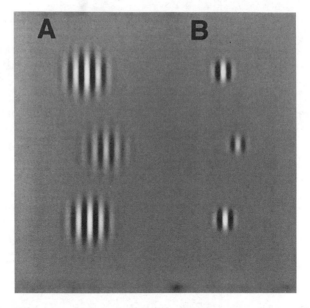

FIG. 8.3. A task used to test spatial uncertainty in amblyopes. The task is to line up the middle Gabor patch between the upper and lower ones. [Reprinted from Hess, R. F., & Holliday, I. E. (1992). *Vision Research, 32*, 1319–1339. Copyright 1992, with permission from Elsevier.]

needs a stimulus that is devoid of local vernier cues. Hess and Holliday used a triplet of Gabor patches (Fig. 8.3), with the task being to line up the middle one between the upper and lower ones. Anisometropic amblyopes showed no deficit when the elements were set to the same fraction above threshold for both the normal and amblyopic eye.

In sum, different anisometropes show different amounts of loss in acuity and contrast sensitivity, depending on the extent of their anisometropia. However, losses in other parameters, such as vernier acuity and spatial localization, are scaled in proportion to their acuity loss. The system acts as though the connections between the retina and cortex are imprecise, causing a blurring of information transfer that affects all aspects of visual performance equally.

2. Effect of Cataracts

Amblyopia resulting from cataract is called stimulus-deprivation amblyopia. In untreated cases, the effect is much worse than in anisometropia or strabismus. In unilateral cataract, much of the input from the deprived eye to the cortex is lost, whereas in anisometropia this input is reduced a little and is not as precise as normal. Consequently, many children with congenital untreated unilateral cataract have an acuity of less than 20/200 (1/10 normal) and are legally blind [Maurer & Lewis, 1993; see Fig. 8.4(A)]. The therapy is to remove the cataract surgically, provide optical correction to compensate for the loss of the lens, and then to patch the good eye for 40% to 50% of

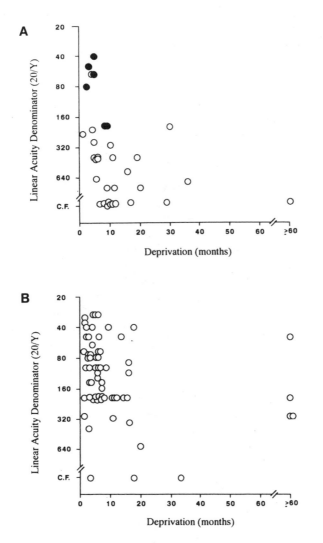

FIG. 8.4. (A) Linear letter acuity for children with unilateral cataract as a function of the duration of deprivation. In some cases the good eye was patched 40% to 50% of waking time (•) and in some cases it was not (○). (B) Linear letter acuity as a function of the duration of deprivation in children treated for bilateral congenital cataracts. [Reprinted with permission from Maurer, D., & Lewis, T. L. (1993). *Early visual development, normal and abnormal* (pp. 454–484). Figures 26.10 and 26.12.]

each day to force the child to use the poor eye. Even this is not totally effective [Fig. 8.4(A)]. Children with congenital bilateral cataract are better off, but their vision is still substantially below normal [Fig. 8.4(B)].

Interestingly, while acuity in the deprived eye in unilateral cataract is generally worse than in bilateral cataract, even after patching, some motion and spatial vision is better (Ellemberg, Lewis, Maurer, Brar, & Brent, 2002; Lewis, Ellemberg, Maurer, Wilkinson, Wilson, Dirks, & Brent, 2002). The assumption is that connections for motion and spatial vision develop in unilateral cataract under the influence of the nondeprived eye, and can subsequently be accessed through the deprived eye, whereas these connections do not develop in bilateral cataract where both eyes are deprived. These connections for motion and spatial vision may be at a higher level than V1, for example, in V4 or V5 (MT), but this is not certain. The main point is that motion and spatial vision can develop independent of acuity.

3. Amblyopia from Strabismus

The deficits caused by strabismus are more complicated. Sometimes the angle of deviation is quite small. In these cases the result is not very different from that in anisometropia: There will be poor acuity and poor contrast sensitivity in the wandering eye.

Sometimes a new point of fixation is created away from the fovea. This occurs mainly in cases of esotropia, where the angle of deviation is not too large, and remains constant during early development, which allows the new fixation point to be established. Connections may form from the new point of fixation to higher areas of cortex that deal with central vision, creating anomalous retinal correspondence, as discussed in previous chapters.

Acuity at the new point of fixation is limited by the density of ganglion cells in the retina and the size of the center of their receptive fields. The center of the receptive field gets larger and the density per unit area of retina gets lower as one moves away from the fovea (Fig. 8.5). This limits the acuity that can be obtained. No matter how precisely the connections between retina and cortex are rearranged, acuity can never be better than

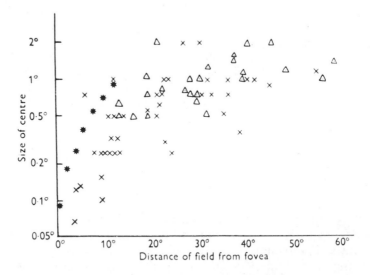

FIG. 8.5. Decrease in spatial summation away from the fovea, related to the increase in the size of the center of receptive fields in the retina. X indicates ON center units, and △ indicates OFF center cells. (From Hubel & Wiesel, 1960). * represent minimum of the Westheimer function (a measurement of summation area) in normal human eyes. [From Enoch, J. M., et al. (1970). *Documenta Opthalmologica, 29,* 127–153. Reprinted by permission of Kluwer Academic Publishers.]

the spacing of the ganglion cells in the retina. However, acuity is frequently worse than permitted by this limit, showing that there is also a muddling of connections between the new point of fixation and the cortex (Hess, 1977).

Despite the visual center having changed, the fovea still exists with a high density of receptors, ganglion cells, and lateral geniculate cells per unit area of retina. Consequently, vision is clearest away from the point of fixation in the direction of the fovea. This is illustrated in Figure 8.6, from Pugh (1962). The subject was amblyopic in the left eye with esotropia and some hypotropia. Thus, the fovea was to the left and above the point of fixation, and the direction of clearest vision was to the right and below. Therefore, the right-hand side of objects was seen more clearly than the left-hand side.

Many different rearrangements of the connections between retina and cortex can occur to compensate for strabismus. Presumably, the extent and nature of the rearrangements are related to the direction and extent of the deviation of the eye during the first few months of life and to whether this deviation is constant or not. One can only discover the variability of visual experience by asking the patient what he or she sees—something that, with one or two exceptions, is rarely reported in the scientific literature. Some of the variations are illustrated neatly by Hess, Campbell, and Greenhalgh (1978), who both measured contrast sensitivity curves in a number of patients and asked them what the gratings looked like.

Some patients who saw distorted gratings reported normal contrast sensitivity (Fig. 8.7). For others who had normal contrast sensitivity, part of the grating disappeared at fine spatial frequencies (Fig. 8.8). Presumably, in these cases enough fine-grain foveal connections were still present to give normal acuity. However, there is some scrambling of connections in areas of central vision, and the nature of these varies from case to case.

In other cases, patients reported degraded contrast sensitivity and a variety of deficits in the detailed perception of the grating. An example is given in Figure 8.9: In this case, the lines in the grating appeared to be broken up. Obviously, the results also depend on the size and position of the test grating. A large grating will cover a large area of retina, and the orientation of the grating can be detected by any part of the field of view that is included. Results with a small grating will depend on where it is placed in the field of view. This point is particularly relevant when the part of the retina that is amblyopic is large (Fig. 8.10).

The results of Hess and colleagues help to explain why letter acuity is worse than grating acuity—a phenomenon that has been known for decades (Gstalder & Green, 1971). This is not just an example of the crowding phenomenon (see below) because acuity for single letters is worse than grating acuity, as well as acuity for letters in a line (Katz & Sireteanu, 1990; see Fig. 8.11). Two factors combine to produce this result. One is simply that a grating can be detected if it is visible in any part of the field of view that it covers. The other is that local distortions of the image make the details of letters hard to see.

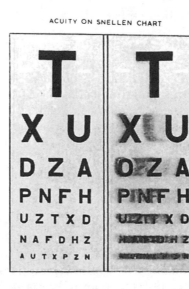

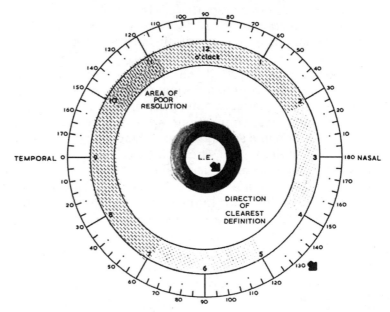

FIG. 8.6. Illustration of an amblyope's visual perception for a subject with esotropia and hypotropia in the left eye. Objects were clearer on their right edge than on their left. A second letter was seen between the large letters on the Snellen chart (anomalous retinal correspondence). The smaller letters on the chart tended to run together. Consequently, acuity for single letters was better than acuity for letters in a line (crowding phenomenon). [Reprinted with permission from Pugh, M. G. (1962). *British Journal of Ophthalmology, 46,* 193–211. Published by BMJ Publishing Group.]

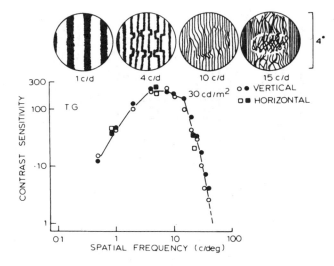

FIG. 8.7. Results from an amblyope with normal contrast sensitivity and distorted vision. Results from the amblyopic eye are denoted by the *filled symbols*, and from the normal eye by *open symbols*. Contrast sensitivity curves are shown at the bottom. A representation of what the amblyope saw is shown at the top. [Reprinted with permission from Hess, R. F., et al. (1978). *Pfluger's Archives fur gesamte Physiologie, 377,* 201–207. Copyright 1978 Springer-Verlag.]

3.1. Crowding

As illustrated in Figure 8.6, the small letters on the Snellen chart tend to run together. This is called separation difficulty or the crowding effect (Irvine, 1948; Stuart & Burian, 1962). As a result, acuity for single letters is better than

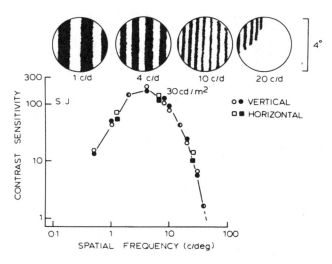

FIG. 8.8. Results from an amblyope with normal contrast sensitivity but poor acuity in one part of the field of view. [Reprinted with permission from Hess, R. F., et al. (1978). *Pfluger's Archives fur gesamte Physiologie, 377,* 201–207. Copyright 1978 Springer-Verlag.]

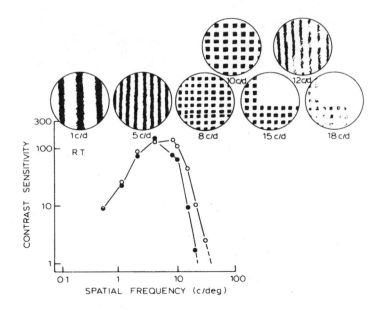

FIG. 8.9. An amblyope with loss of contrast sensitivity where the lines of the grating appeared to be broken up. [Reprinted with permission from Hess, R. F., et al. (1978). *Pfluger's Archives fur gesamte Physiologie, 377*, 201–207. Copyright 1978 Springer-Verlag.]

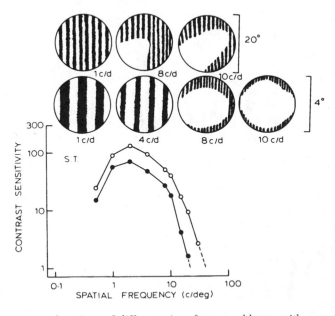

FIG. 8.10. Appearance of gratings of different sizes for an amblyope with a scotoma in central vision. [Reprinted with permission from Hess, R. F., et al. (1978). *Pfluger's Archives fur gesamte Physiologie, 377*, 201–207. Copyright 1978 Springer-Verlag.]

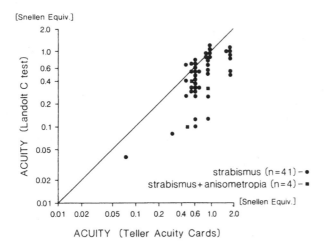

FIG. 8.11. Letter acuity measured with the Landolt C test compared with grating acuity measured with Teller acuity cards. In the Landolt C test, the task is to detect the gap in a C, when it is presented in one of four different orientations. With Teller acuity cards, the patient is presented with a grating and a uniform card, and the investigator determines which card the patient spends the most time looking at. Acuity with the Landolt C test is frequently worse, and never significantly better than with the Teller acuity cards. [Reprinted from Katz, B., & Sireteanu, R. (1990). *Clinical Vision Sciences, 5,* 307–323. Copyright 1985, with permission from Elsevier.]

acuity for letters in a line. As Irvine says, "others describe a crowding together of the letters on a line as if the macular area and a portion of the retina to one side of it project in almost the same direction."

The crowding phenomenon occurs in normal people as well as in amblyopes (Stuart & Burian, 1962; Flom, Weymouth, & Kahneman, 1963). For anybody, the presence of an object affects the visibility of an object nearby. This probably occurs because the cells in the visual cortex that analyze the orientation of edges and form, for one location, interact with similar cells for a neighboring location. In the case of anisometropic amblyopes, the magnitude of the crowding effect is proportional to the degradation in acuity (Levi & Klein, 1985). In the case of strabismic amblyopes, as expected from the nature of the rearrangement of the connections between retina and cortex, the crowding deficit can be much greater than the acuity deficit (Levi & Klein, 1985).

A similar point can be made using stimuli where the bars flanking a target are varied in contrast (Hess, Dakin, Tewfik, & Brown, 2001; see Fig. 8.12). The physics of the stimulus predicts that there should be contour interactions when the flanking bars have the same contrast as the target, but not when the flanking bars are of opposite contrast. This effect is seen in people with normal vision when perception in the fovea is tested, but both the same and opposite contrasts give contour interactions and crowding in normal people in the periphery of the field of view. About half the strabismic amblyopes tested had central vision perception that was like that seen in the peripheral visual field in normal people, and half had a smaller effect. Other experiments have also shown that the extent of crowding scales with the target size in

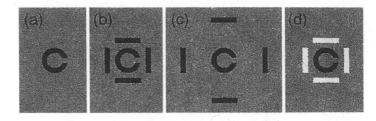

FIG. 8.12. Stimuli used to compare the effect of contours of opposite contrast with contours of the same contrast on the ability to detect the orientation of a Landolt C. [Reprinted from Hess, R. F., et al. (2001). *Vision Research, 41,* 2285–2296. Copyright 2001, with permission from Elsevier.]

the normal fovea, but not in the normal periphery or the amblyopic fovea (Tripathy & Cavanagh, 2002).

3.2. Vernier Acuity

Similar points can be seen in studies of vernier acuity. One can express vernier acuity as a percentage of the resolution limit, as measured with a grating. For normal eyes, this percentage is about 16%. If the vernier acuity is measured with a pair of gratings offset from each other (see Fig. 3.7), there is an increase in this percentage when the gratings are fine, within one octave (a factor of 2) of the resolution limit (Levi & Klein, 1982; see Fig. 8.13). Results

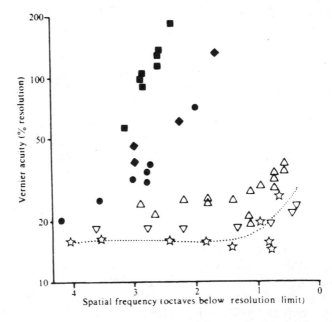

FIG. 8.13. Vernier acuity tested with two gratings offset from each other as a function of the fundamental frequency of the grating. Both the abscissa and the ordinate have been scaled to take account of each subject's grating resolution. Results from normal eyes are shown by the *dotted line*. Results from anisometropic amblyopes are denoted by *open symbols*. Results from strabismic amblyopes are denoted by *filled symbols*. Vernier acuity, when scaled like this, is close to normal for anisometropic amblyopes, and far from normal for strabismic amblyopes. [Reprinted with permission from Levi, D.M., & Klein, S. (1982). *Nature, 298,* 268–270. Copyright 1982 MacMillan Magazines Limited.]

in anisometropic amblyopes are similar to normal. However, results in strabismic amblyopes are very different: Vernier acuity is substantially more than 16% of grating acuity when the spatial frequency of the display is less than three octaves below the resolution limit.

Interestingly, vernier acuity improves with practice in adults with amblyopia (Levi & Polat, 1996) and normal people (McKee & Westheimer, 1978). The improvement can be substantial, up to 60% to 70% in both cases. Novice observers improve more than experienced ones. Practice with vernier acuity leads to an improvement in Snellen acuity as well. This should be considered in evaluating how much recovery is seen in amblyopia with treatment.

3.3. Spatial Uncertainty

This loss of vernier acuity is a form of spatial uncertainty at a fine level, in the sense that amblyopes cannot tell where one grating is in relation to the other. Spatial uncertainty at a coarse level is also worse in strabismic amblyopes than in anisometropic amblyopes. This deficit can be seen in a bisection task, where the amblyope is asked to line up a short line with markers above and below it, or place it midway between two others on each side of it [Flom & Bedell, 1985; see Fig 8.14(A)]. It can also be seen in a placing task, where the amblyope is asked to place a sequence of dots equidistant from a central fixation point. The result can be distinctly asymmetric [Fig. 8.14(B)],

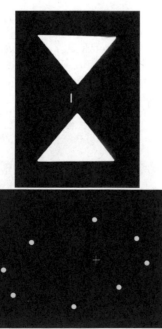

FIG. 8.14. (Top) Spatial localization task. The subject is asked to line up the line between the points of the two triangles. (Bottom) Spatial distortion in a strabismic amblyope. The patient attempted to set the dots to be equidistant from the central cross. The rightmost dot was 1.5° from the cross. [Reprinted with permission from Flom, M. C., & Bedell, H. E. (1985). *American Journal of Optometry and Physiological Optics, 62*, 153–160.]

although deficits of this magnitude are fairly rare. While spatial uncertainty in anisometropic amblyopes can be accounted for by their contrast sensitivity deficit (Hess & Holliday, 1992), both spatial uncertainty and vernier acuity are distinctly worse in strabismic amblyopes than their contrast sensitivity deficit would predict.

Spatial uncertainty may be due to undersampling (Levi & Klein, 1986) or distorted sampling, also known as neural disarray (Hess et al., 1978). Undersampling covers the situation where cells in the visual cortex receive projections from the correct part of the retina, but these projections are either fewer than normal or spread more widely than normal, so the receptive fields of the cells in the cortex are larger than normal. Distorted sampling covers the situation where cells in the visual cortex receive projections from the wrong part of the retina. In the case of undersampling, when the patient is tested, he or she will, on average, place the stimulus in the correct position, but the errors are larger than normal. In the case of distorted sampling, the patient will, on average, place the stimulus in an incorrect position. Logically speaking, undersampling should be involved in anisometropic amblyopia, and both undersampling and distorted sampling in strabismic amblyopia, depending on the nature and history of the strabismus. Different results may be obtained in different patients, but distorted sampling is certainly a factor in strabismus (Demanins, Wang, & Hess, 1999).

3.3.1. Shape Discrimination

Various stimuli have been devised to test the ability of amblyopes to detect shapes. Some involve the detection of curves or lines of Gabor patches embedded in a sea of patches around the curve or line (Fig. 3.10). Others involve distinguishing an irregular circle from a regular circle (Fig. 8.15). The latter task has been used with strabismic amblyopes, where the deficit affects low as well as high radial frequencies of the stimulus to about the same

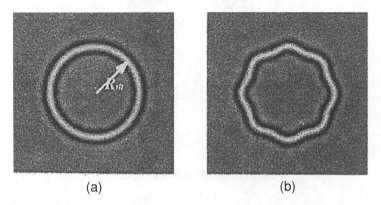

(a)   (b)

FIG. 8.15. Stimuli used to test discrimination of an irregular circle from a regular circle. [Reprinted from Hess, R. F., et al. (1999). *Vision Research, 39,* 901–914. Copyright 1999, with permission from Elsevier.]

degree (Hess, Wang, Demanins, Wilkinson, & Wilson, 1999). The deficit does not depend critically on the contrast of the pattern. At suprathreshold levels, the performance of the amblyopic and its fellow eye are comparable. This task has also been used with stimulus-deprivation amblyopes (Jeffrey, Wang, & Birch, 2004). The results suggest that both undersampling and distorted sampling may play a role. Thus, a variety of results are seen in different types of amblyopia.

3.3.2. Deficits in Movement and Direction Perception

Some tests of movement perception in amblyopes show significant deficits and others show little. For example, Simmers, Ledgeway, Hess, and McGraw (2003) used a test of global motion perception consisting of detecting the movement of a pattern of dots in which varying numbers of the dots moved in the same direction. The dots were either a different luminance from the background or the same luminance and a different contrast. There were deficits that were unrelated to the contrast sensitivity of the amblyope, and the deficits were more extensive for the contrast-defined stimuli than for the luminance-defined stimuli. The authors suggest that this can be accounted by deficits in the extrastriate cortex. On the other hand, if one measures visually evoked potentials (VEPs) and compares the results from the onset of movement with the reversal of a pattern, there is little effect on the former compared with the latter in amblyopic eyes (Kubova, Kuba, Juran, & Blakemore, 1996). Experiments with other tests show a similar variety of results. In total, the results suggest that amblyopes do have motion deficits, but the appropriate test is required to reveal them.

3.3.3. Border Distinctness

When amblyopes are asked to match an edge of variable blur seen in their amblyopic eye with an edge of variable blur seen in their normal eye, they do very well (Hess, Pointer, Simmers, & Bex, 2003). Indeed, the conclusion is that they see a sharp edge as sharp, not blurred, just as normal people do in the periphery of the field of view. Presumably edges that adequately stimulate the highest spatial frequency filters will be seen as maximally distinct.

3.3.4. Counting Features

Another deficit found in amblyopes is that they are poor at counting features. This has been tested with a set of Gabor spots, and with features missing from a 7 × 7 array (Sharma, Levi, & Klein, 2000). Normal observers count up to four briefly presented items without error, and make errors if more items are presented. Strabismic amblyopes perform substantially worse. This is not due to feature visibility, crowding, positional jitter, or abnormal temporal integration. Presumably it is due to a deficit at a higher level of processing: The authors speculate that the deficit is somewhere in parietal cortex.

3.4. Suppression

The image in the good eye of an amblyope suppresses the image in the amblyopic eye to avoid double vision (diplopia). There are different types of suppression in different types of amblyopia, and also in different parts of the visual field of the same amblyope (Harrad, 1996). Anisometropic amblyopes and amblyopes with small-angle strabismus essentially have an in-focus image that falls on the fovea of the good eye, and a displaced image that is blurred by the amblyopia that falls near the fovea of the amblyopic eye. The displaced image gets suppressed by a mechanism akin to dichoptic masking, which is seen in normal people when an in-focus image is presented to one eye and a slightly displaced out-of-focus image to the other (Daw, 1962). With large-angle strabismus and alternating fixation, the contours of the images in the two eyes may have different orientations, and a process akin to binocular rivalry takes place, with an alternation between one image and the other. This distinction was illustrated well by Schor (1977), who showed that strabismic subjects will suppress one image when gratings of similar orientation are presented and will experience the image alternation caused by binocular rivalry when gratings of different orientation are presented.

3.4.1. Components of the Loss in Acuity in Various Strabismics

It should be clear from the preceding discussion that there are several components to the reduction in visual acuity in strabismic amblyopes. While everybody who deals with strabismic amblyopes is aware of this point, there have been few published attempts to quantify it. One of the few is Freeman, Nguyen, and Jolly (1996). They measured monocular losses due to amblyopia, defined as the loss in the amblyopic eye due to poor or scrambled connections to the visual cortex; strabismic deviation, defined as loss due to shifting of the image away from the fovea to the more peripheral retina; and binocular losses due to suppression and masking. The results from nine amblyopes can be seen in Figure 8.16. Interestingly, strabismic deviation was the largest component, amblyopia the next largest, and suppression and masking the smallest.

3.4.2. Detailed Comparison of Groups of Amblyopes

A more detailed comparison of the deficits in a large number of amblyopes has been made by McKee, Levi, and Movshon (2003). They measured performance in a set of acuity tests (Snellen, vernier, and grating) and in a set of contrast sensitivity tests (Pelli–Robson and edge contrast sensitivity). They were able to classify the subjects into four groups: those with high acuity and moderate sensitivity (normals and refractives); those with moderate acuity and high sensitivity (strabismics, former strabismics, and inconstant strabismics); those with moderate acuity and low sensitivity (anisometropes, inconstant strabismic anisometropes, deprivationals, and other abnormals); and those with low acuity and moderate or low sensitivity (strabismic anisometropes and eccentric fixators). The reader should go to the original paper

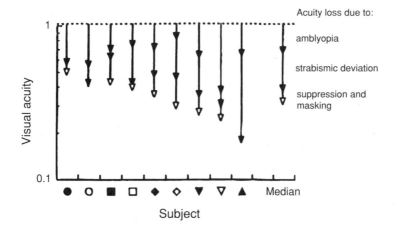

FIG. 8.16. Components of acuity loss in nine strabismic subjects. The *dashed line* gives the mean acuity in normal subjects. Amblyopic loss was determined from the acuity during monocular viewing compared with normal subjects. Loss due to strabismic deviation was the additional loss due to eccentric viewing. Loss due to suppression and masking was found by comparing acuity in binocular viewing with acuity in monocular viewing. [Reprinted from Freeman, A. W., et al. (1996). *Vision Research, 36*, 765–774. Copyright 1996, with permission from Elsevier.]

for the definition of these groups and descriptions of the tests. Two interesting findings were the high sensitivity in the second group and the poor vision in strabismic anisometropes as compared with strabismics and anisometropes. Nonbinocular subjects with mild-to-moderate acuity deficits had, on average, better monocular contrast sensitivity than binocular subjects with the same acuity loss.

3.4.3. The Peripheral Field of View

Eye doctors are concerned primarily with acuity in the central field of view. The clinical aim is to get the two eyes to look in the same direction to avoid double vision. This requires the establishment of the fovea as the fixation point, which in turn requires improvement of the acuity in the foveal region until it is as close as possible to normal. Yet, strabismus leads to mismatches in the images in the peripheral retina as well as in the center, and anisometropia, if severe, leads to a significant blurring of the image in the peripheral as well as the central retina. Very few studies have considered this question.

Acuity is reduced out to 20° from the fovea in strabismic amblyopes (Sireteanu & Fronius, 1981). There is considerable variability in the extent of the deficit in this region from one case to another (Hess & Jacobs, 1979; see Fig. 8.17). Generally speaking, acuity is reduced more in the nasal part of the retina for esotropes and more in the temporal part of the retina for exotropes. These parts of the retina are close to the fovea, and therefore the mismatch between the two images is likely to have more effect because the size of the receptive fields of the cells involved is smaller. Anisometropic amblyopes have reduced acuity over a wider area of retina than do strabismic

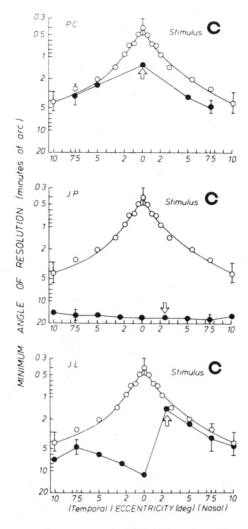

FIG. 8.17. Acuity as a function of eccentricity in three strabismic amblyopes. *Open circles* represent the acuity from four normal subjects. *Filled circles* show the acuity from the amblyopes. *Arrow* marks the point of fixation. Amblyope PC had central fixation and a small symmetric reduction in acuity. Amblyope JP had fixation 2° away from the fovea and a large reduction in acuity at all eccentricities. Amblyope JL was an exotrope, and acuity was reduced substantially more in the temporal field of view than in the nasal. [Reprinted from Hess, R. F., & Jacobs, R. J. (1979). *Vision Research, 19,* 1403–1408. Copyright 1979, with permission from Elsevier.]

amblyopes (Hess & Pointer, 1985). For some reason, the diffusion of the image is a stronger influence than the lateral displacement of the image on cells with large receptive fields at large eccentricities.

Binocular interaction has been studied in the peripheral field of view in amblyopes using tests of binocular summation, and transfer of the tilt aftereffect (Sireteanu, Fronius, & Singer, 1981). Generally, results from these tests showed deficiencies in the areas of reduced acuity. That is, binocular interactions were present in the peripheral field of view of strabismic amblyopes,

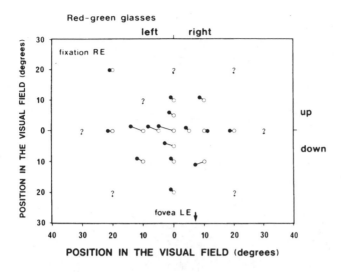

FIG. 8.18. Subjective localization by an untreated strabismic amblyope. Red stimulus presented to one eye and green stimulus to the other through red–green glasses. *Open circles*: normal eye; *filled circles*: amblyopic eye. *Question marks*: no decision about the relative localization of the stimuli was possible. [Reprinted with permission from Sireteanu, R., & Fronius, M. (1989). *Investigative Ophthalmology and Visual Science, 30*, 2023–2033.]

but not anisometropic amblyopes. However, the results varied considerably from case to case, depending on the extent of the amblyopia.

There can also be interesting variations in retinal correspondence between the center and periphery of the field of view. The easiest to explain occurs in strabismics with an angle of deviation that is too large to have anomalous retinal correspondence in the central field of view. Compensation in such cases occurs through the suppression of the image in the deviating eye. However, anomalous retinal correspondence may occur in the *peripheral* field of view, where the receptive fields of the cells are larger, and the anatomical distance in the cortex over which connections must be rearranged to get anomalous correspondence is smaller (Sireteanu & Fronius, 1989). As a result, subjective localization in the central field of view differs in the two eyes, whereas subjective localization in the peripheral field of view is the same (Fig. 8.18).

The general conclusion is that the reduction in acuity depends on the extent of the binocular mismatch in relation to the size of the receptive fields of the part of the retina involved. A moderate mismatch will have a large effect where the receptive fields are small, near the fovea, and a small effect where the receptive fields are large, in the periphery. Binocular interactions are affected much like acuity is. In some cases acuity, binocular interactions, and subjective localization are all degraded severely near the fovea, yet are normal in the peripheral part of the field of view.

3.4.4. A Rapid Test for Amblyopia

Basing their idea on theoretical grounds, Pelli and colleagues have proposed a rapid test for amblyopia (Pelli, Levi, & Chung, 2004). The subject is

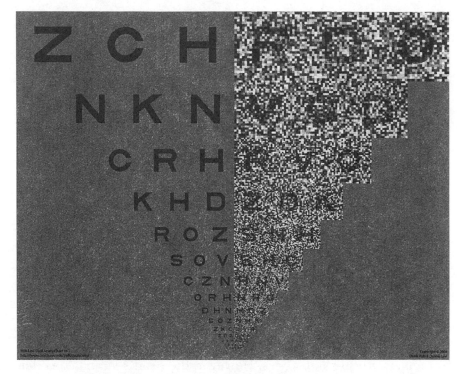

FIG. 8.19. Pelli–Levi dual acuity chart. Normal people show the same acuity on both sides of the chart and amblyopes show a one- to two-line difference. [Reprinted with permission from http://psych.nyu.edu/pelli/dualacuity/.]

asked to read all six letters on each row (Fig. 8.19), continuing down until he or she gets all three no-noise letters wrong. Partial credit is given for each letter that is correctly identified in the last triplet in which any letters were correctly read. The score of interest is the difference in lines between the two sides. There is generally no difference in normal subjects, and a one- or two-line difference in amblyopes. The chart may be used at any distance. Various models for amblyopia have been ruled out by experiments, resulting in this chart.

4. Summary

Amblyopia includes a variety of deficits. In nearly all cases there is a loss of acuity and contrast sensitivity, although in two cases described by Hess and colleagues (1978) this was not true. Vernier acuity is degraded. Spatial localization is distorted. The details of objects are distorted. Shapes are not recognized properly. There are some deficits in motion perception. The number of objects is not counted as accurately as in people with normal vision.

In anisometropia, most of these factors are degraded in proportion to each other. Vernier and Snellen acuities are reduced in proportion to the loss of resolution measured by grating acuity. Spatial uncertainty can be explained by the loss of contrast sensitivity. In strabismus, vernier and Snellen acuities are reduced more than grating acuity. If the angle of deviation of the eye is constant and not too large, there will be a new point of fixation. In this case, vision will be clearest in the peripheral field of view nearest to the projection of the fovea. If the angle of deviation is large, the image in one eye will be suppressed because it is not possible for the anatomical connections to be rearranged over the large distance required to compensate for the deficit. In bilateral cataract, the result is like a bad case of anisometropia. In unilateral cataract, the situation is much worse: spatial vision is almost totally lost in one eye.

There have been discussions in the literature as to whether amblyopia is due to a loss of connections between the retina and cortex (undersampling), lack of precision of these connections (spatial uncertainty), or rearrangement of these connections (spatial scrambling) (Hess, Field, & Watt, 1990; Levi & Klein, 1990; Wilson, 1991). It should be clear from this chapter that all three occur in different forms of amblyopia, and all three could occur in a single case of amblyopia. The clearest case of loss of connections between retina and cortex is in monocular deprivation, or stimulus-deprivation amblyopia, where these connections are radically reduced. However, some reduction in the strength of connections has been documented in animal models of anisometropia and strabismus. From the anatomical point of view, the lack of precision of connections and rearrangement of connections are the same fundamental phenomenon. It is just a question of whether the connections are rearranged in a circularly symmetric fashion, as in anisometropia, or in a bipolar fashion, as in anomalous retinal correspondence from strabismus, or something in between. It seems likely that, in severe cases of strabismus with anomalous retinal correspondence, several forms of rearrangement will occur: (a) the formation of two sets of connections between retina and cortex, one from the new point of fixation to the part of cortex that handles central vision, and one from the new point of fixation to its normal location; (b) a blurring of the precise topography around each of these locations; and (c) some loss in the density of the connections from the amblyopic eye. In addition to these forms of anatomical rearrangement, there is also the physiological suppression of the image in the amblyopic eye by the image in the normal eye.

The variety of results that can occur is illustrated clearly in the classic paper of Hess, Campbell, and Greenhalgh (1978). What this paper also illustrates is that measurement of the contrast sensitivity curve can obscure the details of the loss of vision in the patient. The contrast sensitivity curve lumps together a number of different conditions because the stimulus covers a large area of the retina, and the patient detects the grating on the basis of whatever part of the retina has the most distinct vision. Moreover, the contrast sensitivity curve does not detect errors in spatial localization. To understand the full nature of the deficit, a variety of tests must be performed.

References

Bradley, A., & Freeman, R. D. (1981). Contrast sensitivity in anisometropic amblyopia. *Investigative Ophthalmology, 21*, 467–476.

Daw, N. W. (1962). Why after-images are not seen in normal circumstances. *Nature, 196*, 1143–1145.

Demanins, R., Wang, Y. Z., & Hess, R. F. (1999). The neural deficit in strabismic amblyopia: sampling considerations. *Vision Research, 39,* 3575–3585.

Ellemberg, D., Lewis, T. L., Maurer, D., Brar, S., & Brent, H. P. (2002). Better perception of global motion after monocular than after binocular deprivation. *Vision Research, 42,* 169–179.

Enoch, J. M., Berger, R., & Birns, R. (1970). A static perimetric technique believed to test receptive field properties: extension and verification of the analysis. *Documenta Ophthalmologica, 29,* 127–153.

Flom, M. C., & Bedell, H. E. (1985). Identifying amblyopia using associated conditions, acuity, and nonacuity features. *American Journal of Optometry and Physiological Optics, 62,* 153–160.

Flom, M. C., Weymouth, F. W., & Kahneman, D. (1963). Visual resolution and contour interaction. *Journal of the Optical Society of America A, 53,* 1026–1032.

Freeman, A. W., Nguyen, V. A., & Jolly, N. (1996). Components of visual acuity loss in strabismus. *Vision Research, 36,* 765–774.

Gstalder, R. J., & Green, D. G. (1971). Laser interferometric acuity in amblyopia. *Journal of Pediatric Ophthalmology and Strabismus, 8,* 251–256.

Harrad, R. (1996). Psychophysics of suppression. *Eye, 10,* 270–273.

Hess, R. F. (1977). On the relationship between strabismic amblyopia and eccentric fixation. *British Journal of Ophthalmology, 61,* 767–773.

Hess, R. F., & Holliday, I. E. (1992). The spatial localization deficit in amblyopia. *Vision Research, 32,* 1319–1339.

Hess, R. F., & Jacobs, R. J. (1979). A preliminary report of acuity and contour interaction across the amblyope's visual field. *Vision Research, 19,* 1403–1408.

Hess, R. F., & Pointer, J. S. (1985). Differences in the neural basis of human amblyopia: the distribution of the anomaly across the visual field. *Vision Research, 25,* 1577–1594.

Hess, R. F., Campbell, F. W., & Greenhalgh, T. (1978). On the nature of the neural abnormality in human amblyopia: neural aberrations and neural sensitivity loss. *Pfluger's Archives fur gesamte Physiologie, 377,* 201–207.

Hess, R. F., Dakin, S. C., Tewfik, M., & Brown, B. (2001). Contour interaction in amblyopia: scale selection. *Vision Research, 41,* 2285–2296.

Hess, R. F., Field, D. J., & Watt, R. J. (1990). The puzzle of amblyopia. In C. Blakemore (Ed.), *Vision: coding and efficiency.* pp. 267–280. Cambridge, UK: Cambridge University Press.

Hess, R. F., Pointer, J. S., Simmers, A., & Bex, P. J. (2003). Border distinctness in amblyopia. *Vision Research, 43,* 2255–2264.

Hess, R. F., Wang, Y. Z., DeManins, R., Wilkinson, F., & Wilson, H. R. (1999). A deficit in strabismic amblyopia for global shape detection. *Vision Research, 39,* 901–914.

Hubel, D. H., & Wiesel, T. N. (1960). Receptive fields of optic nerve fibres in the spider monkey. *Journal of Physiology, 154,* 572–580.

Irvine, S. R. (1948). Amblyopia ex anopsia. Observations on retinal inhibition, scotoma, projection, light difference discrimination and visual acuity. *Transactions of the American Ophthalmological Society, 66,* 527–575.

Jeffrey, B. G., Wang, Y. Z., & Birch, E. E. (2004). Altered global shape discrimination in deprivation amblyopia. *Vision Research, 44,* 167–177.

Katz, B., & Sireteanu, R. (1990). The Teller acuity card test: a useful method for the clinical routine? *Clinical Vision Sciences, 5,* 307–323.

Kubova, Z., Kuba, M., Juran, J., & Blakemore, C. (1996). Is the motion system relatively spared in amblyopia? Evidence from cortical evoked responses. *Vision Research, 36,* 181–190.

Levi, D. M., & Klein, S. A. (1982). Hyperacuity and amblyopia. *Nature, 298,* 268–270.

Levi, D. M., & Klein, S. A. (1985). Vernier acuity, crowding and amblyopia. *Vision Research, 25,* 979–991.

Levi, D. M., & Klein, S. A. (1986). Sampling in spatial vision. *Nature, 320,* 360–362.

Levi, D. M., & Klein, S. A. (1990). Equivalent intrinsic blur in amblyopia. *Vision Research, 30,* 1995–2022.

Levi, D. M., & Polat, U. (1996). Neural plasticity in adults with amblyopia. *Proceedings of the National Academy of Sciences of the United States of America, 93,* 6830–6834.

Lewis, T. L., Ellemberg, D., Maurer, D., Wilkinson, F., Wilson, H. R., Dirks, M., & Brent, H. P. (2002). Sensitivity to global form in glass patterns after early visual deprivation in humans. *Vision Research, 42,* 939–948.

Maurer, D., & Lewis, T. L. (1993). Visual outcomes after infantile cataract. In K. Simons (Ed.), *Early visual development, normal and abnormal* (pp. 454–484). New York: Oxford University Press.

McKee, S. P., & Westheimer, G. (1978). Improvement in vernier acuity with practice. *Perception & Psychology, 24*, 258–262.

McKee, S. P., Levi, D. M., & Movshon, J. A. (2003). The pattern of visual deficits in amblyopia. *Journal of Vision, 3*, 380–405.

Pelli, D. G., Levi, D. M., & Chung, S. T. L. (2004). Using visual noise to characterize amblyopic letter identification. *Journal of Vision, 4*, 904–920.

Pugh, M. (1962). Amblyopia and the retina. *British Journal of Ophthalmology, 46*, 193–211.

Schor, C. M. (1977). Visual stimuli for strabismic suppression. *Perception, 6*, 583–588.

Sharma, V., Levi, D. M., & Klein, S. A. (2000). Undercounting features and missing features: evidence for a high-level deficit in strabismic amblyopia. *Nature Neuroscience, 3*, 496–501.

Simmers, A. J., Ledgeway, T., Hess, R. F., & McGraw, P. V. (2003). Deficits to global motion processing in human amblyopia. *Vision Research, 43*, 729.

Sireteanu, R., & Fronius, M. (1981). Naso-temporal asymmetries in human amblyopia: consequence of long-term interocular suppression. *Vision Research, 21*, 1055–1063.

Sireteanu, R., & Fronius, M. (1989). Different patterns of retinal correspondence in the central and peripheral visual field of strabismics. *Investigative Ophthalmology and Visual Science, 30*, 2023–2033.

Sireteanu, R., Fronius, M., & Singer, W. (1981). Binocular interaction in the peripheral visual field of humans with strabismic and anisometropic amblyopia. *Vision Research, 21*, 1065–1074.

Stuart, J. A., & Burian, H. M. (1962). A study of separation difficulty. *American Journal of Ophthalmology, 53*, 471–477.

Tripathy, S. P., & Cavanagh, P. (2002). The extent of crowding in peripheral vision does not scale with target size. *Vision Research, 42*, 2357–2369.

Wilson, H. R. (1991). Model of peripheral and amblyopic hyperacuity. *Vision Research, 31*, 967–982.

9

Critical Periods

In the previous chapter we discussed amblyopia and the various deficits that can occur. There are critical periods for these deficits, defined as periods during which some property of the system can be changed. In their pioneering experiments, Wiesel and Hubel (1963a) used the term *critical period* to describe the period during which the ocular dominance of cells in the visual cortex of cats can be changed by monocular deprivation; in other words, the period during which ocular dominance can be disrupted. This was clearly different from the initial period of development of ocular dominance, and authors have become increasingly aware that there are critical periods for other properties as well. Considering acuity, Wick, Wingard, Cotter, and Scheiman (1992) talk about the critical period for development versus the plastic period for treatment. There is also the period during which a property can recover after it has been disrupted, and investigators have become increasingly aware that these periods are not necessarily identical either. Thus, Hardman Lea, Loades, and Rubinstein (1989) talk about the sensitive period for the development of amblyopia versus the sensitive period for its treatment.

Consequently, we have to distinguish three periods: the initial period for development of a property, discussed in Chapter 3; the critical period for disruption of the property; and the critical period for recovery of the property after it has been disrupted. For some properties these may be the same, but for others they are clearly not. The prime purpose of this chapter is to discuss in which cases there are similar time courses and in which the time courses are different. In most people's minds, the terms *critical period* and *sensitive period* are probably interchangeable. I will use the term *critical period* and will discuss here the initial period of development, and the critical periods for disruption and recovery.

The crucial visual factor for humans is the quality of vision as measured by acuity. Measurements of acuity show that it develops in normal children to adult levels in 3 to 5 years. However, acuity can be disrupted by strabismus or anisometropia until 7 or 8 years of age. After it has been disrupted, acuity can be improved by effective therapy in teenagers, and sometimes even in adults with maintained therapy. This supports the observation that the critical period for disruption of a property lasts longer than the period of initial development, and the period during which recovery is possible lasts longer still.

Experiments with animals also show that there are a variety of critical periods, and that the time course of any given critical period depends on the part of the visual system being studied. Monocular deprivation has little effect on the retina, a very small effect on the lateral geniculate nucleus, and a major effect on the primary visual cortex. Within the primary visual cortex, the critical period for the effect on cells in layer IV ends earlier than the critical period for cells in layers outside IV. Furthermore, the critical period for the direction of movement ends earlier than the critical period for monocular deprivation. Moreover, rearing an animal in the dark delays both the onset and the end of the critical period for monocular deprivation.

Thus, one cannot talk about the critical period as a single entity. One has to talk about the critical period for a particular function in a particular part of the nervous system after a particular history of visual exposure with a particular kind of visual deprivation. This chapter will discuss the evidence for these variations in the critical period and consider the general hypotheses that may be drawn from the evidence.

1. General Principles from Experiments with Animals

1.1. The System Is Plastic between Eye Opening and Puberty

The manipulation that has been carried out most often in animals, and is easiest to use for a comparison between species, is monocular deprivation. In the cat, the critical period for monocular deprivation lasts from 3 weeks to 8 months of age (Olson & Freeman, 1980; Jones, Spear, & Tong, 1984; Daw, Fox, Sato, & Czepita, 1992). The eyes open at 3 to 12 days of age, and puberty occurs at 6 months of age. In the rat, the critical period lasts from before 3 to about 7 weeks of age (Fagiolini, Pizzorusso, Berardi, Domenici, & Maffei,1994; Guire, Lickey, & Gordon, 1999). The eyes open at 10 to 12 days, and puberty occurs at 8 to 12 weeks, later for males than females. For mice, the critical period is before 18 to more than 35 days of age (Gordon & Stryker, 1996), with eye opening at 10 to 12 days and puberty at 6 to 8 weeks. Macaque monkeys are born with their eyes open, and the critical period for monocular deprivation lasts from close to birth to nearly 1 year of age. Puberty is at 3 to 3.5 years for males and 2 to 3 years for females. Humans are also born with their eyes open, with a critical period for unilateral cataract that lasts from 6 to 8 weeks to 10 years of age (Vaegan & Taylor, 1979; Birch, Stager, Leffler, & Weakley, 1998).

It is often difficult to judge the start of the critical period because experiments with infants can be very difficult, and so can physiological recordings in young animals. Similarly, the end of the critical period depends on the severity of the deprivation, as described in the next section, and the technique used: for example, single unit recording versus visually evoked potentials. Thus, comparisons are difficult to make. Nevertheless, the generalization that the critical period starts soon after eye opening and ends around puberty seems to be broadly true with exceptions to be noted below. The one exception seems to be the macaque, where current evidence shows that the critical period ends at about 1 to 2 years of age, and puberty occurs some time after that.

One consequence of this generalization is that the end of the critical period could vary with gender in species where puberty varies with gender, such as rat and macaque monkey. Experiments to test a direct relationship between the end of the critical period and levels of steroids that increase around puberty have been either negative (Daw, Baysinger, & Parkinson, 1987) or equivocal (Daw, Sato, Fox, Carmichael, & Gingerich, 1991). However, the relationship might be indirect, and the possibility of a relationship between gender and the end of the critical period in rats and macaques, where the difference in puberty between the two genders is most striking, has never been tested.

Within the critical period, the susceptibility to monocular deprivation increases to a peak during which the system is extremely sensitive, then declines. At the peak, 1 to 2 days of deprivation can have an effect in species like mouse and cat, and 1 week can have an effect in primates, for example, macaque and human. The peak sensitivity is at 4 to 6 weeks in cat, around 4 weeks in rat and mouse, around 6 weeks in macaque, and around 6 months in human, although it is not very well defined in the last two species.

1.2. More Severe Deprivations Have a Larger Effect

Numerous studies, starting with the first papers by Wiesel and Hubel (1963a) on cats and LeVay, Wiesel, and Hubel (1980) on macaques, have shown that the extent of the ocular dominance shift from monocular deprivation depends on both the length of deprivation and the time at which it is applied. During the most sensitive part of the critical period in the cat, 1 day of deprivation has a slight effect, 2.5 to 3.5 days has a large effect, and after 6 to 10 days of deprivation nearly all cells in the cortex are totally dominated by the eye that remained open (Hubel & Wiesel, 1970; Olson & Freeman, 1975).

The first experiment that tested the effect of a constant period of monocular deprivation at various ages was done in the cat (Olson & Freeman, 1980). The authors used approximately 10 days of deprivation and showed a small ocular dominance shift for deprivation between 8 and 19 days of age, a substantial one with deprivation between 18 and 27 days of age, and significant shifts for deprivation at ages up to between 109 and 120 days of age, when the shift was again very small. The conclusion was that the critical period lasted from 3 weeks to 3.5 months of age. Subsequent experiments with 1 month (Jones et al., 1984) and 3 months of deprivation (Daw et al., 1992) showed that these longer periods of deprivation were effective even at 9 months of age in the cat. Thus, the end and the length of the critical period both depend on how long the deprivation lasts (Fig. 9.1).

Deprivations that are more severe than suturing the eyelids shut can have an effect even in the adult (Gilbert & Wiesel, 1992). If large lesions are made in the retinas of both eyes so that the cortex has no input in this part of the field of view, cells in the cortex representing the area of the lesion will start responding to areas in the retina outside the lesion. There is a short-term

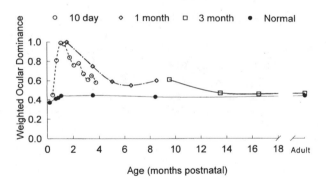

FIG. 9.1. Critical period for monocular deprivation in the cat. Weighted ocular dominance is calculated as $n_7 + 5/6n_6 + 4/6n_{5+} 3/6n_4 + 2/6n_3 + 1/6n_2$, where n_i is the number of cells in ocular dominance group i, divided by the total number of cells recorded. Weighted ocular dominance for normal animals is 0.43 because there is a slight dominance by the contralateral eye. Points for 10 days of deprivation from Olson & Freeman (1980); for 1 month from Jones, Spear, & Tong (1984); for 3 months from Daw, Fox, Sato, & Czepita (1992). [Reprinted with permission from Daw, N. W. (1994). *Investigative Opthalmology, 35*, 4168–4179.]

physiological change and a long-term anatomical change through sprouting of lateral connections within the cortex (Darian-Smith & Gilbert, 1994). The physiological change can be produced with an artificial scotoma as well as a lesion (Pettet & Gilbert, 1992).

1.3. Higher Levels of the System Have a Later Critical Period

As pointed out above, visual deprivation has larger effects in the cortex than in retina and lateral geniculate nucleus. Monocular deprivation has very little effect in the retina (Wiesel & Hubel, 1963a; Sherman & Stone, 1973) on any of the cell types found there (Cleland, Mitchell, Crewther, & Crewther, 1980). There is also little effect on the physiological properties of cells in the lateral geniculate nucleus (Wiesel & Hubel, 1963b; Shapley & So, 1980; Derrington & Hawken, 1981). Cells in the lateral geniculate nucleus driven by the deprived eye are smaller (Wiesel & Hubel, 1963b), but this almost certainly occurs because they support reduced endings in the cortex, particularly in the part of the field of view that is binocular where competition between the two eyes occurs (Guillery & Stelzner, 1970).

The most noticeable effects of monocular deprivation occur in primary visual cortex, where cells are completely dominated by the open eye, and most cannot be driven at all by the closed eye after long periods of deprivation. This is true particularly of cells in the extragranular layers (layers II, III, V, and VI), which are the output layers of the cortex. Some cells in the input layer, layer IV, can still be driven by the deprived eye (Shatz & Stryker, 1978). When deprivation occurs late in the critical period, the ocular dominance of cells in layers II, III, V, and VI is altered, whereas the ocular dominance of cells in layer IV is not (Mower, Caplan, Christen, & Duffy, 1985; Daw et al., 1992). Thus, the critical period for the input layer ends earlier than the critical period for the output layers.

The primary visual cortex projects to the inferior temporal cortex, where faces and objects are recognized. Here plasticity continues for a substantial period of time (Rodman, 1994). Visual memories are also stored in the temporal cortex, and plasticity presumably continues for them indefinitely. Temporal cortex projects to the hippocampus, which is known to be plastic in the adult.

1.4. Different Properties Have Different Critical Periods

The first experiment comparing critical periods for different properties was done with ocular dominance and direction selectivity in the cat visual cortex. Kittens were reared in a drum moving continually in one direction, then the drum's direction was reversed and the cortex was assayed for the percentage of cells preferring the direction seen first compared with the percentage preferring the direction seen second (Daw & Wyatt, 1976). The results were compared with data on ocular dominance where one eye was open first, then closed and the other eye opened (Blakemore & Van Sluyters, 1974). With ocular dominance, the eye that was opened second dominated if the switch was made before 7 weeks of age, and the eye that was open first dominated if the switch was made later. With direction selectivity, the direction seen second dominated if the switch was made before 4 weeks, and the direction seen first dominated for a later switch in direction, implying that the critical period for direction selectivity ends earlier than the critical period for ocular dominance (Fig. 9.2). Interestingly, when one eye was open until 5 weeks of age looking at a drum moving in one direction, then both eyes and direction were switched, the majority of cells preferred the direction seen first and the eye open second (Daw, Berman, & Ariel, 1978), as expected for critical periods

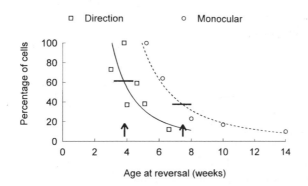

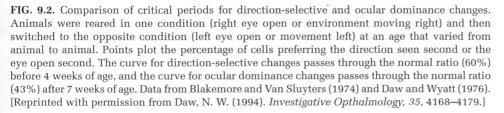

FIG. 9.2. Comparison of critical periods for direction-selective and ocular dominance changes. Animals were reared in one condition (right eye open or environment moving right) and then switched to the opposite condition (left eye open or movement left) at an age that varied from animal to animal. Points plot the percentage of cells preferring the direction seen second or the eye open second. The curve for direction-selective changes passes through the normal ratio (60%) before 4 weeks of age, and the curve for ocular dominance changes passes through the normal ratio (43%) after 7 weeks of age. Data from Blakemore and Van Sluyters (1974) and Daw and Wyatt (1976). [Reprinted with permission from Daw, N. W. (1994). *Investigative Opthalmology, 35,* 4168–4179.]

ending at different times. The general point is supported by the observation that orientation selectivity becomes fixed before ocular dominance in ferrets (Chapman & Stryker, 1993; Issa, Trachtenberg, Chapman, Zahs, & Stryker, 1999).

To fit this result in with the previous generalization that critical periods end earlier at lower levels of the system, as defined in Chapter 2, one has to argue that directional selectivity is created at a lower level than ocular dominance. This is partly true in the cat. Many cells in layer IV of the visual cortex (the input layer) are directionally selective, and many are also monocular. Thus, direction selectivity is a property created at the initial level of primary visual cortex, at least in the cat where these experiments were conducted, whereas binocularity is a property created primarily at higher levels of the system (output layers of primary visual cortex).

Interestingly, stereoscopic acuity develops rapidly between 5 and 7 weeks of age in the cat (Timney, 1981), when direction and orientation are no longer plastic and while ocular dominance can still be changed. Presumably stereoscopic vision needs cells that are well tuned for the same orientation and direction of movement in the two eyes, and the development of stereoscopic acuity depends on continued ocular dominance development (Daw, 1994).

Another example of different critical periods for different properties occurs in layer IV of the primary visual cortex in the macaque monkey. There are two parallel pathways for processing different properties within the geniculostriate projections in the macaque. Form and color are processed in the P pathway, which projects to the parvocellular layers of the lateral geniculate nucleus and layer IVCβ in primary visual cortex. Movement is processed in the M pathway, which projects to the magnocellular layers of the lateral geniculate nucleus and layer IVCα in primary visual cortex. Monocular deprivation leads to a reduction in the extent of the geniculocortical endings in the visual cortex. In animals where one eye is open until 3 weeks of age, then closed and the other eye opened, layer IVCα is dominated by the endings from the eye that was open first, while layer IVCβ is dominated by the endings from the eye that was opened second (LeVay et al., 1980; Fig. 9.3). Thus, the critical period for the magnocellular endings comes to a close before the critical period for the parvocellular endings. Connections for movement get wired into place while connections for form and color are still plastic.

A further example comes from experiments with monocular deprivation in the macaque monkey (Harwerth, Smith, Duncan, Crawford, & Von Noorden, 1986). Monocular deprivation can affect a variety of behavioral measures, such as sensitivity to light in the dark-adapted state, sensitivity to increments of light in the light-adapted state, sensitivity to contrast at high spatial frequencies, and binocular summation. Dark-adapted sensitivity is affected by monocular deprivation before 3 months of age, increment sensitivity before 6 months, contrast sensitivity at high spatial frequencies before 18 months, and binocular summation before 24 months (Fig. 9.4). This sequence of effects also fits in with the generalization that properties dealt with at a higher level of the system have critical periods that end later.

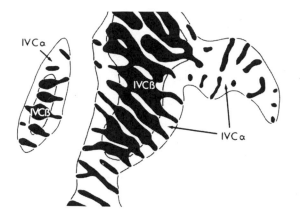

FIG. 9.3. Effect of reverse suture at 3 weeks of age on labeling pattern in the right cortex. Right eye sutured first, then opened and left eye sutured. Injection was into the right eye. Right eye (*black area*) dominated in layer IVCß because this layer was still plastic at 3 weeks of age; left eye (*white area*) dominated in layer VICα, because the critical period for this layer was over at 3 weeks of age. [From LeVay, S., et al. (1980). The development of ocular dominance columns in normal and visually deprived monkeys. *Journal of Comparative Neurology, 191*, 1–51. Copyright © 1980. Reprinted by permission of John Wiley & Sons, Inc.]

1.5. The Critical Period Depends on the Previous Visual History of the Animal

As described above, rearing an animal in the dark affects the critical period. Monocular deprivation changes the ocular dominance in dark-reared animals at several months of age, when there is little effect in light-reared animals of the same age (Cynader & Mitchell, 1980). Early in the critical period, monocular deprivation has a larger effect on light-reared animals than on dark-reared animals (Mower, 1991; Beaver, Ji, & Daw, 2001). Thus, rearing in the dark delays both the start and the end of the critical period. This leads to the interesting result that dark-reared cats are less plastic than light-reared cats at 5 to 6 weeks of age, equally plastic at 8 to 9 weeks, and more plastic at 12 to 20 weeks (Fig. 9.5). This result can be used to distinguish factors that are related to plasticity, as opposed to factors that simply increase or decrease with age during the development of the visual cortex (see Chapter 11).

1.6. Procedures Affect the Critical Period

Monocular deprivation has an effect in adult mice if urethane is used as an anesthetic rather than barbiturate, and the measure is the visually evoked potential (VEP) rather than single unit recordings (Sawtell, Frenkel, Philpot, Nakazawa, Tonegawa, & Bear, 2003; Pham, Graham, Suzuki, Barco, Kandel, Gordon, & Lickey, 2004). The VEP from stimulation of the nondeprived eye increases rather than the VEP from stimulation of the deprived eye decreasing. The effect of deprivation is less persistent over time in adults than in juveniles. The mechanism of plasticity in adults may also be different from that in juveniles (Pham et al., 2004). This plasticity in adult animals is a recent finding, and much remains to be discovered about it. We need to know

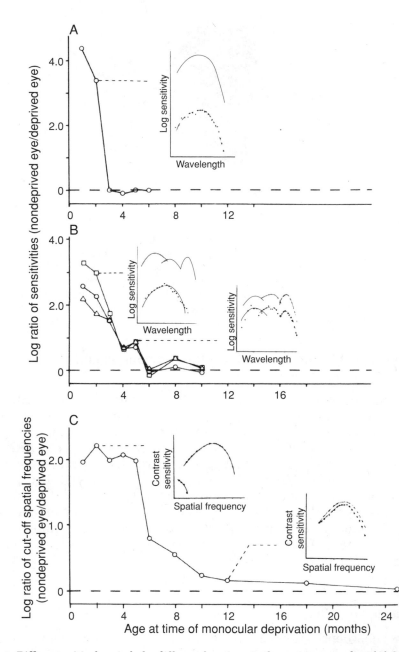

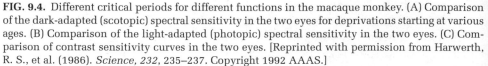

FIG. 9.4. Different critical periods for different functions in the macaque monkey. (A) Comparison of the dark-adapted (scotopic) spectral sensitivity in the two eyes for deprivations starting at various ages. (B) Comparison of the light-adapted (photopic) spectral sensitivity in the two eyes. (C) Comparison of contrast sensitivity curves in the two eyes. [Reprinted with permission from Harwerth, R. S., et al. (1986). *Science, 232*, 235–237. Copyright 1992 AAAS.]

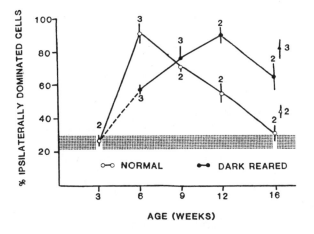

FIG. 9.5. Dark-reared cats are less plastic than normal at 6 weeks of age, equally plastic at 9 weeks of age, and more plastic at 12 to 16 weeks of age. Percentage of ipsilaterally dominated cells is plotted after 2 days of monocular deprivation at these ages for both rearing regimes. Shaded region indicates the percentage in cats without monocular deprivation. At 16 weeks, data from cats who experienced prolonged deprivation is also plotted. Numbers indicate the number of cats. [Reprinted from Mower, G. D. (1991). *Developmental Brain Research, 58,* 151–158. Copyright 1991, with permission from Elsevier.]

if it is seen in other species, and more about the differences in time course and mechanism.

1.7. The Periods of Development, Disruption, and Recovery May Be Different

There are several examples of differences in the critical periods for the disruption of a developing property and for its recovery after the disruption. These examples are from animal experiments. As an example of anatomical changes, consider the geniculocortical endings in layer IV of the visual cortex, which are initially overlapping and come to be segregated into separate bands of left and right eye endings. This segregation is assayed by the transport of substances injected into the eye and carried through the lateral geniculate nucleus to the terminals in the visual cortex. This process of ocular dominance segregation is complete in the macaque monkey by 6 to 8 weeks of age (LeVay et al., 1980) or earlier (Horton & Hocking, 1996). Nevertheless, the pattern of ocular dominance can be affected by monocular deprivation up to 10 to 12 weeks of age (Horton & Hocking, 1997). Moreover, geniculocortical endings that have been induced to retract by monocular deprivation can be made to expand again by opening the initially closed eye, and closing the initially open eye (Swindale, Vital-Durand & Blakemore, 1981). Recent experiments in the ferret have shown that the segregation of ocular dominance columns in the cortex initially occurs between P 15 and P 20. However, monocular deprivation between P 40 and P 65 can modify these columns, supporting a distinction between the period of initial development and the period of plasticity (Crowley & Katz, 2000). Furthermore, ferrets that are monocularly deprived for 3 weeks from P49 can recover binocularity when the deprived eye is reopened after the end of the critical period for monocular deprivation (Liao, Krahe, Prusky, Medina, & Ramoa, 2004).

A more clear-cut example comes from the ocular dominance histograms assembled from recordings of cells in all layers of primary visual cortex. In normal animals, the histogram contains a large percentage of binocular cells and is slightly dominated by the contralateral eye at all ages. The histogram changes as the geniculocortical afferents change, becoming slightly less binocular and slightly less dominated by the contralateral eye (Albus & Wolf, 1984; Hubel & Wiesel, 1970). By 6 weeks of age, in both cats and macaque monkeys, the histogram is indistinguishable from that recorded in adults. Nevertheless, monocular deprivation has a dramatic influence on the histogram for many months after this.

In terms of behavioral responses, the acuity of kittens develops to maturity at 3 months of age (Giffin & Mitchell, 1978). Both reductions in acuity after deprivation by occlusion of one eye and increases in acuity when the occluded eye is opened and the other eye is occluded (reverse occlusion) can be obtained up to 1 year of age (Mitchell, 1988, 1991). In some cases increases were also seen in the previously occluded eye without reductions in acuity in the previously open eye, but this point was not stringently tested because the purpose of the experiments was to obtain recovery, not cause amblyopia (Mitchell, 1991).

That the effect of deprivation can be reversed for some time after the critical period for the creation of the deficit has ended is most clear in relation to strabismus in humans. The comparable experiments in macaque monkeys or cats have yet not been done. The experiments that have been done will be discussed below, after the human data are presented.

2. Critical Periods in Humans

2.1. Disruption of Acuity

The study of patients with spontaneous and traumatic cataract has provided detailed information on the critical period for stimulus deprivation in humans (Vaegan & Taylor, 1979). This critical period lasts from a few weeks after birth to 10 years of age (Fig. 9.6). Susceptibility declines with age: for example, patient SH who was monocularly deprived for about a year starting at age 1 year was completely blind in the deprived eye; patient LF, who was monocularly deprived for about the same period from 4 to 5 years of age had acuity reduced to one tenth of normal; and patient AN, who was monocularly deprived for the same period from 8 to 9 years of age, had normal acuity. Longer periods of deprivation have a greater effect, as shown by comparing patient SD, who was deprived for 6 months at 3 years of age, and had an acuity 1/20 of normal at the end of the deprivation, with patients SR and AB who were deprived for 3 years, and had acuity of 1/160 normal. Similar results have been obtained by other investigators (Von Noorden, 1981). All of these results agree with the general principles determined in animal experiments.

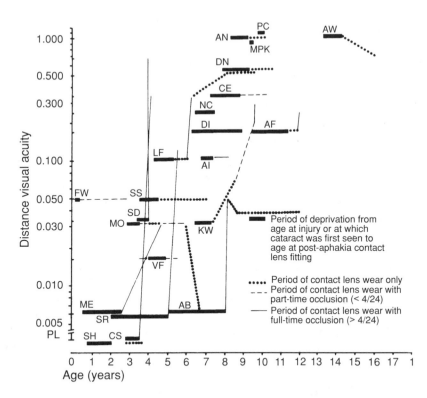

FIG. 9.6. Cases of unilateral cataract in man, in which the beginning and end of deprivation are well defined. Heavy horizontal bars span the period of deprivation and are set at the level of the first visual acuity score obtained after adequate correction after taking out the cataract. [Reprinted with permission from Vaegen, & Taylor, D. (1979). *Transactions of the Ophthalmology Society (UK)*, *99*, 432–439. Published by BMJ Publishing Group.]

Bilateral cataract has less severe consequences than unilateral cataract. The comparison is most easily made in patients who have had cataract from birth because cases of bilateral cataract, with dense cataracts in both eyes that develop and are treated at the same time, rarely occur later in life (Maurer & Lewis, 1993). After treatment, acuity in cases of bilateral cataract reaches somewhere between 20/30 and 20/200 in most cases (see Fig. 8.4). Acuity in cases of unilateral cataract rarely gets better than 20/200, and reaches this value only when the patient follows the patching procedure well. Interestingly, the duration of the deprivation does not make a large difference in cases of bilateral cataract, and compliance with patching is much more important than duration of deprivation in cases of unilateral cataract.

The difference between unilateral and bilateral congenital cataracts is apparent only when treatment is started after 2 months of age (Birch et al., 1998). With treatment started before 6 to 8 weeks of age, there is very little difference. Thus, the effects of competition between the two eyes does not make itself felt until after 2 months of age. The competition could be due to a reduction in the connections from the deprived eye to the visual cortex, or to suppression of the signals from the deprived eye by signals from the good eye, or both. Whatever the mechanism, competition does not develop in the first 2 months of life.

An interesting comparison of similar deprivations at different ages is provided by surgery for eyelids that turn inwards (Awaya, Sugawara, & Miyake, 1979). This is usually binocular, so surgery is done on one eye, then the other. Each eye has to be patched for 1 week after the surgery. As far as a study of critical periods is concerned, the procedure is complicated because strabismus often results from the operation. Thus, the deprivation involves stimulus deprivation followed by a less well-defined period of strabismus. In all cases, it is the eye closed second that becomes amblyopic. Good recovery of acuity is obtained if the operation is performed after 18 months of age. Before this time, there is poor recovery in 50% to 70% of the cases. Thus, the critical period for short-term occlusion is over by 18 months of age. However, the interpretation is uncertain because of the unknown period of strabismus occurring after the short-term occlusion.

The critical period for disruption of acuity by anisometropia is much less well defined (Hardman Lea et al., 1989). Cases rarely occur in which the anisometropia starts after birth with a known starting date, and in which the anisometropia is not treated for long enough that amblyopia results. The onset is almost always under the age of 5 years, and amblyopia does not result unless the anisometropia persists for 3 or more years (Abrahamsson, Andersson & Sjostrand, 1990; Von Noorden, 1990). There is no significant correlation between the age at which treatment starts and the initial acuity before treatment (Hardman Lea et al., 1989).

Testing for the degradation of acuity caused by strabismus requires a prospective study. Such a study has been done by Dobson & Sebris (1989) on infants with or at risk for esotropia. There was no significant difference in grating acuity between esotropic and normal infants at 6, 9, 12, 18, or 24 months of age. There was a significant difference at 30 and 36 months of age, by which time most subjects had had a surgical procedure for eye alignment (could the degradation of acuity be a result of surgery rather than esotropia?!).

The clinical experience is that amblyopia from strabismus does not develop after 6 to 8 years of age (Von Noorden, 1990). Keech and Kutsche (1995) investigated the age after which visual deprivation does not produce amblyopia in a series of patients that included 17 with strabismus, 27 with corneal lacerations, 31 with cataract, and 7 others. None had amblyopia if the visual deprivation started after 73 months of age. Unfortunately, the data do not give the length of deprivation for each patient as is given in Figure 9.6. Quite possibly the investigators might have seen some reduction in acuity for a deprivation lasting 2 years at a later age, as for patient AF in Figure 9.6.

Most researchers would consider that monocular deprivation is the most severe form of deprivation, with strabismus and anisometropia both being milder. The data from Vaegan and Taylor (1979) show a critical period lasting until 10 years of age for monocular deprivation. The critical period for disruption of acuity by strabismus and anisometropia almost certainly ends earlier than this, making a general clinical estimate of 6 to 8 years reasonable.

Whereas acuity is not disrupted by stimulus deprivation, strabismus, or anisometropia after the age of 10, recovery can still be obtained after this age with appropriate therapy, although, to come to this conclusion, one has to pay more attention to the successes in the literature than to the failures. Therapy can be very time consuming for the patient, parent, and eye care practitioner. The nonamblyopic eye must be patched to bring up the acuity in the amblyopic eye before eye muscle surgery in the case of strabismus, but patching cannot be continued for so long that acuity in the nonamblyopic eye is reduced. Exercises may be required to get the eyes to move together, particularly after strabismus surgery. Use of the amblyopic eye in visual tasks helps the improvement. Continual monitoring is required to assess progress. Failure can easily be due to lack of persistence in the therapy rather than to an inability of the visual system to recover.

A review of the literature shows that considerable improvement is possible after 7 years of age (Birnbaum, Koslowe, & Sanet, 1977). Indeed, using an improvement of four lines on the acuity chart as the criterion, success was more than 50% for children in the 7-to-10 year and 11-to-15 year groups, and dropped to 40% in the over-15-year group. Lack of compliance may be one of the reasons for failure in older groups of children. In anisometropic amblyopes, large improvements can be obtained at all ages with full refractive correction, added lenses or prisms to improve alignment of the visual axes, 2 to 5 h/day of patching, and active vision therapy (Wick et al., 1992). The vision therapy included visual stimulation during patching, binocular anti-suppression therapy, and stimulation of vergence eye movements. With these treatments, the results in older patients were much better than with refractive correction and patching alone (Fig. 9.7), although improvements were obtained in previous studies with less extensive therapy in teenagers (Meyer, Mizrah, & Perlman, 1991).

A study of 407 strabismic children treated by patching suggested that some recovery can be obtained up to 12 years of age (Epelbaum, Milleret, Buisseret, & Dufier, 1993). Acuity in the patched eye was reduced temporarily over the same age range, suggesting that the critical period for the induction of amblyopia by stimulus deprivation is coextensive with the critical period for the recovery from amblyopia caused by strabismus (Fig. 9.8).

Recovery after strabismus is more complicated than recovery after anisometropia. Acuity may be degraded by several factors: reduced vision in the foveal area; fixation with an area outside the fovea where acuity is limited by the coarser connections between the photoreceptors and the visual cortex; suppression of vision in the amblyopic eye by signals from the nonamblyopic eye; and masking when the nonamblyopic and amblyopic eyes view different scenes (Freeman, Nguyen, & Jolly, 1996). Most studies do not distinguish these factors, which may have different critical periods. One of the few that did distinguish them included 14 patients from 13 to 54 years old, but did not follow the various components during treatment and recovery. There did not seem to be any correlation between age and the magnitude of any of the components.

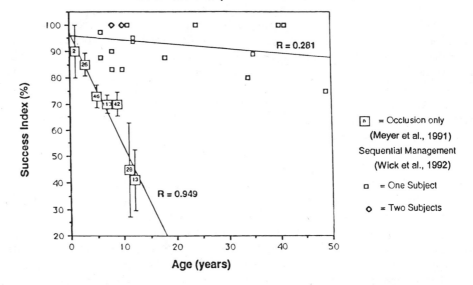

FIG. 9.7. Comparison of success in anisometropic amblyopes treated with occlusion only (Meyer et al., 1991) and those treated with full refractive correction, prisms, or lenses to improve alignment, and visual therapy (Wick et al., 1992). Success index is defined as initial acuity—final acuity/initial acuity—test distance × 100. [Reprinted with permission from Wick, B., et al. (1992). *Optometry and Vision Science, 69,* 866–878.]

The effect on Snellen acuity in strabismus is interesting. Grating acuity and Snellen acuity are degraded in proportion to each other in anisometropes, but Snellen acuity is degraded more than grating acuity in strabismics (Levi & Klein, 1982). This is partly due to eccentric fixation in the strabismics. During treatment, grating acuity improves faster than Snellen acuity (Stuart & Burian, 1962; Pasino & Cordella, 1959). The authors describe this as an increase in

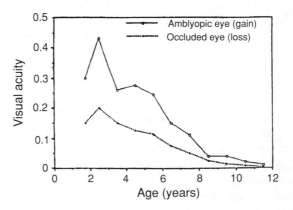

FIG. 9.8. Comparison between the gain in acuity (expressed in decimal units) of the amblyopic eye and the loss in acuity of the occluded eye, measured at the end of the occlusion, as a function of the age of initiation of therapy in strabismic children. [Reprinted with permission from Epelbaum, M., et al. (1993). *Ophthalmology, 100,* 323–327.]

separation difficulty during treatment. This explanation needs further study, with careful attention to changes in the point of fixation during recovery.

In a number of reported cases, acuity is improved in the amblyopic eye after a loss of function in the nonamblyopic eye. A review of the literature that considered loss of function from vascular causes, glaucoma, tumors, macular degeneration, and retinal detachment, showed significant improvements in the amblyopic eye (Vereecken & Brabant, 1984). Patients who get macular degeneration in their nonamblyopic eye can also have dramatic and sustained improvements in the amblyopic eye (Tierney, 1989; El Mallah, Chakravarthy, & Hart, 2000). Even elderly patients with cataract can have large improvements in acuity in their amblyopic eye that can be maintained after the cataract is removed, and the vision is restored in that eye (Wilson, 1992). The assumption is that the degradation in the nonamblyopic eye leads to a removal of suppression of the amblyopic eye. All of these cases reinforce the point that recovery can be obtained over a long period of time.

2.3. Binocularity

Binocular function can be tested in the human by a phenomenon called *interocular transfer of the tilt after-effect* (Banks, Aslin, & Letson, 1975). If one stares at slanted lines for a period of time, then looks at vertical lines, the vertical lines appear to be tilted in the opposite direction. The amount of tilt can be quantified. To measure interocular transfer, the subject stares at the slanted lines with one eye, and the after-effect in that eye is measured and compared with the size of the after-effect in the other eye. No after-effect in the other eye implies that the cells in the visual cortex do not have binocular input. Modeling of the results from this test in early- and late-onset strabismus patients suggests a critical period that starts at 3 to 6 months of age, peaks at 1 to 2 years of age, and declines over 2 to 8 years of age (Fig. 9.9).

Binocular fusion, tested with FPL and checkerboards or random dot displays, develops rapidly between 2 and 6 months of age (Birch, Shimojo, & Held, 1985). It can also be tested by measuring the VEP response to a dynamic random dot correlogram (Eizenman, Westfall, Geer, Smith, Chatterjee, Panton, Kraft, & Skarf, 1999). The authors tested esotropes before surgery (4.4 to 33 months of age), and compared the results to esotropes after surgery (13 to 102 months of age) and to normal children. Five out of the 13 subjects in the first group had detectable responses, compared with 11 out of 13 in the second. In another study, Von Noorden (1988) showed that binocular vision can be obtained in a number of cases with alignment after 2, or even 4, years of age, but stereopsis was rare. The results suggested that binocular fusion is more robust than stereopsis to abnormal visual experience, and has a later critical period.

2.4. Stereopsis

In infants with infantile esotropia, stereopsis develops until 4 months of age, then declines (Birch, 1993). After 6 months of age, only 20% of patients have any stereopsis when tested at the initial visit prior to treatment

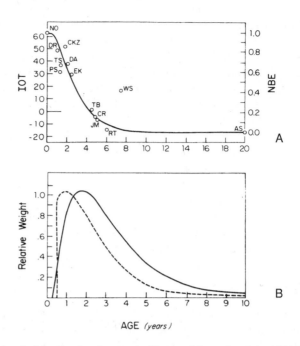

FIG. 9.9. Sensitive period for the development of human binocular vision. (A) Interocular transfer of the tilt after-effect for 12 congenital esotropes, plotted as a function of the age at which corrective surgery was done. Esotropes identified by their initials. (B) Weights given to binocular experience at various ages that provided the best fit to the measurements in (A) (———), and to measurements made from 12 late-onset esotropes (- - - -). [Reprinted with permission from Banks, M. S., et al. (1975). *Science, 190*, 675–677. Copyright 1975 AAAS.]

(Fig. 9.10). The criterion was a disparity of 45′ of arc, representing a coarse level of stereopsis; the graph shows the percentage of infants passing this test. Thus, the results show a degradation of coarse stereopsis over the same period of time that development takes place. However, stereopsis can also be degraded after the initial period of development in cases, for example, of accommodative esotropia (Fawcett, Leffler, & Birch, 2000).

Some recovery can be obtained up to at least 2 years of age. When the results are tallied according to the time at which eye alignment is achieved, binocularity is seen in nearly all cases up to 2 years of age, and coarse stereopsis is found in over 40% of the cases. For those treated before 6 months of age, stereopsis is found in three quarters of the cases, while for those treated after 6 months of age, fewer than half have detectable stereopsis (Birch, Fawcett, & Stager, 2000b). Taylor (1972) found that most of his patients (30/50) who were treated with surgery before 23 months of age and had their tropia converted to a phoria had stereopsis. Stereoscopic acuity after treatment varied from 40″ to 400″ of arc, and the stereoscopic acuity depended on the size of the area of suppression in the macula. Patients with a suppression scotoma of 1° or less had acuities of 40″ to 60″ of arc. When the eyes were aligned after 2 years of age, less than 50% had binocularity and less than 30% had stereopsis (Ing, 1983).

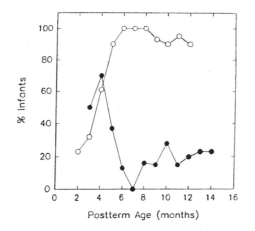

FIG. 9.10. Percent of normal (○) and esotropic (●) infants who reached criterion (45′ of arc) for stereopsis. All esotropic infants were diagnosed by the age of 6 months, had no known neurological or neuromuscular disorders, and were tested at the initial visit prior to any treatment. [Reprinted with permission from Stager & Birch, (1986).]

Whether fine stereopsis can ever be achieved after strabismus is uncertain. In 1988 von Noorden stated: "The noteworthy isolated case of Parks (1984) notwithstanding, there is universal agreement between strabismologists that complete restoration of normal binocular vision with normal random dot stereopsis is unattainable in infantile esotropia." Since von Noorden's summary, Wright, Edelman, McVey, Terry, and Lin (1994) have reported two patients (out of a group of 7) who achieved stereo of 40″ to 70″ of arc, after surgery at 13 and 19 weeks of age. There are few other cases, because surgery at this age is controversial. It is difficult to achieve correct alignment, and some alignment might be achieved without the surgery, making the surgery unnecessary. In theory, early alignment should help if good stereopsis is desired as well as good acuity (Helveston, 1993). However, alignment is the operative word. Early surgery is not enough if it does not lead to alignment. Unless practice evolves to where good alignment can be achieved and maintained by 4 months of age, this point will not be tested.

In summary, stereopsis can be degraded after the initial period of development. Some recovery can be obtained after this time, adequate to drive vergence eye movements and achieve binocular fusion. What happens in the case of fine stereopsis is largely unknown. Nobody knows whether fine stereopsis can be degraded in the period 6 months to 2 years of age, after coarse stereopsis is established, without affecting coarse stereopsis. All the evidence suggests that recovery of fine stereopsis once it has been disrupted is difficult at all ages, and almost impossible after the age of 2, which is before it finally finishes developing in normal people. Thus, fine stereopsis may be an exception to the generalization that the critical periods for development, degradation, and recovery are different. If anything, the critical period for recovery may end earlier than the critical period for development for this visual property. However, the real answers can only be obtained from experiments with animals.

2.5. Movement

The asymmetry of eye movements in following a rotating drum disappears between birth and 3 to 5 months of age (see Chapter 6). This symmetry does not develop in infantile esotropes, depending on the age of onset of the esotropia. In patients studied by Demer and Von Noorden (1988), 58% of patients with onset before 6 months showed asymmetry, as did 22% of those with onset at 6 to 12 months, 9% of those with onset at 12 to 24 months, and 5% of those with onset after 24 months. In patients studied by Bourron-Madignier, Ardoin, and Cypres (1987), the numbers were 92% of those with onset under 6 months, 64% of those with onset at 6 to 12 months, 33% of those with onset at 12 to 24 months, and 23% of those with onset after 24 months. Whether the difference in the numbers is due to different techniques or different populations of patients is not clear, but it is clear that the symmetry in the monocular optokinetic nystagmus can be disrupted for some time after it develops in normal infants (Fig. 9.11).

There is also an asymmetry in the response to motion assayed by VEPs. This is in the opposite direction from the optokinetic nystagmus (OKN) asymmetry: with VEPs, nasotemporal movement produces a better response. The motion VEP is not seen at 0.5 to 1 month of age, is asymmetric when it appears, and eventually becomes symmetric. The time course of this maturation was reported to be between 2 and 10 months of age in normal infants in one study (Birch, Fawcett, & Stager, 2000a), between 5 months and 2 years in another (Norcia, 1996), and between 6 and 15 weeks in a third (Mason, Braddick, Wattam-Bell, & Atkinson, 2001). The asymmetry depends on cortical mechanisms and its period of development lasts longer than the period of development for OKN asymmetry because different mechanisms are involved;

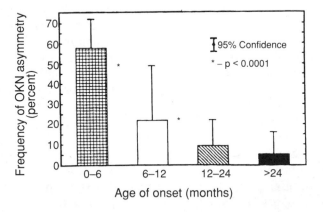

FIG. 9.11. Histogram showing the prevalence of clinical monocular optokinetic nystagmus (OKN) asymmetry in esotropic patients with various ages of onset of strabismus. The asterisks indicate statistically significant differences in prevalence between adjacent columns, and the error bars indicate 95% confidence intervals for mean prevalence. Thus, there was a significantly greater prevalence of asymmetry in esotropic patients with onset before the age of 6 months than those with onset between 6 and 12 months, and these patients in turn had a significantly greater prevalence than in those with even later onset. [Reprinted with permission from Demer, J. L., & Von Noorden, G. K. (1988). *Journal of Pediatric Opthalmology and Strabismus, 25,* 286–292.]

the motion VEP is obviously a purely cortical response, whereas OKN has subcortical components. The development of a symmetrical motion VEP is related to the ability to fuse an image with the two foveas (bifoveal fusion) rather than to stereoscopic vision (Fawcett & Birch, 2000). For infants with infantile esotropia, the asymmetry is within normal limits at 4 to 6 months of age, and becomes abnormal at 7 to 9 months of age (Birch et al., 2000a). Seventy-three percent of infants with infantile esotropia show asymmetry in this response, compared with 20% of infants with onset after 2 years (Hamer, Norcia, Orel-Bixler, & Hoyt, 1993). The latter figure shows that motion VEPs, like monocular OKN, can be disrupted by strabismus after the initial period of development is over. This general point has been confirmed for OKN and for perceptual and motion VEP direction biases in a more recent summary of the data (Brosnahan, Norcia, Schor, & Taylor, 1998).

The critical period for recovery is determined by looking at asymmetry as a function of the age of alignment. Infants whose eyes were aligned at 11 to 18 months had asymmetry indices for motion VEPs that were significantly worse than those of infants whose eyes were aligned by 10 months of age (Birch et al., 2000a). Those with eyes aligned after 2 years of age had asymmetry that was significantly worse than those whose eyes were aligned before (Norcia, Hamer, & Jampolsky, 1995). Moreover, alternate occlusion therapy between 35 and 60 weeks of age can reduce the asymmetry significantly (Norcia, 1996). All these results show that the critical period for recovery also lasts longer than the initial period of development for infantile esotropia. To know whether the critical period for recovery extends beyond the critical period for disruption needs further data or further analysis of data that have already been collected.

3. Summary

This description and analysis of critical periods is summarized in Figure 9.12 and Table 9.1: the figure shows the periods over which different properties develop; the table shows whether the critical period for disruption of a property and/or the critical period for recovery lasts longer than the initial period of development.

Acuity develops between birth and 3 to 5 years of age; vernier acuity between a few months and age 10 years; binocularity between 2 and 6 months of age; stereopsis between 3 and 5 months of age and more slowly after that; monocular OKN between birth and 3 to 5 months of age; motion VEP between 2 months and 2 years of age; and contrast sensitivity between birth and 7 years of age (Fig. 9.12). The period of development for suppression is unknown. The time course for the development of these various visual functions definitely supports the idea that functions handled by lower levels of the system develop earlier.

Disruption of acuity can certainly occur after acuity has first developed in cases of stimulus deprivation (Fig. 9.6). How far this is true in cases of strabismus and anisometropia is unclear. There are few tabulations of the clinical data and a variety of measures of acuity are used. Thus, many comparisons are

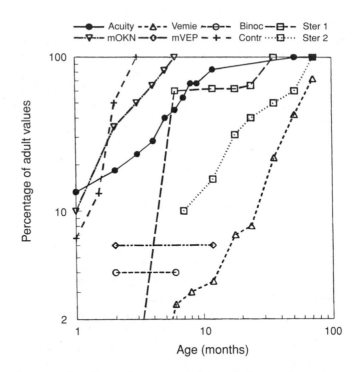

FIG. 9.12. Development of grating acuity, stereopsis, binocularity, vernier acuity, monocular OKN, motion VEP, and contrast sensitivity as a function of age. Stereopsis measurements for projected patterns and line stereograms (stereo 1), and for random dot stereocards (stereo 2). There are few numerical values for binocularity or motion VEPs, so the horizontal line simply shows the period over which these develop. [Reprinted with permission from Daw, N. W. (2003). *Neurobiology of infant vision* (pp. 43–103).]

like apples and oranges. Binocularity can be disrupted over several years with a critical period similar to that for acuity. Stereopsis is disrupted by strabismus over the same period as it develops, and also afterwards. Monocular OKN and the motion VEP can both be disrupted after the period of development is

TABLE 9.1. Summary of Whether the Critical Period (CP) for Disruption of a Property is Later Than the Period of Development of that Property, and Whether the Critical Period for Recovery Lasts Longer Than the Critical Period for Disruption.

Property	Is CP for disruption later?	Is CP for recovery later?
Acuity	Maybe	Yes
Vernier acuity	?	Yes
Binocularity	Yes	?
Stereopsis	Yes	No
Monocular OKN	Yes	Yes
Motion VEP	Yes	Yes
Suppression	?	?
Myopia	Yes	?
Contrast sensitivity	No	No

over. Myopia can certainly be induced after the eyeball is fully grown. There is not a lot of information on the disruption of vernier acuity and changes in suppressive effects as a function of the age of onset of the deprivation.

Recovery of acuity can occur for anisometropia long after the period of disruption has passed, and for strabismus in cases where the nonamblyopic eye loses function. With stimulus deprivation, there is not a lot of recovery later on. Vernier acuity can be improved in the adult, in normal as well as stimulus-deprived people, but the improvement is much larger in deprived people. Recovery of stereopsis is difficult after 2 years of age, which is still within the period of development of fine stereopsis, although coarse stereopsis is probably fully developed by then. There is recovery for both monocular OKN and motion VEPs, when they have been disrupted, after the initial period of development.

All of this emphasizes the point that we started off with: one has to define the visual property, the previous visual history, and the type of visual deprivation when discussing a critical period. Strabismus and anisometropia change the critical period in humans just as rearing in the dark does in animals. The critical period for disruption differs for strabismus, anisometropia, and stimulus deprivation, and so does the critical period for recovery. These three types of deprivation have different effects on different properties. Not all the critical periods have been worked out because of limitations in the data available from humans, and the difficulty and tediousness of the experiments required to find the answer from animals. However, the general rule that the critical period for disruption of a property lasts longer than the initial period of development, and that recovery can be obtained at a time when disruption no longer occurs, seems to be true for most properties with the exception of contrast sensitivity.

References

Abrahamsson, M., Andersson, A. K., & Sjostrand, J. (1990). A longitudinal study of a population based sample of astigmatic children I. Refraction and amblyopia II. The changeability of anisometropia (Fabian). *Acta Ophthalmologica Copenhagen, 68*, 428–434.

Albus, K., & Wolf, W. (1984). Early postnatal development of neuronal function in the kitten's visual cortex: a laminar analysis. *Journal of Physiology, 348*, 153–185.

Awaya, S., Sugawara, M., & Miyake, S. (1979). Observations in patients with occlusion amblyopia. *Transactions of the Ophthalmological Society (UK), 99*, 447–454.

Banks, M. S., Aslin, R. N., & Letson, R. D. (1975). Sensitive period for the development of human binocular vision. *Science, 190*, 675–677.

Beaver, C. J., Ji, Q.-H., & Daw, N. W. (2001). Layer differences in the effect of monocular vision in light- and dark-reared kittens. *Visual Neuroscience, 18*, 811–820.

Birch, E. E. (1993). Stereopsis in infants and its developmental relation to visual acuity. In K. Simons (Ed.), *Early visual development, normal and abnormal* (pp. 224–236). New York: Oxford University Press.

Birch, E. E., Fawcett, S., & Stager, D. R. (2000a). Why does early surgical alignment improve stereoacuity outcomes in infantile esotropia? *Journal American Association of Pediatric Ophthalmology and Strabismus, 4*, 10–14.

Birch, E. E., Fawcett, S., & Stager, D. R. (2000b). Co-development of VEP motion response and binocular vision in normal infants and infantile esotropes. *Investigative Ophthalmology and Visual Science, 41*, 1719–1723.

Birch, E. E., Shimojo, S., & Held, R. (1985). Preferential-looking assessment of fusion and stereopsis in infants aged 1–6 months. *Investigative Ophthalmology, 26*, 366–370.

Birch, E. E., Stager, D. R., Leffler, J., & Weakley, D. R. (1998). Early treatment of congenital unilateral cataract minimizes unequal competition. *Investigative Ophthalmology and Visual Science, 39*, 1560–1566.

Birnbaum, M. H., Koslowe, K., & Sanet, R. (1977). Success in amblyopia therapy as a function of age: a literature survey. *American Journal of Optometry and Physiological Optics, 54*, 269–275.

Blakemore, C., & Van Sluyters, R. C. (1974). Reversal of the physiological effects of monocular deprivation in kittens: further evidence for a sensitive period. *Journal of Physiology, 237*, 195–216.

Bourron-Madignier, M., Cypres, C., & Vettard, S. (1987). Study of optokinetic nystagmus in children. *Bulletin des Societes d'Ophtalmologie de France, 87*, 1269–1272.

Brosnahan, D., Norcia, A. M., Schor, C., & Taylor, D. G. (1998). OKN, perceptual and VEP direction biases in strabismus. *Vision Research, 38*, 2833–2840.

Chapman, B., & Stryker, M. P. (1993). Development of orientation selectivity in ferret visual cortex and effects of deprivation. *Journal of Neuroscience, 13*, 5251–5262.

Cleland, B. G., Mitchell, D. E., Crewther, S. G., & Crewther, D. P. (1980). Visual resolution of retinal ganglion cells in monocularly deprived cats. *Brain Research, 192*, 261–266.

Crowley, J. C., & Katz, L. C. (2000). Early development of ocular dominance columns. *Science, 290*, 1321–1325.

Cynader, M. S., & Mitchell, D. E. (1980). Prolonged sensitivity to monocular deprivation in dark-reared cats. *Journal of Neurophysiology, 43*, 1026–1040.

Darian-Smith, C., & Gilbert, C. D. (1994). Axonal sprouting accompanies functional reorganization in adult cat striate cortex. *Nature, 368*, 737–740.

Daw, N. W. (1994). Mechanisms of plasticity in the visual cortex. *Investigative Ophthalmology, 35*, 4168–4179.

Daw, N. W. (2003). Critical periods in the visual system. In B. Hopkins & S. P. Johnson (Eds.), *Neurobiology of infant vision* (pp. 43–103). Westport, CT: Praeger.

Daw, N. W., & Wyatt, H. J. (1976). Kittens reared in a unidirectional environment: evidence for a critical period. *Journal of Physiology, 257*, 155–170.

Daw, N. W., Baysinger, K. J., & Parkinson, D. (1987). Increased levels of testosterone have little effect on visual cortical plasticity in the kitten. *Journal of Neurobiology, 18*, 141–154.

Daw, N. W., Berman, N. J., & Ariel, M. (1978). Interaction of critical periods in the visual cortex of kittens. *Science, 199*, 565–567.

Daw, N. W., Fox, K. D., Sato, H., & Czepita, D. (1992). Critical period for monocular deprivation in the cat visual cortex. *Journal of Neurophysiology, 67*, 197–202.

Daw, N. W., Sato, H., Fox, K. D., Carmichael, T., & Gingerich, R. (1991). Cortisol reduces plasticity in the kitten visual cortex. *Journal of Neurobiology, 22*, 158–168.

Demer, J. L., & Von Noorden, G. K. (1988). Optokinetic asymmetry in esotropia. *Journal of Pediatric Ophthalmology and Strabismus, 25*, 286–292.

Derrington, A. M., & Hawken, M. J. (1981). Spatial and temporal properties of cat geniculate neurones after prolonged deprivation. *Journal of Physiology, 316*, 1–10.

Dobson, V., & Sebris, S. L. (1989). Longitudinal study of acuity and stereopsis in infants with or at-risk for esotropia. *Investigative Ophthalmology, 30*, 1146–1158.

Eizenman, M., Westfall, C. A., Geer, I., Smith, K., Chatterjee, S., Panton, C. M., Kraft, S. P., & Skarf, B. (1999). Electrophysiological evidence of cortical fusion in children with early-onset esotropia. *Investigative Ophthalmology and Visual Science, 40*, 354–362.

El Mallah, M. K., Chakravarthy, U., & Hart, P. M. (2000). Amblyopia: is visual loss permanent? *British Journal of Ophthalmology, 84*, 952–956.

Epelbaum, M., Milleret, C., Buisseret, P., & Dufier, J. L. (1993). The sensitive period for strabismic amblyopia in humans. *Ophthalmology, 100*, 323–327.

Fagiolini, M., Pizzorusso, T., Berardi, N., Domenici, L., & Maffei, L. (1994). Functional postnatal development of the rat primary visual cortex and the role of visual experience: dark rearing and monocular deprivation. *Vision Research, 34*, 709–720.

Fawcett, S., & Birch, E. E. (2000). Motion VEPs, stereopsis, and bifoveal fusion in children with strabismus. *Investigative Ophthalmology and Visual Science, 41*, 411–416.

Fawcett, S., Leffler, J., & Birch, E. E. (2000). Factors influencing stereoacuity in accommodative esotropia. *Journal American Association of Pediatric Ophthalmology and Strabismus, 4*, 15–20.

Freeman, A. W., Nguyen, V. A., & Jolly, N. (1996). Components of visual acuity loss in strabismus. *Vision Research, 36*, 765–774.

Giffin, F., & Mitchell, D. E. (1978). The rate of recovery of vision after early monocular deprivation in kittens. *Journal of Physiology, 274*, 511–537.

Gilbert, C. D., & Wiesel, T. N. (1992). Receptive field dynamics in adult primary visual cortex. *Nature, 356*, 150–152.

Gordon, J. A., & Stryker, M. P. (1996). Experience-dependent plasticity of binocular responses in the primary visual cortex of the mouse. *Journal of Neuroscience, 16*, 3274–3286.

Guillery, R. W., & Stelzner, D. J. (1970). The differential effects of unilateral eye closure on the monocular and binocular segments of the dorsal lateral geniculate nucleus in the cat. *Journal of Comparative Neurology, 139*, 413–422.

Guire, E. S., Lickey, M. E., & Gordon, B. (1999). Critical period for the monocular deprivation effect in rats: assessment with sweep visually evoked potentials. *Journal of Neurophysiology, 81*, 121–128.

Hamer, R. D., Norcia, A. M., Orel-Bixler, D., & Hoyt, C. S. (1993). Motion VEPs in late-onset esotropia. *Clinical Vision Sciences, 8*, 55–62.

Hardman Lea, S. J., Loades, J., & Rubinstein, M. P. (1989). The sensitive period for anisometropic amblyopia. *Eye, 3*, 783–790.

Harwerth, R. S., Smith, E. L., Duncan, G. C., Crawford, M. J., & Von Noorden, G. K. (1986). Multiple sensitive periods in the development of the primate visual system. *Science, 232*, 235–238.

Helveston, E. M. (1993). The origins of congenital esotropia. *Journal of Pediatric Ophthalmology and Strabismus, 30*, 215–232.

Horton, J. C., & Hocking, D. R. (1996). An adult-like pattern of ocular dominance columns in striate cortex of newborn monkeys prior to visual experience. *Journal of Neuroscience, 16*, 1791–1807.

Horton, J. C., & Hocking, D. R. (1997). Timing of the critical period for plasticity of ocular dominance columns in macaque striate cortex. *Journal of Neuroscience, 17*, 3684–3709.

Hubel, D. H., & Wiesel, T. N. (1970). The period of susceptibility to the physiological effects of unilateral eye closure in kittens. *Journal of Physiology, 206*, 419–436.

Ing, M. R. (1983). Early surgical alignment for congenital esotropia. *Ophthalmology, 90*, 132–135.

Issa, N. P., Trachtenberg, J. T., Chapman, B., Zahs, K. R., & Stryker, M. P. (1999). The critical period for ocular dominance plasticity in the ferret's visual cortex. *Journal of Neuroscience, 19*, 6965–6978.

Jones, K. R., Spear, P. D., & Tong, L. (1984). Critical periods for effects on monocular deprivation: differences between striate and extrastriate cortex. *Journal of Neuroscience, 4*, 2543–2552.

Keech, R. V., & Kutsche, P. J. (1995). Upper age limit for the development of amblyopia. *Journal of Pediatric Ophthalmology and Strabismus, 32*, 89–93.

LeVay, S., Wiesel, T. N., & Hubel, D. H. (1980). The development of ocular dominance columns in normal and visually deprived monkeys. *Journal of Comparative Neurology, 191*, 1–51.

Levi, D. M., & Klein, S. (1982). Hyperacuity and amblyopia. *Nature, 298*, 268–270.

Liao, D. S., Krahe, T., Prusky, G. T., Medina, A. E., & Ramoa, A. S. (2004). Recovery of cortical binocularity and orientation selectivity after the critical period for ocular dominance plasticity. *Journal of Neurophysiology, 92*, 2113–2121.

Mason, A. J. S., Braddick, O. J., Wattam-Bell, J., & Atkinson, J. (2001). Directional motion asymmetry in infant VEPs—which direction? *Vision Research, 41*, 201–211.

Maurer, D., & Lewis, T. L. (1993). Visual outcomes after infantile cataract. In K Simons (Ed.), *Early visual development, normal and abnormal* (pp. 454–484). New York: Oxford University Press.

Meyer, E., Mizrahi, E., & Perlman, I. (1991). Amblyopia success index: a new method of quantitative assessment of treatment efficiency; application in a study of 473 anisometropic amblyopic patients. *Binocular Vision Quarterly, 6*, 83–90.

Mitchell, D. E. (1988). The extent of visual recovery from early monocular or binocular visual deprivation in kittens. *Journal of Physiology, 395*, 639–660.

Mitchell, D. E. (1991). The long-term effectiveness of different regimens of occlusion on recovery from early monocular deprivation in kittens. *Philosophical Transaction of the Royal Society. Series B. Biological sciences, 333*, 51–79.

Mower, G. D. (1991). The effect of dark rearing on the time course of the critical period in cat visual cortex. *Developmental Brain Research, 58,* 151–158.

Mower, G. D., Caplan, C. J., Christen, W. G., & Duffy, F. H. (1985). Dark rearing prolongs physiological but not anatomical plasticity of the cat visual cortex. *Journal of Comparative Neurology, 235,* 448–466.

Norcia, A. M. (1996). Abnormal motion processing and binocularity: infantile esotropia as a model system for effects of early interruptions of binocularity. *Eye, 10,* 259–265.

Norcia, A. M., Hamer, R. D., & Jampolsky, A. (1995). Plasticity of human motion processing mechanisms following surgery for infantile esotropia. *Vision Research, 35,* 3279–3296.

Olson, C. R., & Freeman, R. D. (1975). Progressive changes in kitten striate cortex during monocular vision. *Journal of Neurophysiology, 38,* 26–32.

Olson, C. R., & Freeman, R. D. (1980). Profile of the sensitive period for monocular deprivation in kittens. *Experimental Brain Research, 39,* 17–21.

Parks, M. M. (1984). Congenital esotropia with a bifixation result: report of a case. *Documenta Ophthalmologica, 58,* 109–114.

Pasino, L., & Cordella, M. (1959). Il comportamento della difficoltà di separazione durante il trattamento dell'ambliopia strabica. *Istituto di clinica oculistica dell'università di Sassari, 25,* 111–115.

Pettet, M. W., & Gilbert, C. D. (1992). Dynamic changes in receptive-field size in cat primary visual cortex. *Proceedings of the National Academy of Sciences of the United States of America, 89,* 8366–8370.

Pham, T. A., Graham, S. J., Suzuki, S., Barco, A., Kandel, E. R., Gordon, B., & Lickey, M. E. (2004). A semi-persistent adult ocular dominance plasticity in visual cortex is stabilized by activated CREB. *Learning and Memory, 11,* 738–747.

Rodman, H. R. (1994). Development of inferior temporal cortex in the monkey. *Cerebral Cortex, 5,* 484–498.

Sawtell, N. B., Frenkel, M. Y., Philpot, B. D., Nakazawa, K., Tonegawa, S., & Bear, M. F. (2003). NMDA receptor-dependent ocular dominance plasticity in adult visual cortex. *Neuron, 38,* 977–985.

Shapley, R. M., & So, Y. T. (1980). Is there an effect of monocular deprivation on the proportion of X and Y cells in the cat lateral geniculate nucleus? *Experimental Brain Research, 39,* 41–48.

Shatz, C. J., & Stryker, M. P. (1978). Ocular dominance in layer IV of the cat's visual cortex and the effects of monocular deprivation. *Journal of Physiology, 281,* 267–283.

Sherman, S. M., & Stone, J. (1973). Physiological normality of the retina in visually deprived cats. *Brain Research, 60,* 224–230.

Stager, D. R., & Birch, E. E. (1986). Preferential-looking acuity and stereopsis in infantile esotropia. *Journal of Pediatric Ophthalmoglogy and Strabismus, 23,* 160–165.

Stuart, J. A., & Burian, H. M. (1962). A study of separation difficulty. *American Journal of Ophthalmology, 53,* 471–477.

Swindale, N. V., Vital-Durand, F., & Blakemore, C. (1981). Recovery from monocular deprivation in the monkey. III. Reversal of anatomical effects in the visual cortex. *Proceedings of the Royal Society. Series B. Biological sciences, 213,* 435–450.

Taylor, D. M. (1972). Is congenital esotropia functionally curable? *Transactions of the American Ophthalmological Society, 70,* 529–576.

Tierney, D. W. (1989). Vision recovery in amblyopia after contralateral subretinal hemorrhage. *Journal of the American Optometric Association, 60,* 281–283.

Timney, B. N. (1981). Development of binocular depth perception in kittens. *Investigative Ophthalmology, 21,* 493–496.

Vaegan & Taylor, D. (1979). Critical period for deprivation amblyopia in children. *Transactions of the Ophthalmological Society (UK), 99,* 432–439.

Vereecken, E. P., & Brabant, P. (1984). Prognosis for vision in amblyopia after loss of the good eye. *Archives of Ophthalmology, 102,* 220–224.

Von Noorden, G. K. (1981). New clinical aspects of stimulus deprivation amblyopia. *American Journal of Ophthalmology, 92,* 416–421.

Von Noorden, G. K. (1988). A reassessment of infantile esotropia. *American Journal of Ophthalmology, 105,* 1–10.

Von Noorden, G. K. (1990). *Binocular vision and ocular motility.* St. Louis: Mosby.

Wick, B., Wingard, M., Cotter, S., & Scheiman, M. (1992). Anisometropic amblyopia: is the patient ever too old to treat? *Optometry and Vision Science, 69*, 866–878.

Wiesel, T. N., & Hubel, D. H. (1963a). Single cell responses in striate cortex of kittens deprived of vision in one eye. *Journal of Neurophysiology, 26*, 1003–1017.

Wiesel, T. N., & Hubel, D. H. (1963b). Effects of visual deprivation on morphology and physiology of cells in the cat's lateral geniculate body. *Journal of Neurophysiology, 26*, 978–993.

Wilson, M. E. (1992). Adult amblyopia reversed by contralateral cataract formation. *Journal of Pediatric Ophthalmology and Strabismus, 29*, 100–102.

Wright, K. W., Edelman, P. M., McVey, J. H., Terry, A. P., & Lin, M. (1994). High-grade stereo acuity after early surgery for congenital esotropia. *Archives of Ophthalmology, 112*, 913–919.

III

Mechanisms of Plasticity

10

Concepts of Plasticity

The fundamental questions that many scientists in the field of visual development are tackling today are: What are the mechanisms that underlie plasticity in the visual cortex? How can the system adapt to abnormalities in the visual environment, and readapt when the abnormality is corrected? How do infants and children have this capability, and why do adults lack it? In this section, we will discuss the mechanisms of sensory-dependent plasticity.

In sensory-dependent plasticity, the connections in the visual cortex change in response to an altered sensory input. The change is specific to the input. Ocular dominance is altered by an abnormal balance in the input from the two eyes; orientation selectivity is altered by an emphasis on lines of a particular orientation in the input; direction selectivity is altered by continued motion in one direction, and so on. All these signals are carried to the cortex by electrical activity. Consequently, blocking electrical activity from reaching the cortex with tetrodotoxin prevents sensory-dependent plasticity (Stryker & Harris, 1986; Chapman & Stryker, 1993; see Chapter 4).

The cortex responds to sensory input with long-term changes in the physiological properties of the cells. In most cases, this probably reflects a rearrangement of the anatomical connections. Certainly this is true for monocular deprivation, where the connections between the lateral geniculate and cortex are altered. Probably it is also true for orientation changes, in loss of acuity, and anomalous retinal correspondence, but this point has not been specifically tested. The suppression found in strabismus may involve a change in the connections of inhibitory cells, or it may just involve a long-term change in the physiological properties of the synapses. Again, the proof awaits technical advances.

Given our current understanding, we can restate the fundamental question: How does a change in the pattern of electrical activity reaching the visual cortex lead to a rearrangement of anatomical connections or long-term changes in the physiological properties of the synapses, and a long-term change in the physiological properties of the cells?

There are bound to be a number of steps leading to these anatomical and physiological changes. Electrical activity leads to release of synaptic transmitters, which leads to changes in second messengers within the cell and changes in protein synthesis for the formation of new cell membranes, new cell processes, and new synaptic proteins. So there are really two fundamental questions: (1) What steps lead to the final cortical alterations? (2) Which steps that enable the cortices of young animals to be plastic are absent or reduced in adults?

1. The Hebb Postulate

Many years ago Donald Hebb (1949) proposed that learning takes place by strengthening the transmission at a single synapse. He postulated: "When an axon of cell A is near enough to excite cell B and repeatedly or persistently takes part in firing it, some growth process or metabolic change takes place in one or both cells such that A's efficiency, as one of the cells firing B, is increased" (p. 62).

We can expand on this proposition in various respects to take account of current knowledge. First, there must be a weakening of inactive synapses, as well as a strengthening of active ones (Stent, 1973). There has to be forgetting as well as memory. A single synapse cannot be strengthened indefinitely. The process cannot go in only one direction.

Second, one has to take account of the idea of competition. Active synapses drive out inactive ones not only in the visual cortex, but also in other systems where the question has been closely studied, such as the neuromuscular junction and various ganglia (Purves & Lichtman, 1980). Hebb's postulate considers what happens at a single synapse rather than what happens at one synapse compared with others on the same postsynaptic cell.

To illustrate the competition aspect, let us consider ocular dominance changes, where the phenomenon of competition is most clearly established. In monocular deprivation, when inputs from the intact eye fire together without inputs from the deprived eye, connections from the deprived eye to the cortex are weakened. With strabismus, inputs from the left and right eyes are not in synchrony, so some cells become totally driven by the left eye, and some totally by the right eye; very few binocular cells are left. The same result occurs if one eye is open, then the other, but both eyes are never open together (Hubel & Wiesel, 1965; Blasdel & Pettigrew, 1979). It also happens if natural activity is abolished with tetrodotoxin and the eyes are stimulated electrically out of synchrony with each other (Stryker & Strickland, 1984).

To explain competition, it is important to consider that there are several inputs to the postsynaptic cell and to assume that the postsynaptic cell is only activated if a number of inputs are active at once. In Figure 10.1, four synapses are shown. One could postulate that the postsynaptic cell fires only when two presynaptic inputs arrive at the same time. The postsynaptic cell will then fire in conjunction with the presynaptic input only if two left eye inputs arrive at the same time, two right eye inputs arrive at the same time, or a left eye input and a right eye input arrive at the same time. Synapses that are passive or only weakly activated will degenerate. Binocularity will be maintained only if left and right eye inputs arrive together. The left eye will take over if the left eye is active and the right eye is not. If the two eyes rarely

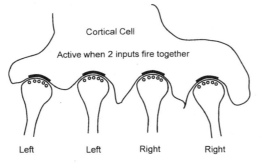

FIG. 10.1. Hebb synapse drawn to take account of the competition between the left and right eyes in the visual cortex. In this example, the hypothesis is that some process in the postsynaptic cell is activated when two or more inputs arrive together; this process strengthens active synapses and weakens inactive ones. [Reprinted with permission from Daw, N. W. (1994). *Investigative Ophthalmology and Visual Science, 35*, 4168–4179.]

fire in synchrony with each other, then postsynaptic cells initially dominated by the left eye will tend to be taken over by the left eye, and cells initially dominated by the right eye will tend to be taken over by the right eye.

Third, the process that Hebb referred to as *firing* may not in reality require firing of an action potential. The question of what voltage change is required for strengthening the synapse is important but unresolved. The voltage change leads to entry of calcium into the postsynaptic cell, and it could be that a particular level of calcium in the dendritic spine is important for this process (Zador, Koch, & Brown, 1990). The voltage change and/or the calcium change must then trigger a storage process that changes the state of the synapse so that it becomes potentiated and remains potentiated over a long period of time. The synaptic alteration could be stored by a molecule, such as calcium/calmodulin-dependent kinase (CaM-KII) that has two stable states and a threshold for conversion from one state to the other (Lisman, 1985). All these hypotheses are consistent with the Hebb postulate, in the sense that there is a switch in the postsynaptic cell that gets turned on when a sufficient number of presynaptic inputs arrive at the same time.

Fourth, the Hebb synapse model does not consider the formation of new synapses, only potentiation of existing ones. Sprouting of processes almost certainly occurs, and presumably some of these processes form new synapses. So the postulate has to be expanded to include some factor for the generation of these new synapses, which may be random, or could be under the guidance of some molecular cue.

2. How Electrical Activity Can Strengthen Some Synapses and Weaken Others

The idea that synapses can be weakened as well as strengthened leads to a problem. Signals are carried to the visual cortex by electrical activity. Electrical activity is always a positive parameter: it can increase from zero, but cannot be negative. It is possible that there is a certain level of electrical activity above which synapses are strengthened and below which they are weakened (Bienenstock, Cooper, & Munro, 1982). This could happen if a low level of input were to activate some processes in the postsynaptic cell, and a high level of input were to activate others. However, the phenomenon of competition must be taken into account along with the reality that all the results cannot be accounted for on the basis of what happens at a single synapse.

To realistically model the actual events, one has to consider what happens in the postsynaptic cell, where electrical activity will affect one or more substances that in turn affect synaptic strength. In one model, the crucial factor is the state of phosphorylation of CaM-KII (Lisman, 1989). All levels of electrical activity lead to entry of calcium into the cell, and to phosphorylation of CaM-KII. Low levels of calcium activate a calcineurin cascade, leading to dephosphorylation of CaM-KII. High levels of calcium activate cyclic AMP and turn off the dephosphorylation. Thus, high levels of electrical activity lead to highly phosphorylated CaM-KII and increase synaptic efficacy, and low levels of electrical activity reduce this effect. The appealing feature of this model is that it puts clothes onto what are frequently rather bare and theoretical discussions of the problem. However, many issues will have to be resolved before this model, or any other, can be proved. These issues include the subcellular location of the enzymes, how gradients of calcium within the cell affect the outcome, and what the physical location of the left and right eye inputs are in relation to each other and to the enzymes, among others. Clearly, the problem is not a simple one. Some more detailed hypotheses will be dealt with in Chapter 11.

3. Feedback from the Postsynaptic Cell to the Presynaptic Terminal

The Hebb synapse model requires activation of the postsynaptic cell for the synapse to be strengthened. However, changes also occur in the presynaptic terminals. The best evidence for this comes from monocular deprivation. When one eye is closed, the endings in the visual cortex coming from that eye retract. As pointed out before, this is not simply a degeneration of input from the deprived eye: monocular deprivation, involving competition between active inputs from the normal eye and inactive inputs from the deprived eye, has a much stronger effect on the deprived eye inputs than binocular deprivation, where there is simply inactive input from both eyes. This is evidence that competition for synaptic space on the postsynaptic cell, where binocular convergence occurs, leads to strengthening of some presynaptic terminals, and weakening of others. While the postsynaptic cell must be involved because there would be no competition without it, the result of the competition is carried back to the presynaptic terminals, and shows up there as a change in the presynaptic terminal arborization.

The point that the postsynaptic cell is involved in electrical effects on synaptic efficacy is reinforced by experiments on orientation-selective deprivation (Rauschecker & Singer, 1979). To test for postsynaptic involvement in synaptic efficacy, kittens were reared in the dark until 5 weeks of age. One eye was then closed for 9 days, and the kitten had unrestricted vision through the other eye. Next, the open eye was closed, and the closed eye opened and looked at horizontal contours (vertical contours were blurred by a strong cylindrical lens) for another 10 days. Only the postsynaptic cells in the visual cortex are specific for orientation. During the reverse suture, the cells in the visual cortex specific for horizontal lines were driven through the re-opened eye, but the cells specific for vertical lines were not. Thus, if the postsynaptic cell were involved, one would expect ocular dominance to be reversed by the second exposure for horizontal lines but not for vertical ones. This is what occurred.

Thus, the Hebb model, with modifications, fits the general results obtained in the visual cortex from sensory deprivation. When pre- and postsynaptic cells are activated together, the synapse between them is strengthened. When they are not activated together, the synapse is weakened. The postsynaptic cell is not activated unless several presynaptic inputs arrive at the same time. Consequently the pattern of presynaptic inputs is important. The presynaptic inputs compete with each other for space on the postsynaptic cell. The final result is not only a change in synaptic efficacy, but also a change in the terminal arbor of the presynaptic cell, implying a feedback signal from the postsynaptic cell to the presynaptic terminal.

4. Criteria for Critical Factors in the Critical Period

This discussion of the Hebb synapse shows that there must be a series of processes and reactions between the electrical activity that guides plastic changes in the visual cortex and the axonal and dendritic alterations that eventually result. The electrical activity leads to release of the synaptic transmitter glutamate, activation of glutamate receptors, activation of second messengers, various biochemical reactions within the postsynaptic cell, and the feedback signal from the postsynaptic cell to the presynaptic terminals. In nearly all studies, the model for this has been monocular deprivation (Fig. 10.2). A number of factors and substances have been shown to affect these processes.

In determining whether or not a factor is actually important in plasticity, the first test is usually to see if removing the factor or applying its antagonist reduces or abolishes plasticity. In the monocular deprivation model, this means: Are the ocular dominance changes that normally occur after monocular deprivation disrupted? Such experiments have led to the generation of a long list of putative factors. Some items on the list definitely represent important contributors to the regulation of plasticity. The prime example of this has already been discussed: tetrodotoxin, which abolishes electrical activity, also abolishes plasticity in the visual cortex because the signals that guide plasticity are carried by the neurons in the visual pathway.

Other items on the list influence plasticity but do not contribute directly to it. One example is the reduction of the noradrenaline and acetylcholine

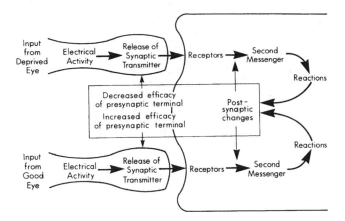

FIG. 10.2. Steps involved in plasticity in the visual cortex, using ocular dominance changes as a model.

input to the cortex (Bear & Singer, 1986). The afferents that use these transmitters come from the brainstem and carry signals about the sleep/wake cycle and the general state of attention. Interruption of both these pathways with a combination of lesions and antagonists affects ocular dominance changes. Nobody knows exactly how this might occur, but probably acetylcholine and noradrenaline affect the state of depolarization and/or second messengers of the cells in the visual pathway, and thereby accentuate or reduce the signals in those pathways. Another example is that lesions of the intermedullary lamina and medial dorsal nucleus of the thalamus reduce ocular dominance changes (Singer, 1982). These are areas that also have to do with attention and with eye movements. Nobody has yet determined whether the effect of the lesions on attention or their effect on eye movements is the crucial factor, but in either case, these areas modulate the visual pathway rather than being directly on it. To emphasize this point, Singer describes these results as showing there is gating control of plasticity. The signals are not on the pathway for sensory-dependent control of connections in the visual cortex, but they may gate those signals.

Other items on the list have general nonspecific actions on the nervous system and affect all aspects of activity there. One example is anesthesia and paralysis (Freeman & Bonds, 1979): because anesthesia is a general depressant of activity in all parts of the nervous system, it is no surprise that it abolishes plasticity. Another example is infusion of glutamate directly into the cortex (Shaw & Cynader, 1984). Glutamate excites all cells in the nervous system to such an extent that it can kill them. This is another general nonspecific action. Consequently, the fact that a factor or substance reduces or abolishes plasticity is suggestive, but certainly not conclusive, that it is directly involved in plasticity. Other pieces of supporting evidence must also be assembled before direct involvement can be established.

The complete series of reactions that are directly involved in plasticity will involve some, such as electrical activity, that are present at all ages, and others that are more abundant or more active in young animals than in

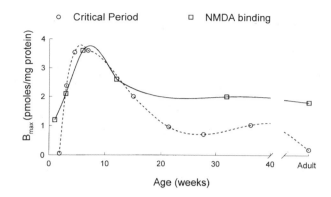

FIG. 10.3. B_{max} for the binding of MK801 to NMDA channels in cat visual cortex as a function of age, compared with the critical period for ocular dominance plasticity. The curve for the critical period was taken from Figure 9-1 and scaled to be the same height as B_{max} for MK801 binding at the peak. [Reprinted with permission from Daw, N. W. (1994). *Investigative Ophthalmology and Visual Science, 35,* 4168–4179.]

adults. The latter can be said to be crucial or critical for plasticity because it is their presence in young animals that makes them more plastic. Factors or substances that are crucial for plasticity should have a time course of expression that follows the critical period for plasticity. Moreover, this time course should vary with cortical layer, just as the critical period varies by layer. The factor or substance should disappear from layer IV earlier than it disappears from layers II, III, V, and VI.

As an example, consider the class of glutamate receptors called NMDA receptors. Infusion of an NMDA antagonist abolishes ocular dominance plasticity (Kleinschmidt, Bear, & Singer, 1987), and the total number of NMDA receptors in the visual cortex follows the critical period quite closely (Gordon, Daw, & Parkinson, 1991; see Fig. 10.3), particularly the NR2A subunit (Chen, Cooper, & Mower, 2000). As a counter-example, there is a growth-associated protein called GAP-43 that is associated with plasticity in the hippocampus (Lovinger, Akers, Nelson, Barnes, McNaughton, & Routtenberg, 1985), and is therefore a candidate to be involved in plasticity in the visual cortex. However, this protein has a concentration that is high shortly after birth in cat visual cortex, and declines to values that are close to adult at the peak of the critical period (McIntosh, Daw, & Parkinson, 1990; see Fig. 10.4). GAP-43 is also associated with growth cones (Skene, Jacobson, Snipes, McGuire, Norden, & Freeman, 1986), suggesting another function: the time at which it is high is when axons are finding their way to their targets, rather than after they have formed synapses, or when synapses are being modified in response to sensory input. Both of these substances are clearly involved in development, but the time course of their change with age suggests that NMDA receptors may be critically involved in sensory-dependent plasticity, whereas GAP-43 is primarily involved in events that occur before sensory-dependent plasticity.

One treatment that can alter the time course of the critical period is rearing animals in the dark. This causes the critical period to last longer (Cynader &

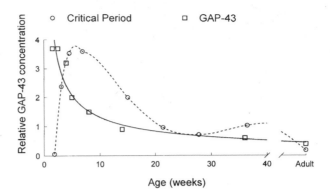

FIG. 10.4. Levels of GAP-43 in the cat visual cortex, compared with the critical period for ocular dominance plasticity. [Reprinted with permission from Daw, N. W. (1994). *Investigative Ophthalmology and Visual Science, 35*, 4168–4179.]

Mitchell, 1980), and delays its onset as well (Mower, 1991; Beaver, Ji, & Daw, 2001). Thus, at 5 to 6 weeks of age, light-reared animals are more plastic than dark-reared animals; at 8 to 9 weeks of age they are equally plastic; and at 12 to 20 weeks of age, dark-reared animals are more plastic than light-reared animals. If a factor or substance is critically involved in plasticity, its concentration should vary similarly between light- and dark-reared animals. This is an important criterion to distinguish factors related to activity, which simply increase or decrease with age, from factors related to plasticity. This distinction has, unfortunately, not been recognized by a number of workers in the field.

Very few factors have so far been discovered that follow this stringent criterion. One is the NR2A subunit of the NMDA receptor (Chen et al., 2000). A second is ibotenate-stimulated phosphoinositide turnover, which is related to the activation of metabotropic glutamate receptors (Dudek & Bear, 1989). A third is the level of cAMP driven by the metabotropic glutamate agonist ACPD (Reid, Daw, Gregory, & Flavin, 1996). cAMP activates protein kinase A, which, as we will see in Chapter 11, is definitely involved in ocular dominance plasticity. A fourth is Munc 13-3, which is a mammalian analog of the *Caenorhabditis elegans* uncoordinated gene Unc 13, and plays a role in synaptic vesicle release (Yang, Zheng, Li, & Mower, 2002). A fifth is the immediate early gene c-Fos (Mower & Kaplan, 1999). These substances need careful attention in terms of their role in ocular dominance plasticity.

Finally, a substance that is critically involved in plasticity might bring back plasticity in adult animals. However, there are some caveats to this possibility. First, there may be more than one critical factor in plasticity. If so, then introducing one of them into the adult without also introducing the others may not help. Second, there may be an irreversible process of development that depends on the critical factors, and that, when set in place, becomes set forever.

The possibility that plasticity could be brought back after the critical period has rarely been tested, at least partly because of these caveats. It may not be possible to test it adequately until the complete series of reactions that is directly involved in plasticity has been defined. Nevertheless, this is the possibility that most people in the field are working toward. The hope is that after the whole process is understood, it will be practical to regenerate a plastic state in older animals.

5. Summary

Electrical activity in the afferents to the visual cortex leads to a series of reactions in cells in the cortex. These reactions affect the strength of the synapses between the presynaptic terminals and the postsynaptic cell. Active synapses are strengthened and inactive ones are weakened. A combination of inputs may be required to drive the reactions in the postsynaptic cell so that inputs that arrive together will strengthen each other, and inputs that do not will be weakened. The series of reactions includes feedback to the presynaptic terminals and morphological changes in these terminals. Some of the steps in the series of reactions will be found in the cortex at all ages. Others will be found at a higher level, or with higher activity, at the peak of the critical period for plasticity. The latter are the steps that are critical for plasticity.

We can define three criteria for a factor or substance that is critical for plasticity: (1) removing the factor, or providing antagonists to the substance should reduce or abolish plasticity; (2) the presence or activity of the factor or substance should follow the time course of the critical period for plasticity; (3) treatments that affect the critical period for plasticity should affect the factor or substance similarly.

In addition, it is possible that reintroducing the critical factors or substances after the critical period is over may return the system to a plastic state. After all the steps directly involved in plasticity have been defined, this criterion will also need to be fulfilled.

References

Bear, M. F., & Singer, W. (1986). Modulation of visual cortical plasticity by acetylcholine and nora-drenaline. *Nature, 320*, 172–176.

Beaver, C. J., Ji, Q. H., & Daw, N. W. (2001). Layer differences in the effect of monocular vision in light- and dark-reared animals. *Visual Neuroscience, 18*, 811–820.

Bienenstock, E. L., Cooper, L. N., & Munro, P. W. (1982). Theory for the development of neuron selectivity: orientation specificity and binocular interaction in visual cortex. *Journal of Neuroscience, 2*, 32–48.

Blasdel, G. G., & Pettigrew, J. D. (1979). Degree of interocular synchrony required for maintenance of binocularity in kitten's visual cortex. *Journal of Neurophysiology, 42*, 1692–1710.

Chapman, B., & Stryker, M. P. (1993). Development of orientation selectivity in ferret visual cortex and effects of deprivation. *Journal of Neuroscience, 13*, 5251–5262.

Chen, L., Cooper, N. G. F., & Mower, G. D. (2000). Developmental changes in the expression of NMDA receptor subunits (NR1, NR2A, NR2B) in the cat visual cortex and the effects of dark rearing. *Molecular Brain Research, 78*, 196–200.

Cynader, M. S., & Mitchell, D. E. (1980). Prolonged sensitivity to monocular deprivation in dark-reared cats. *Journal of Neurophysiology, 43*, 1026–1040.

Daw, N. W. (1994). Mechanisms of plasticity in the visual cortex. *Investigative Ophthalmology and Visual Science, 35*, 4168–4179.

Dudek, S. M., & Bear, M. F. (1989). A biochemical correlate of the critical period for synaptic modification in the visual cortex. *Science, 246*, 673–675.

Freeman, R. D., & Bonds, A. B. (1979). Cortical plasticity in monocularly deprived immobilized kittens depends on eye movement. *Science, 206*, 1093–1095.

Gordon, B., Daw, N. W., & Parkinson, D. (1991). The effect of age on binding of MK-801 in the cat visual cortex. *Developmental Brain Research, 62*, 61–68.

Hebb, D. O. (1949). *The organization of behaviour.* New York: Wiley.

Hubel, D. H., & Wiesel, T. N. (1965). Binocular interaction in striate cortex of kittens reared with artificial squint. *Journal of Neurophysiology, 28*, 1041–1059.

Kleinschmidt, A., Bear, M. F., & Singer, W. (1987). Blockade of "NMDA" receptors disrupts experience-dependent plasticity of kitten striate cortex. *Science, 238*, 355–358.

Lisman, J. E. (1985). A mechanism for memory storage insensitive to molecular turnover: a bistable autophosphorylating kinase. *Proceedings of the National Academy of Sciences of the United States of America, 82*, 3055–3057.

Lisman, J. E. (1989) A mechanism for the Hebb and the anti-Hebb processes underlying learning and memory. *Proceedings of the National Academy of Sciences of the United States of America, 86*, 9574–9578.

Lovinger, D. M., Akers, R. F., Nelson, R. B., Barnes, C. A., McNaughton, B. L., & Routtenberg, A. (1985). A selective increase in phosphorylation of protein F1, a protein kinase C substrate, directly related to three day growth of long term synaptic enhancement. *Brain Research, 344*, 137–143.

McIntosh, H., Daw, N. W., & Parkinson, D. (1990). GAP-43 in the cat visual cortex during postnatal development. *Visual Neuroscience, 4*, 585–594.

Mower, G. D. (1991). The effect of dark rearing on the time course of the critical period in cat visual cortex. *Developmental Brain Research, 58*, 151–158.

Mower, G. D., & Kaplan, I. V. (1999). Fos expression during the critical period in visual cortex: differences between normal and dark reared cats. *Molecular Brain Research, 64*, 264–269.

Purves, D., & Lichtman, J. W. (1980). Elimination of synapses in the developing nervous system. *Science, 210*, 153–157.

Rauschecker, J. P., & Singer, W. (1979). Changes in the circuitry of the kitten visual cortex are gated by postsynaptic activity. *Nature, 280*, 58–60.

Reid, S. M., Daw, N. W., Gregory, D. S., & Flavin, H. J. (1996). cAMP levels increased by activation of metabotropic glutamate receptors correlate with visual plasticity. *Journal of Neuroscience, 16*, 7619–7626.

Shaw, C., & Cynader, M. S. (1984). Disruption of cortical activity prevents ocular dominance changes in monocularly deprived kittens. *Nature, 308*, 731–734.

Singer, W. (1982). Central core control of developmental plasticity in the kitten visual cortex: I. Diencephalic lesions. *Experimental Brain Research, 47*, 209–222.

Skene, J. H. P., Jacobson, R. D., Snipes, G. J., McGuire, C. B., Norden, J. J., & Freeman, J. A. (1986). A protein induced during nerve growth (GAP43) is a major component of growth-cone membranes. *Science, 233*, 783–786.

Stent, G. S. (1973). A physiological mechanism for Hebb's postulate of learning. *Proceedings of the National Academy of Sciences of the United States of America, 70*, 997–1001.

Stryker, M. P., & Harris, W. A. (1986). Binocular impulse blockade prevents the formation of ocular dominance columns in cat visual cortex. *Journal of Neuroscience, 6*, 2117–2133.

Stryker, M. P., & Strickland, S. L. (1984). Physiological segregation of ocular dominance columns depends on the pattern of afferent electrical activity. *Investigative Ophthalmology Supplement, 25*, 278.

Yang, C. B., Zheng, Y. T., Li, G. Y., & Mower, G. D. (2002). Identification of Munc 13-3 as a candidate gene for critical period neuroplasticity in visual cortex. *Journal of Neuroscience, 22*, 8614–8618.

Zador, A., Koch, C., & Brown, T. H. (1990). Biophysical model of a Hebbian synapse. *Proceedings of the National Academy of Sciences of the United States of America, 87*, 6718–6722.

11

Mechanisms of Plasticity in the Visual Cortex

Nearly all experiments on plasticity in the visual cortex of animals *in vivo* have been done with monocular deprivation. This is the easiest paradigm to apply and gives results that can be readily quantified and tested for significance. One approach to such experiments is to infuse an antagonist to the putative factor directly into the visual cortex of a cat with an osmotic minipump at a concentration that is above threshold for antagonism 2 to 4 mm away from the minipump, and below threshold 5 to 6 mm away. The effect of the antagonist is determined by making statistical comparisons between the ocular dominance histogram for a group of cells recorded near the minipump and the ocular dominance histogram for a group of cells recorded far from the minipump. Another approach is to test mice that are mutant for a factor of interest. In this case the comparison is made between the ocular dominance histogram for a group of experimental animals and the ocular dominance histogram for a group of control animals. A significant difference denotes ocular dominance plasticity (ODP).

We will first discuss instructive factors, that is, factors that are directly on the pathway between activation of the visual cortex by sensory signals and the physiological and anatomical changes that make the deprived eye less effective and the nondeprived eye more effective in driving the visual cortex. These factors include electrical activity coming from the retina, neurotransmitter receptors (NMDA receptors, metabotropic glutamate receptors, and GABA), second messengers (calcium and cyclic AMP), protein kinases (CaM kinase, protein kinase A and several others), protein phosphatases (calcineurin), anchoring proteins (A kinase anchoring protein), growth factors (brain derived neurotrophic factor, BDNF), nuclear binding proteins (cyclic AMP responsive binding protein, CREB), immediate early genes (IEGs), and genes that are turned on and their products.

Next, we will discuss modulatory factors that may affect the steps of the instructive pathway at various levels. These include sleep, environmental enrichment, noradrenaline, acetylcholine, serotonin, and nerve growth factor (NGF).

One factor that affects plasticity and does not fit neatly into either of these categories is the immune system's Class I major histocompatibility antigens (Class I MHCs).

It is important to distinguish, particularly for factors on the instructive pathway, between factors that simply carry the signal from one step to the next, and factors that are crucial or critical for plasticity in the sense that they are more abundant or more active during the critical period for plasticity than before or afterwards. Here, factors will be evaluated by this criterion where evidence is available.

Finally, we will discuss factors that are found on the pathway for making the deprived eye less effective but not on the pathway for making the nondeprived eye more effective, or vice versa. We will also discuss factors that are found on the pathway for ocular dominance plasticity but not on the pathway for recovery from ocular dominance plasticity. Unfortunately, there are very few such factors that have been discovered so far.

1. Electrical Activity

Electrical activity governs sensory-dependent plasticity, as discussed in Chapter 10. The question to be addressed here is: Is there anything different about the electrical activity in young animals that affects the maturation of the system?

We now know that the pattern of electrical activity is important rather than the overall level. It is the pattern of electrical activity that distinguishes vertical lines from horizontal, leftward movement from rightward, and signals generated by one eye from those generated by the other. The pattern of electrical activity is also important before the eyes open. At this stage, there are no sensory-dependent signals but there is an important developmental change that does not occur when electrical activity is abolished by tetrodotoxin: the lamination of the lateral geniculate nucleus (Shatz & Stryker, 1988). During this period the ganglion cells in the retina, particularly those near each other, tend to fire in synchrony in an oscillating pattern (Wong, Meister, & Shatz, 1993; Fig. 11.1). The hypothesis is that left-eye cells firing in synchrony with each other, and out of synchrony with right-eye cells, leads to the endings of the left- and right-eye cells in the lateral geniculate nucleus segregating from one another, just as endings from the left- and right-eye projections to layer IV of the cortex segregate from each other later on. The tendency for neighboring ganglion cells to fire together may also help to refine the topographic map.

After the eyes open, sensory input becomes important, and the left- and right-eye afferents from the lateral geniculate to layer IV of the visual cortex segregate from each other. This process does not occur when electrical activity is abolished, as pointed out in Chapter 4. Synchrony of activity within each eye would tend to cause the afferents to segregate and synchrony of activity between the eyes would tend to retain binocularity. Presumably there is substantial synchrony of activity within each eye at 3 weeks of age to start the

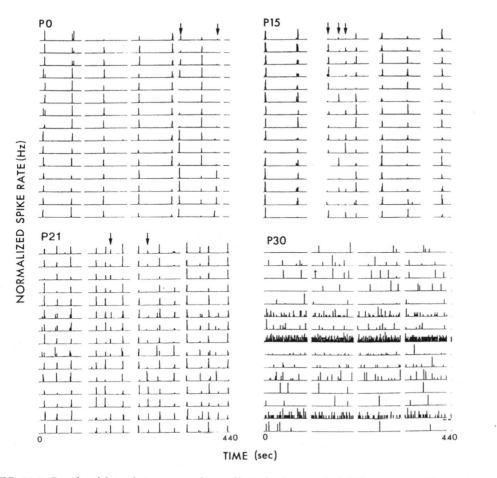

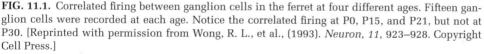

FIG. 11.1. Correlated firing between ganglion cells in the ferret at four different ages. Fifteen ganglion cells were recorded at each age. Notice the correlated firing at P0, P15, and P21, but not at P30. [Reprinted with permission from Wong, R. L., et al., (1993). *Neuron, 11*, 923–928. Copyright Cell Press.]

process of segregation. Between 3 and 6 weeks of age synchrony within each eye is reduced and synchrony between the eyes increases. No quantitative measurements of synchrony of activity within each eye as compared with synchrony between the eyes has been made over this period of time. However, the process seems likely to be organized as suggested above, given the Hebbian mechanism, and the fact that segregation of afferents from the retinas to the lateral geniculate nucleus is complete, while segregation of afferents to the cortex from the lateral geniculate is not.

Although it is clear that electrical activity plays an instructive role in both the formation of layers in the lateral geniculate nucleus and the formation of columns for ocular dominance and orientation in the visual cortex, there may also be molecular factors involved. The experiments and arguments are complicated, and have been reviewed by Sengpiel and Kind (2002). The true test of the existence of molecular factors will be their identification, and so far none have been identified.

2. Polarization of the Postsynaptic Neuron

The state of depolarization of the postsynaptic neurons within the visual cortex is likely to be important. Both the orientation sensitivity and the ocular dominance of cells can be changed by coupling one stimulus with depolarization of the neuron, and another stimulus with hyperpolarization (Fregnac, Shulz, Thorpe, & Bienenstock, 1992). After several dozen couplings, the cell becomes more responsive to the stimulus coupled with depolarization, and less responsive to the stimulus coupled with hyperpolarization (Fig. 11.2). Indeed, the orientation preference of the cell can be reversed. Moreover, high-frequency stimulation can produce either long-term potentiation (LTP) or long-term depression (LTD) in the visual cortex, depending on the state of depolarization of the postsynaptic neuron (Artola, Brocher, & Singer, 1990;

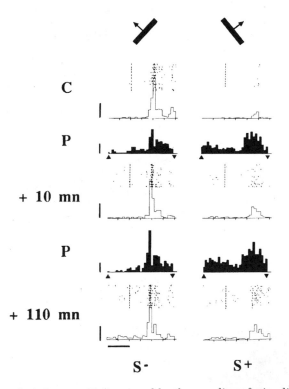

FIG. 11.2. Change in orientation sensitivity caused by the coupling of stimuli with polarization of the cell. In the control situation (C), the cell preferred movement up and to the left. After the investigators paired movement up and to the right with depolarization, and movement up and to the left with hyperpolarization, this orientation preference was reversed (P). Ten minutes later, the cell had reverted to its original orientation preference (10 mn). Two hours after a second pairing (110 mn), some shift in orientation preference persisted. [Reprinted with permission from Fregnac, Y., et al. (1992). *Journal of Neuroscience, 12,* 1280–1300. Copyright 1992 Society for Neuroscience.]

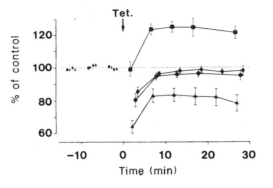

FIG. 11.3. Long-term potentiation (LTP) and LTD in slices of rat visual cortex. A tetanus (a burst of high frequency stimulation) was given at time 0. In normal conditions, there was no long-term effect. With a low level of the GABA antagonist bicuculline (0.1–0.2 μM), which blocks inhibitory signals and depolarizes the neuron, the tetanus produced LTD (▲) and with a higher level of bicuculline (0.3 μM) the tetanus produced LTP (■). [Reprinted with permission from Artola, A., et al. (1990). *Nature, 347*, 69–72. Copyright 1990 MacMillan Magazines Limited.]

see Fig. 11.3). Putting these two results together suggests that the state of the cellular properties of the neuron may affect what kind of long-term changes result from the visual input impinging on the cortical cell.

A number of cellular properties change with age in the rat (McCormick & Prince, 1987). Among them, the resting potential becomes slightly more hyperpolarized and the input resistance drops substantially. Both these changes could result in the afferent input having a larger effect in young animals. A larger input resistance in young animals would lead to a larger voltage change for the same current input, by Ohm's law. A more depolarized resting potential would bring the membrane potential closer to threshold for action potentials and closer to the potential required to activate NMDA currents, so that a smaller change in voltage would activate these currents. Moreover, the inhibitory transmitter GABA actually excites neurons in young animals, leading to a calcium influx, because its reversal potential is more positive than the membrane potential of the cell at that age (Yuste & Katz, 1991; Lin, Takahashi, Takahashi, & Tsumoto, 1994). Unfortunately, these experiments have not been carried out in the cat visual cortex, where the time course of the critical period is well defined. Consequently, we do not know if these changes are complete before the critical period or take place during and after it.

3. NMDA Receptors

Electrical activity releases the transmitter glutamate in the visual cortex, and glutamate activates three types of glutamate receptor in the postsynaptic neuron: AMPA/kainate receptors, *N*-methyl-D-aspartate (NMDA) receptors, and metabotropic glutamate receptors. *N*-methyl-D-aspartate receptors have been hypothesized for some time to play a role in plasticity because they are voltage dependent. Thus, they open channels when the postsynaptic neuron is depolarized and accentuate the transmission of the signal in a multiplicative fashion. This makes it more likely that the postsynaptic cell will fire when the presynaptic cell fires. They also let calcium into the cell through their channels, and calcium is believed to be involved in plasticity.

Antagonists to the NMDA receptor abolish the ocular dominance plasticity that normally occurs after monocular deprivation (Bear, Kleinschmidt, Gu, & Singer, 1990; Fig. 11.4). There was some question as to whether this result was due to an effect of the antagonist on the activity of cells in the visual cortex, making it like a low dose of tetrodotoxin. This question was resolved by further experiments with different techniques, showing that plasticity is abolished even when activity is not significantly affected (Roberts, Meredith, & Ramoa, 1998; Daw, Gordon, Fox, Flavin, Kirsch, Beaver, Ji, Reid, & Czepita, 1999).

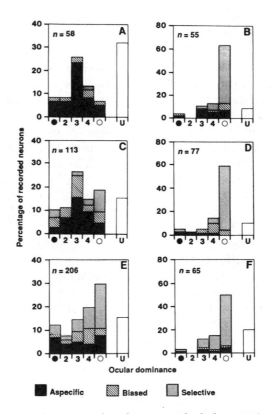

FIG. 11.4. Ocular dominance histograms from kittens in which the experimental hemisphere was infused with APV (A, C, and E), compared with histograms from the control hemisphere (B, D, and F). (A and B) Dark-reared until treatment; (C–F), reared normally. (A and C) Treated with 50 mM APV; (E) treated with 5 mM. The differences between (A) and (B), and between (C) and (D) were substantially greater than the difference seen in monocularly deprived animals that were not treated with an antagonist, and significantly greater than the difference between the hemispheres ipsilateral and contralateral to the open eye. Fewer cells were specific for the orientation of the stimulus in APV-treated animals. Thus, treatment with APV reduced both the ocular dominance shift and the orientation specificity. [Reprinted with permission from Kleinschmidt, A., et al. (1987). *Science 238*, 355–358. Copyright 1987 AAAS.]

The NMDA receptor consists of an NR1 subunit in combination with various NR2 subunits. In the visual cortex at birth, the secondary subunits are primarily NR2B and this switches during development to NR2A. At least in the ferret, this switch occurs at the start of the critical period for ocular dominance plasticity (Roberts & Ramoa, 1999). As the switch takes place, the duration of the open time for the NMDA channels becomes shorter (Carmignoto & Vicini, 1992; Roberts & Ramoa, 1999), making it less likely that NMDA responses in the postsynaptic neuron will overlap with each other. The hypothesis is that a lack of overlap between deprived eye responses and nondeprived eye responses is required for a shift in ocular dominance.

N-methyl-D-aspartate receptors, along with their subunits NR1, NR2A, and NR2B, all peak with the critical period and decline thereafter (Gordon, Daw, & Parkinson, 1991; Chen, Cooper, & Mower, 2000). Thus, the start of the critical period is related to an overall increase in NMDA receptors, as well as the shift from NR2B to NR2A, whereas the end of the critical period is related to a decline in NMDA receptors without any shift in subunits. In dark-reared animals there is less NR2A than normal at 5 weeks of age and more at 20 weeks of age, but no change at either age in NR2B or NR1 (Fig. 11.5). By this criterion, the subunit most related to plasticity is NR2A. Moreover, mice mutant for the NR2A subunit show reduced ocular dominance plasticity (Fagiolini, Katagiri, Miyamoto, Mori, Grant, Mishina, & Hensch, 2003).

A physiological parameter that represents the contribution of NMDA receptors to the visual response can be measured. This is done by recording from cells in the visual cortex while iontophoresing the NMDA antagonist APV. The amount by which the visual response is reduced represents the NMDA contribution to the visual response in relation to the contribution from AMPA/kainate receptors. This NMDA contribution remains high in layers II and III of the visual cortex at all ages (Fox, Sato, & Daw, 1989). However, it drops in layers IV, V, and VI between 3 and 6 weeks of age. This is the period during which ocular dominance columns segregate in layer IV. Dark-rearing

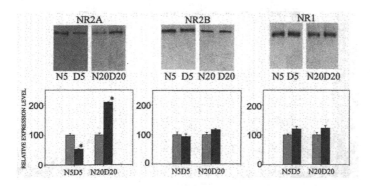

FIG. 11.5. The effects of dark rearing on the level of expression of NMDA receptor subunits NR2A (left), NR2B (middle), and NR1 (right). Levels of expression were compared at 5 weeks of age in normal (N5) and dark-reared cats (D5) and at 20 weeks of age in normal (N20) and dark-reared cats (D20). The top of each panel shows Western blot results. The bottom of each panel summarizes the relative level of expression at each age and rearing condition. [Reprinted from Chen, L., et al. (2000). *Brain Research, 78*, 196–200. Copyright 2000, with permission from Elsevier.]

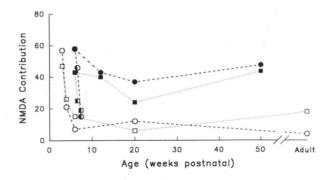

FIG. 11.6. Effect of rearing in the dark on the NMDA contribution to the visual response. NMDA contribution remains high in dark-reared animals in layer IV (●) and layers V and VI (■), compared with animals reared in the light (○ and □). When animals are reared in the dark until 6 weeks of age, then brought into the light, the drop in the NMDA contribution to the visual response proceeds (◐ and ◨). [Used with permission from Czepita, D., et al. (1994). *Journal of Neurophysiology, 72,* 1220–1226.]

postpones the reduction in the NMDA contribution to the visual response in layers IV, V, and VI (Fox, Daw, Sato, & Czepita, 1992): even after several months in the dark, the contribution remains high (Fig. 11.6). If animals are brought into the light after being in the dark until 6 weeks of age, the reduction in the NMDA contribution to the visual response proceeds. Thus, the change in the NMDA contribution to the visual response is definitely under the control of light.

Treatment with NMDA antagonists also reduces the specificity of the responses of cells in the visual cortex (Bear et al., 1990). Moreover, application of antisense oligonucleotides, which also suppresses NMDA receptor function, prevents the development of orientation selectivity and stimulus size selectivity (Ramoa, Mower, Liao, & Jafri, 2001).

In summary, NMDA receptor function is related to ocular dominance plasticity by a variety of criteria: the reduction of NMDA receptor function reduces ocular dominance plasticity, NMDA receptors are most abundant during the critical period for ocular dominance plasticity, and dark rearing affects NR2A subunit abundance and plasticity similarly.

4. Metabotropic Glutamate Receptors

Metabotropic glutamate receptors may also mediate plasticity because they release calcium from internal stores in the cell and affect various second messengers such as cAMP and phosphoinositide. Both glutamate stimulation of phosphoinositide turnover (Dudek and Bear, 1989) and production of cAMP by the general metabotropic glutamate agonist ACPD (Reid, Daw, Gregory, & Flavin, 1996) have an expression profile that correlates with the critical period for ocular dominance plasticity in cat visual cortex. Moreover, the production of cAMP is less in dark-reared animals than in normal ones at 6 weeks of age, and is greater than normal at 15 weeks of age (Reid et al., 1996).

There are three groups of metabotropic glutamate receptors. Group I (mGluRs 1 and 5) has facilitatory postsynaptic actions in the visual cortex (Jin, Beaver, Ji, & Daw, 2001), as it does in other parts of the nervous system, and it affects phosphoinositide metabolism and increases cAMP. Groups II (mGluRs 2 and 3) and III (mGluRs 4, 6, 7, and 8) have depressive presynaptic actions (Beaver, Ji, & Daw, 1999), also similar to their actions in other parts of the nervous system, and they decrease cAMP.

The general mGluR antagonist, MCPG, does not affect ocular dominance plasticity (Hensch & Stryker, 1996). However, MCPG is not very potent. It acts as an antagonist against the mGluR agonist ACPD, but is not effective against glutamate-stimulated PI turnover or glutamate-stimulated spike adaptation (Huber, Sawtell, & Bear, 1998). Mice mutant for the Group II receptor mGluR2 show normal ocular dominance plasticity (Renger, Hartman, Tsuchimoto, Yokoi, Nakanishi, & Hensch, 2002). Application of the general Group I agonist PHCCC [*N*-phenyl-7-(hydroxyimimo)cyclopropa(b)chromen-1a-carboxamide] affects plasticity by a small amount, and so does the mGluR1 antagonist LY367385 [(S)-(+)-amino-4-carboxy-2-methylbenzeneacetic acid] but not the mGluR5 antagonist MPEP [2-methyl-6-(phenylethynyl)pyridine] (Fischer, Yang, Beaver, & Daw, 2004). This effect is additive to that of the NMDA antagonists. Thus, it appears that both mGluR1 and NMDA receptors influence ocular dominance plasticity, and probably both need to be blocked to abolish ocular dominance plasticity completely.

5. GABA

The role of the inhibitory neurotransmitter GABA (γ-aminobutyric acid) in ocular dominance plasticity is complicated. If one infuses the GABA agonist muscimol and records the ocular dominance changes as a result of monocular deprivation, the ocular dominance histogram is shifted towards the *deprived* eye, not the nondeprived eye (Reiter & Stryker, 1988). When terminal arborizations of the afferents from the lateral geniculate nucleus to the cortex are measured, afferents from the nondeprived eye are shrunken and afferents from the deprived eye appear normal (Fig. 11.7; Hata, Tsumoto, & Stryker, 1999). This is interpreted in terms of silence in the postsynaptic cell and a resulting lack of a trophic factor, which is needed in greater amounts by the more active afferents. Thus, this result may relate to the state of the postsynaptic cell, rather than to a specific effect of GABA. Presumably any agent that silenced the postsynaptic cell without affecting the presynaptic terminals would have the same result.

There are GABA receptors that open chloride channels (GABA$_A$ and GABA$_C$). There are also metabotropic GABA$_B$ receptors, which act through G proteins, and can affect NMDA receptors, cyclic AMP, and gene expression. Application of the GABA$_B$ receptor agonist baclofen promotes ocular dominance plasticity, while application of the GABA$_B$ receptor antagonist SCH50911 impairs ocular dominance plasticity (Yang, Fischer, & Daw, 2005).

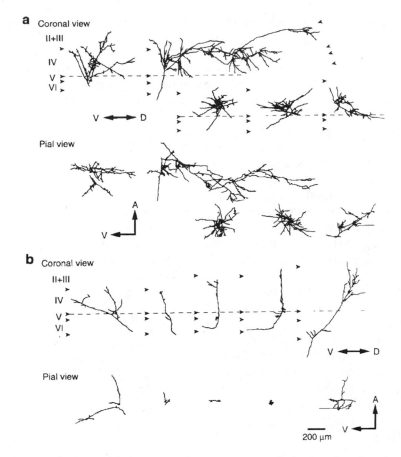

FIG. 11.7. Terminal arbors of thalamocortical axons in cats with the visual cortex silenced with muscimol. (a) Deprived eye arbors. (b) Nondeprived eye arbors. [Reprinted from Hata, Y., et al. (1999). *Neuron, 22*, 375–381. Copyright 1999, with permission from Elsevier.]

Application of the GABA$_A$ receptor antagonist bicuculline also impairs ocular dominance plasticity (Ramoa, Paradiso, & Freeman, 1988). These results can be interpreted in terms of the Hebbian model, with baclofen making the response more transient and synchronous firing less likely, and SCH50911 and bicuculline having the reverse effect. In this interpretation, activation of GABA$_A$ or GABA$_B$ receptors acts just like the switch from NR2B to NR2A.

This hypothesis has been most prominently investigated using mice mutant for the GABA synthesizing enzyme GAD65 (glutamic acid decarboxylase 65). This enzyme synthesizes GABA at synaptic terminals, and there is another enzyme, GAD67, that synthesizes GABA throughout the cell. Ocular dominance plasticity is abolished at all ages in GAD65 mutant mice (Fagiolini & Hensch, 2000). There is a drug, diazepam, that acts at the benzodiazepine site on the GABA receptor and potentiates the receptor response to GABA in the GAD65 mutant mice; diazepam restores ocular dominance plasticity in these mice at all ages (Fagiolini & Hensch, 2000). Indeed, the critical period for ocular dominance plasticity can be initiated early with the use of diazepam. Discharges of cells in the visual cortex are prolonged in the GAD65 mutant mice and shortened in these mice treated with diazepam (Fagiolini & Hensch, 2000). These results have been interpreted to mean that the start of the critical period for ocular dominance plasticity occurs when the balance between excitatory and inhibitory inputs reaches a threshold for inhibition.

More recent work, however, suggests that the situation may be more complicated. There are four types of α subunits for the GABA$_A$ receptor that are sensitive to benzodiazepines: α1, α2, α3, and α5. When the α1 subunit is made insensitive to diazepam, application of diazepam to the receptor shortens the discharge but does not induce early plasticity (Fagiolini, Fritschy, Low, Mohler, Rudolph, & Hensch, 2004). On the other hand, when the α2 subunit is made insensitive to diazepam, application of diazepam to the receptor induces early plasticity but does not shorten the discharge. Thus, shortening of the discharge and accentuating ocular dominance plasticity do not always go along together.

Further complications are found in mice with targeted deletion of the NMDA receptor subunit NR2A. Sensitivity to monocular deprivation is weakened in these mice, but the timing of the critical period for ocular dominance plasticity remains the same (Fagiolini et al., 2003). Ocular dominance plasticity can be increased in these mice by applying diazepam. Thus, the reduction of ocular dominance plasticity through the action of the NR2A subunits of the NMDA receptor can be compensated by an increase in plasticity brought about by the benzodiazepine site of the GABA receptor, but whether this occurs simply through lengthening and shortening the response time is open to question. The results also imply that the mechanism for the increase and decrease of plasticity and the mechanisms for the start of the critical period may not be the same. However, more data will be required to delineate the time course of the critical period in these latest experiments to test these conclusions.

6. Brain Derived Neurotrophic Factor (BDNF)

A variety of neurotrophic factors exist, including nerve growth factor (NGF), brain derived neurotrophic factor (BDNF), neurotrophin-3 (NT-3), and neurotrophin-4/5 (NT-4/5). These factors have a variety of receptors, including trkA for NGF, trkB for BDNF and NT-4/5, and trkC for NT-3. Nerve growth factor is found on the terminals of the acetylcholine afferents from the basal forebrain and is therefore on the modulatory pathway rather than the instructive pathway, and will therefore be discussed below (Silver, Fagiolini, Gillespie, Howe, Frank, Issa, Antonini, & Stryker, 2001). This section will deal primarily with BDNF, whose receptor is found on geniculocortical axons, and is therefore on the instructive pathway (Silver & Stryker, 2001).

The formation of ocular dominance patches in layer IV of the visual cortex, as revealed by autoradiographic transport of [3H] proline from the retina between 3 and 6 weeks of age in the cat, is prevented by treating with BDNF

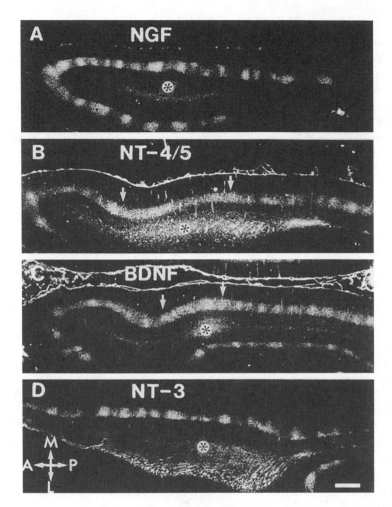

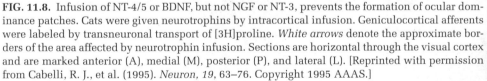

FIG. 11.8. Infusion of NT-4/5 or BDNF, but not NGF or NT-3, prevents the formation of ocular dominance patches. Cats were given neurotrophins by intracortical infusion. Geniculocortical afferents were labeled by transneuronal transport of [3H]proline. *White arrows* denote the approximate borders of the area affected by neurotrophin infusion. Sections are horizontal through the visual cortex and are marked anterior (A), medial (M), posterior (P), and lateral (L). [Reprinted with permission from Cabelli, R. J., et al. (1995). *Neuron, 19,* 63–76. Copyright 1995 AAAS.]

or NT-4/5 in the visual cortex, but not by NGF or NT-3 (Fig. 11.8; Cabelli, Hohn, & Shatz, 1995). It is also prevented by applying a trkB antagonist, but not trkA or trkC antagonists (Cabelli, Shelton, Segal, & Shatz, 1997). Both of these observations can be explained by the requirement for a trophic factor that is taken up by the geniculocortical afferents and is normally in limited supply. In the first case, the trophic factor is abundant, so that both the right and left eye geniculocortical afferents can take up enough of it. In the second case, the antagonist prevents the uptake. Not all evidence supports this explanation (Kohara, Kitamura, Morishima, & Tsumoto, 2001); nevertheless it is the simplest hypothesis. In any case, the experiments clearly distinguish the role of the trkB ligands BDNF and NT-4/5 from the trkA and trkC ligands NGF and NT-3, as expected from their location within the system.

The application of BDNF to the visual cortex during monocular deprivation induces a shift in ocular dominance to the deprived eye, together with a loss of orientation selectivity (Galuske, Kim, Castren, & Singer, 2000). This occurs in kittens but not in cats. Application of NT-4/5 to kittens during monocular deprivation also leads to a loss of orientation selectivity and a lack of an ocular dominance shift (Gillespie, Crair, & Stryker, 2000). The reverse ocular dominance shift with BDNF is reminiscent of the reverse ocular dominance shift seen with the GABA agonist muscimol. The two results are probably related because mice overexpressing BDNF show accelerated maturation of GABAergic innervation and inhibition (Huang, Kirkwood, Pizzorusso, Porciatti, Morales, Bear, Maffei, & Tonegawa, 1999).

The overexpression of BDNF has a number of other results. The critical period for monocular deprivation starts early (Hanover, Huang, Tonegawa, & Stryker, 1999) and ends early as well (Huang et al., 1999). Visual acuity matures early (Huang et al., 1999). The effects of rearing in the dark, such as delayed critical period for monocular deprivation, lack of maturation of visual acuity, and lack of maturation of inhibition, are all reversed in BDNF-overexpressing mice (Gianfranceschi, Siciliano, Walls, Morales, Kirkwood, Huang, Tonegawa, & Maffei, 2003). All of this implies that the overexpression of BDNF and maturation of the GABA system are related to each other, that rearing in the dark has the reverse effect, and that there are numerous consequences for the development of the visual system and for plasticity in the visual cortex.

7. Calcium, α-Calcium/Calmodulin Kinase, and Calcineurin

The activation of NMDA receptors lets calcium into the cell. Calcium has been implicated in synaptic plasticity in the hippocampus by several experiments. The current hypothesis is that small increases of calcium that persist for a long period of time lead to synaptic depression, and large increases that last for a short period of time lead to potentiation (Lisman, 1989; Yang, Tang, & Zucker, 1999). It is therefore almost a tautology that calcium must be involved in ocular dominance plasticity in the visual cortex. Unfortunately, nobody has been able to devise an experiment to test the involvement of calcium in ocular dominance plasticity directly because calcium is involved in so many other cell processes that any disruption of the calcium system would have numerous effects besides altering ocular dominance plasticity that would be hard to control.

Some developmental changes in calcium levels correlate with ocular dominance plasticity, and some do not. Binding sites for voltage-dependent calcium channels in the cat decrease steadily with age, during the period that plasticity is increasing (14–28 days) as well as during the period that plasticity is decreasing (28–70 days), suggesting that the change in the number of binding sites is related to activity rather than to plasticity (Bode-Greuel & Singer, 1988). Rearing in the dark has no effect on the number of these binding sites

(Bode-Greuel & Singer, 1988). Calcium uptake through NMDA receptors in the cat declines steadily between 26 and 90 days of age, and few measurements from before 28 days have been published, unfortunately, for the interpretation of the relationship to plasticity (Feldman, Sherin, Press, & Bear, 1990). Thus, the developmental changes related to calcium binding and uptake do not correlate with plasticity.

Calcium stimulates a number of kinases and the phosphatase calcineurin. One hypothesis is that high levels of calcium stimulate kinases to produce potentiation, and low levels stimulate phosphatases to produce depression (Lisman, 1989, 2001). Experiments done in the visual cortex have primarily focused on α-calcium/calmodulin kinase II (αCaMKII) and calcineurin. In mice mutant for αCaMKII, ocular dominance plasticity was greatly diminished in half the cases, and in the other half it was normal (Gordon, Cioffi, Silva, & Stryker, 1996). A more specific αCaMKII mutant that cannot autophosphorylate shows ocular dominance plasticity for long periods of monocular deprivation, but not for short periods (Fig. 11.9; Taha, Hanover, Silva, & Stryker, 2002). Mice that overexpress the phosphatase calcineurin do not show ocular dominance plasticity (Yang, Fischer, Zhang, Baumgartel, Mansuy, & Daw, 2005). These results are in accordance with the overall hypothesis, but more experiments will be required to fill in the details.

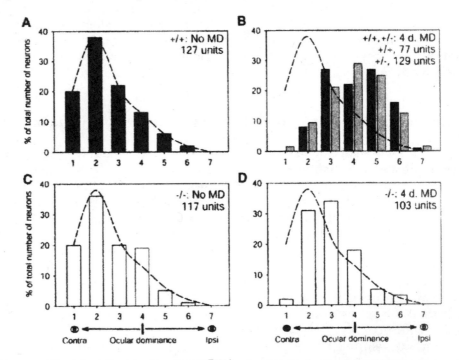

FIG. 11.9. Plasticity is impaired in CaMKII[T286A] mice. (A) Ocular dominance histogram in wild-type mice. The broken line in all panels is a fit to this distribution. (B) Following 4 days of monocular deprivation, wild-type and heterozygous animals show a shift to the right in ocular dominance distribution. (C) Prior to monocular deprivation, the ocular dominance distribution in CaMKII[T286A] homozygous mice was similar to that in wild-type mice. (D) Following 4 days of monocular deprivation, the ocular dominance distribution in CaMKII[T286A] homozygous mice was not shifted. [Reprinted from Taha, S., & Stryker, M. P. (2002). *Neuron, 34*, 425–436. Copyright 2002, with permission from Elsevier.]

In summary, calcium is almost certainly important in plasticity in the visual cortex, where it links the activation of glutamate receptors to the activation of various kinases and phosphatases. However, it is more NMDA receptors that makes the cortex more plastic at the peak of the critical period, not more of some property of calcium or calcium channels. There is no evidence that any property of calcium or calcium channels corresponds to both the rising and falling phases of the critical period, or is affected by dark rearing in the same manner as plasticity. In other words, calcium is a link, but not the factor that makes the cortex plastic.

8. cAMP and Protein Kinase A

cAMP can be produced by NMDA receptors through calcium and calcium-stimulated adenylate cyclases and by metabotropic glutamate receptors, either directly or through calcium released from intracellular stores. cAMP in turn activates protein kinase A, which has been implicated in plasticity in a variety of systems. As pointed out above, cAMP produced in response to the general metabotropic glutamate agonist ACPD mirrors the critical period for ocular dominance plasticity in the cat, and is altered by rearing in the dark, similar to ocular dominance plasticity (Reid et al., 1996). This effect is due largely to developmental changes in cAMP production rather than to developmental changes in the levels of metabotropic glutamate receptors (Daw & Reid, 1996).

Ocular dominance plasticity is abolished by protein kinase A inhibitors (Beaver, Ji, Fischer, & Daw, 2001; Fig. 11.10). This is not due to the action of the inhibitor on activity. Protein kinase A is made of a pair of catalytic subunits and a pair of regulatory subunits, which may be RIα, RIβ, RIIα, or

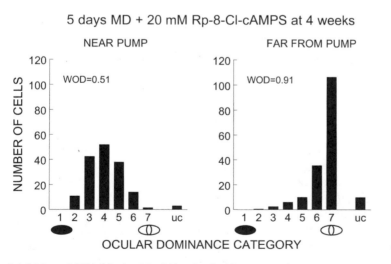

FIG. 11.10. Inhibition of PKA blocks OD shifts. Ocular dominance histograms constructed from four 4-week-old kittens whose left visual cortices were infused with 20 mM Rp-8-Cl-cAMPS during a 5-day period of monocular deprivation. (Right) Cells located far from the tip of the pump cannula. (Left) Cells near the pump cannula. Abbreviations: WOD, weighted ocular dominance scores; UC, uncharacterized. [Reprinted with permission from Beaver, C. J., et al. (2001).]

RIIβ. Experiments with mutant mice show that the RII subunits are involved in ocular dominance plasticity, primarily RIIβ (Fischer, Beaver, Yang, Rao, Jacobsdottir, Storm, McKnight, & Daw, 2004), but also RIIα (Rao, Fischer, Yang, McKnight, LaRue, & Daw, 2004). The RIβ subunit is not involved (Hensch, Gordon, Brandon, McKnight, Iderzda, & Stryker, 1998) nor is the RIα subunit, as far as is known. Treatment with cAMP in conjunction with monocular deprivation can produce ocular dominance changes in the adult cortex, although these changes involve a change in the percentage of cells that are binocularly driven rather than a shift in ocular dominance to the nondeprived eye (Imamura, Kasamatsu, Shirokawa, & Ohashi, 1999). Thus, cAMP and protein kinase A are critical for ocular dominance plasticity by all the criteria listed—inhibitors abolish plasticity, cAMP correlates with the critical period in both light- and dark-reared animals, and amplification of cAMP in adult animals restores plasticity.

9. A Kinase Anchoring Protein at the Postsynaptic Density

Neurotransmitters act on the postsynaptic cell at receptors in the postsynaptic density. Both protein kinase A and calcineurin are found in the postsynaptic density, with protein kinase A held there through its RII subunits by an A kinase anchoring protein, AKAP 79/150 (Coghlan, Perrino, Howard, Langeberg, Hicks, Gallatin, & Scott, 1995). Mice mutant for this AKAP do not show ocular dominance plasticity (Fischer, Yang, Jacobsdottir, McKnight, & Daw, 2005). The proximity of protein kinase A and calcineurin to each other and to the AMPA receptor GluR1 presumably helps their interactions. The AMPA receptor is phosphorylated by protein kinase A and CaM kinase and dephosphorylated by calcineurin in accordance with the general hypothesis given above (Lee, Barbarosie, Kameyama, Bear, & Huganir, 2000).

10. Other Protein Kinases

Protein kinase G and protein kinase C have both been implicated in plasticity in the hippocampus. However, inhibitors of protein kinase G do not affect ocular dominance plasticity, and inhibitors of protein kinase C have not yet been sufficiently well tested, although preliminary evidence suggests that the same may be true for protein kinase C (Beaver et al., 2000; Daw & Beaver, 2001).

Electrical activity, PKA, CaM kinase, calcineurin, and growth factors can all affect the extracellular signal-regulated kinase ERK. ERK inhibitors abolish ocular dominance plasticity in rats (DiCristo, Berardi, Cancedda, Pizzorusso, Putignano, Ratto, & Maffei, 2001). Thus, ERK may be a convergence point for a variety of signals that affect ocular dominance plasticity (Cancedda, Putignano, Impey, Maffei, Ratto, & Pizzorusso, 2003).

11. Cyclic AMP Response Binding Element (CREB)

223

MECHANISMS
OF PLASTICITY
IN THE VISUAL
CORTEX

Calcium, cyclic AMP, BDNF, PKA, CaM kinase, and ERK all act, directly or indirectly, on the calcium/cyclic AMP response binding element (CREB), which is therefore a further downstream convergence point for signals affecting ocular dominance plasticity (Cancedda et al., 2003; Pizzorusso, Ratto, Putignano, & Maffei, 2000). Cyclic AMP response binding element in turn activates gene expression. CRE/CREB gene expression peaks in the thalamus around the time of segregation of the lateral geniculate nucleus into eye-specific layers, and mice mutant for CREB show abnormal segregation (Pham, Rubenstein, Silva, Storm, & Stryker, 2001). Furthermore, CRE-mediated gene expression is activated following monocular deprivation during the critical period for ocular dominance plasticity, but not following monocular deprivation in the adult (Pham, Impey, Storm, & Stryker, 1999). Other experiments have shown that injecting a dominant-negative form of CREB blocks ocular dominance plasticity in the visual cortex of ferrets (Mower, Liao, Nestler, Neve, & Ramoa, 2002). Thus, CREB is an important link between the activation of ocular dominance plasticity by monocular deprivation and the resulting expression of genes.

12. Genes and Protein Synthesis

There are a number of genes that are turned on shortly after a stimulus is applied and are consequently known as immediate early genes (IEGs). These include fos, jun, egr1/zif268, and several others. Most of them are turned off in darkness and turned on in light, so other criteria need to be applied to see if they are related to plasticity rather than to activity. The levels of induced fos are higher in normal than dark-reared cats at 5 weeks of age, comparable at 10 weeks of age, and higher in dark-reared than in normal cats at 20 weeks, a time course that corresponds to the effects of dark-rearing on plasticity (Mower & Kaplan, 2002). Egr1 induction, on the other hand, is higher in dark-reared than normal animals at all ages. Moreover, ocular dominance plasticity is normal in mice mutant for egr1 (Mataga, Fujishima, Condie, & Hensch, 2001). The effect of the loss of fos on ocular dominance plasticity is not known. Thus, fos may be a factor in ocular dominance plasticity, but egr1 is probably not.

Other genes have been identified by the stringent criterion that they are expressed more highly at 5 weeks in normal than dark-reared cats, and more highly at 20 weeks in dark-reared than normal cats (plasticity genes) or vice versa (antiplasticity genes). One antiplasticity gene is Munc 13-3, meaning mouse uncoordinated gene (Yang, Zheng, Li, & Mower, 2002). The protein is located in presynaptic active zones and plays an essential role in synaptic vesicle release. One plasticity-related gene is cpg-15, whose overexpression leads to the exuberant growth of dendritic arbors and promotes the maturation of synapses (Lee & Nedivi, 2002). Several mitochondrial genes have been identified as either plasticity or antiplasticity genes (Yang, Silver, Ellis, & Mower, 2001). The exact role of all these genes in plasticity remains to be determined.

Numerous other genes have been identified by less-stringent criteria using microarrays of cDNA probes to investigate expression in cat visual cortex at various ages (Prasad, Kojic, Li, Mitchell, Hachisuka, Sawada, Gu, & Cynader, 2002). Again, the exact role of most of them is currently unknown. The fundamental questions driving such studies are: What controls the array of genes involved in the formation of axon terminals, dendritic spines, and synapses, as opposed to the array of genes involved in their degradation? How are the levels of calcium, PKA, and other factors that are involved in plasticity related to turning on one set of genes and turning off the other? There is considerable work to be done before these questions will be answered.

Protein synthesis is required for the physiological ocular dominance changes that occur in mouse visual cortex over the first 4 days of monocular deprivation (Taha & Stryker, 2002). This is before any anatomical changes are seen in the geniculocortical afferents. One likely hypothesis is that structural changes in the geniculocortical afferents follow structural changes in layers 2 and 3, and the latter are affected by protein synthesis (Trachtenberg, Trepel, & Stryker, 2000). Proteins may also be synthesized in synaptic areas, which could not be seen by anatomical techniques but would nevertheless show up as physiological changes in ocular dominance. Indeed, a whole array of proteins must be produced for the shift in ocular dominance to happen. This is true for the reduction in the effectiveness of synapses from the deprived eye, the increase in the effectiveness of synapses from the nondeprived eye, the degradation and formation of synapses and of the dendritic spines on which they are found, and the retraction and expansion of axon terminals. Presumably there is a sequence of protein synthesis changes as the cells go through these alterations. The question, therefore, is: Which proteins are synthesized and when does this happen? Not much work has yet addressed this question, except for the observation that protein synthesis in the lateral geniculate nucleus is not required for the initial 4 days of ocular dominance shift in the mouse (Taha & Stryker, 2002).

One molecule that has been studied in some detail is tissue plasminogen activator (tPA). Tissue plasminogen activator is an extracellular serine protease that converts plasminogen into plasmin. Mice treated with tPA inhibitors and mice that are mutant for tPA show deficits in ocular dominance shifts from monocular deprivation (Mataga, Nagai, & Hensch, 2002) and in recovery from these shifts (Muller & Griesinger, 1998). A likely scenario is that dendritic spines fed by the deprived eye become motile due to increased tPA proteolytic activity, and are eventually eliminated (Mataga, Mizuguchi, & Hensch, 2004). Proteolysis by tPA declines with age, and increases with monocular deprivation only in young mice.

Other specific molecules that have received some attention are the chondroitin sulphate proteoglycans, which are components of the extracellular matrix that inhibit axonal sprouting and growth (Pizzorusso, Medini, Berardi, Chierzi, Fawcett, & Maffei, 2002). They condense around the soma and dendrites of a subset of neurons in perineuronal nets during late development, around the end of the critical period. Rearing in the dark prevents the formation of the perineuronal nets. Degradation of chondroitin sulphate proteoglycan chains with chondroitinase ABC in adult rats, after the end of the critical period, allows monocular deprivation to produce an ocular dominance shift. The formation of the perineuronal nets may well be the cause of the closure of plasticity at the end of the critical period (Berardi, Pizzorusso, & Maffei, 2004).

13. Modulatory Factors

A variety of modulatory factors affect ocular dominance plasticity. One has already been mentioned: anesthesia. Another is sleep. Six hours of sleep after 6 h of monocular deprivation produces an ocular dominance shift that is as large as 12 h of monocular deprivation, and rather larger than the shift from 6 h of monocular deprivation (Frank, Issa, & Stryker, 2001). Sleep therefore accentuates the ocular dominance shift. Another modulatory factor is environmental enrichment, as in a cage filled with running wheels and objects to play in. The effect of environmental enrichment on ocular dominance plasticity has not yet been reported, but acuity develops early, as measured at both the cortical and retinal levels (Cancedda, Putignano, Sale, Viegi, Berardi, & Maffei, 2004). A precocious CREB response and increases in BDNF and GAD65/67 expression are also found, so some effect on ocular dominance plasticity would be expected.

Neuronal signals that modulate the state of the nervous system come from the basal forebrain carried by acetylcholine; from the locus coeruleus carried by noradrenaline; from the raphe nuclei carried by serotonin; from the midbrain carried by dopamine; and from the intermedullary nuclei of the thalamus carried by glutamate. In the first four cases, it is quite easy to distinguish the role of the modulatory pathways from the role of the instructive pathways by interrupting these pathways or applying antagonists to their transmitters. An early experiment suggested that the ablation of the noradrenaline pathway by lesioning the dorsal noradrenergic bundle with injections of 6-hydroxydopamine (6-OHDA) abolishes ocular dominance plasticity (Kasamatsu & Pettigrew, 1979). Later experiments showed that this result was due to nonspecific effects induced by the high concentrations of 6-hydroxydopamine used; lower doses of 6-hydroxydopamine, and other treatments more specific to the noradrenaline pathway, do not have the same result (Daw, Videen, Parkinson, & Rader, 1985; Gordon, Allen, & Trombley, 1988). However, antagonists to β-adrenergic receptors do have a very small effect on the ocular dominance shift (Kasamatsu & Shirokawa, 1985).

Antagonists to muscarinic acetylcholine receptors reduce ocular dominance plasticity somewhat, and affect orientation selectivity, probably through their action on M_1 receptors (Gu & Singer, 1993). Lesions of the cholinergic cells in the basal forebrain also reduce ocular dominance plasticity, and a combination of this treatment with lesions of the dorsal noradrenergic bundle from 6-OHDA essentially abolishes ocular dominance plasticity (Bear & Singer, 1986). Bear and Singer also showed that high doses of 6-OHDA antagonize the action of acetylcholine, but it was not certain whether the effects of the combined action of the lesions of the basal forebrain and dorsal noradrenergic bundle could be attributed to acetylcholine alone. Serotonin neurotoxins and a combination of antagonists to the serotonin receptors $5HT_1$ and $5HT_2$ also reduce ocular dominance plasticity (Gu & Singer, 1995). The role of dopamine in visual cortex plasticity has not been studied. Thus, acetylcholine and serotonin afferents definitely have an effect, but evidence about other modulators is uncertain.

Modulatory transmitters act on ion channels and second messengers (Gu, 2002). Potassium channels are affected by several of them. Phospholipase C and phosphoinositides are activated by acetylcholine M_1 and M_3 receptors, noradrenaline α_1 receptors, and serotonin $5HT_2$ receptors together with release of calcium from intracellular stores. Adenylate cyclase is inhibited by acetylcholine M_2 receptors, noradrenaline α_2 receptors, and serotonin $5HT_1$ and $5HT_5$ receptors. Adenylate cyclase is activated by noradrenaline β receptors and serotonin $5HT_4$ and $5HT_6$ receptors. The increase in calcium elicited by glutamate can be enhanced by noradrenaline. All of these are second messengers that are involved in the instructive pathways, onto which the modulatory pathways may also converge.

14. Nerve Growth Factor (NGF)

Nerve growth factor has little effect on plasticity in the visual cortex of the cat. It does not affect the development of geniculocortical endings into ocular dominance columns (Cabelli et al., 1995; Silver et al., 2001), nor does the NGF receptor antagonist, trkA-IgG (Cabelli et al., 1997). Infusion of NGF into the visual cortex does not affect ocular dominance changes caused by monocular deprivation in kittens during the critical period (Galuske et al., 2000; Gillespie et al., 2000; Silver et al., 2001). This treatment does result in the lack of an orientation selectivity map for the deprived eye, presumably because the deprived eye no longer drives cortical cells (Galuske et al., 2000; Silver et al., 2001). Interestingly, the same treatment in adult animals leads to a paradoxical shift towards the deprived eye (Gu, Liu, & Cynader,1994; Galuske et al., 2000). Infusion of NGF into the ventricle can lead to a small reduction in the ocular dominance shift, which could be due to the activation of trkB receptors because of the high concentrations of NGF used (Camignoto, Canella, Candeo, Comelli, & Maffei, 1993). In any case, the results do not add up to a role for NGF in ocular dominance plasticity, particularly because the effects are more noticeable in adult cats than in kittens during the critical period. Results in the rat are different due to technical or species differences (see Daw, 2003).

15. Immune System Molecules

An intriguing finding about the relationship between immune system molecules and plasticity has come from Shatz and colleagues (Corriveau, Huh, & Shatz, 1998). They screened for genes that are expressed in the developing lateral geniculate nucleus during eye-specific layer formation and regulated by spontaneous action potentials in the retinogeniculate pathway. mRNAs coding for Class 1 major histocompatibility complex antigens (class 1 MHC) were found to be decreased in this screen. In mice mutant for class 1 MHC, the refinement of connections between retina and lateral geniculate nucleus was incomplete (Huh, Boulanger, Du, Riquelme, Brotz, & Shatz, 2000). The results from this study suggest that these molecules are located in or near the synapse in a position to affect the connections between cells. How this hypothesis fits with the molecules that have been found to be implicated in ocular dominance plasticity remains to be seen.

16. Different Mechanisms for Different Aspects of Plasticity

The discussion has until now been devoted entirely to mechanisms involved in the ocular dominance shift resulting from monocular deprivation. In many ways recovery from the effects of monocular deprivation is more important. The mechanisms for recovery have not been studied by many authors. Cyclic AMP response binding element is not involved in the recovery of binocularity when both eyes are opened after 6 days of monocular deprivation (Liao, Mower, Neve, Sato-Bigbee, & Ramoa, 2002), whereas it is involved in the initial ocular dominance shift. Phosphorylation of ERK occurs during monocular deprivation, whereas dephosphorylation occurs during recovery (Bittencourt-Navarette, Krahe, & Ramoa, 2004). These are the only two papers in the literature about mechanisms of binocular recovery.

The mechanism for the reverse ocular dominance shift produced by monocular deprivation in the presence of the GABA agonist muscimol is also different from that for the normal ocular dominance shift: the latter involves protein kinase A, whereas the former does not (Shimegi, Fischer, Yang, Sato, & Daw, 2003).

Another possibility that has not yet been studied is that different mechanisms play roles at different stages of the ocular dominance shift. There may be an initial stage with changes in phosphorylation at the postsynaptic density, followed by formation and degradation of synapses, followed by expansion and retraction of dendritic spines and axon terminals. Local protein synthesis may be involved in the early stages, and protein synthesis in the nucleus in the later stages. The reason that NMDA receptor antagonists have been implicated in all aspects of plasticity in the visual cortex is probably that they are on the pathway for all these changes. Further experiments will clearly be needed to work out whether other factors are involved in all these processes or in only some of them.

17. Summary

Putting all these results together, the general hypothesis in the field can be stated as follows (Fig. 11.11): Afferent activity that instructs ocular dominance changes reaches the visual cortex and activates NMDA and metabotropic

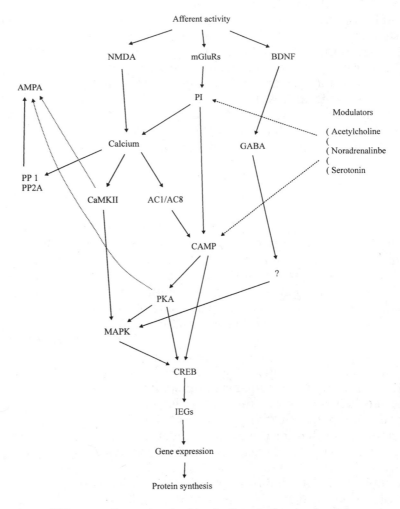

FIG. 11.11. Factors involved in plasticity in the visual cortex.

glutamate receptors. These in turn release calcium and activate phospho-inositides. Low levels of calcium affect calcineurin and high levels affect adenylyl cyclases and CaM kinase. Various pathways converge onto protein kinase A and MAP kinase, which in turn converge onto CREB. Cyclic AMP response binding element activates gene expression and protein synthesis. In parallel with this BDNF and GABA are activated.

However, this is a definite simplification of the steps involved. As pointed out above, some steps may act directly on AMPA receptors and NMDA receptors at the postsynaptic density to change the efficacy of the synapse. Others will act on protein synthesis for synapse, dendrite, and axon terminal production and degradation. There are feedback pathways: for example, activity affects BDNF and BDNF affects activity. Figure 11.11, as complicated as it is, is definitely incomplete.

References

Artola, A., Brocher, S., & Singer, W. (1990). Different voltage-dependent thresholds for inducing long-term depression and long-term potentiation in slices of rat visual cortex. *Nature, 347*, 69–72.

Bear, M. F., & Singer, W. (1986). Modulation of visual cortical plasticity by acetylcholine and noradrenaline. *Nature, 320*, 172–176.

Bear, M. F., Kleinschmidt, A., Gu, Q., & Singer, W. (1990). Disruption of experience dependent synaptic modifications in striate cortex by infusion of an NMDA receptor antagonist. *Journal of Neuroscience, 10*, 909–925.

Beaver, C. J., Ji, Q.-H., & Daw, N. W. (1999). Effect of the Group II metabotropic glutamate agonist, 2R,4R-APDC, varies with age, layer and visual experience in the visual cortex. *Journal of Neurophysiology, 82*, 86–93.

Beaver, C. J., Ji, Q.-H., Fischer, Q. S., & Daw, N. W. (2001). cAMP-dependent protein kinase mediates ocular dominance shifts in cat visual cortex. *Nature Neuroscience, 4*, 159–163.

Berardi, N., Pizzorusso, T., & Maffei, L. (2004). Extracellular matrix and visual cortical plasticity: freeing the synapse. *Neuron, 44*, 905–908.

Bittencourt-Navarrete, R. E., Krahe, T. E., & Ramoa, A. S. (2004). ERK phosphorylation during recovery from the effects of a brief period of monocular deprivation (MD). *Society for Neuroscience Abstracts,* 156.15.

Bode-Greuel, K. M., & Singer, W. (1988). Developmental changes of the distribution of binding sites for organic Ca++ channel blockers in cat visual cortex. *Brain Research, 70*, 266–275.

Cabelli, R. J., Hohn, A., & Shatz, C. J. (1995). Inhibition of ocular dominance column formation by infusion of NT-4/5 or BDNF. *Science, 267*, 1662–1666.

Cabelli, R. J., Shelton, D. L., Segal, R. A., & Shatz, C. J. (1997). Blockade of endogenous ligands of trkB inhibits formation of ocular dominance columns. *Neuron, 19*, 63–76.

Cancedda, L., Putignano, E., Impey, S., Maffei, L., Ratto, G. M., & Pizzorusso, T. (2003). Patterned vision causes CRE-mediated gene expression in the visual cortex through PKA and ERK. *Journal of Neuroscience, 23*, 7012–7020.

Cancedda, L., Putignano, E., Sale, A., Viegi, A., Berardi, N., & Maffei, L. (2004). Acceleration of visual system development by environmental enrichment. *Journal of Neuroscience, 24*, 4840–4848.

Carmignoto, G., & Vicini, S. (1992). Activity-dependent decrease in NMDA receptor responses during development of the visual cortex. *Science, 258*, 1007–1011.

Carmignoto, G., Canella, R., Candeo, P., Comelli, M. C., & Maffei, L. (1993). Effects of nerve growth factor on neuronal plasticity of the kitten visual cortex. *Journal of Physiology, 464*, 343–360.

Chen, L., Cooper, N. G. F., & Mower, G. D. (2000). Developmental changes in the expression of NMDA receptor subunits (NR1, NR2A, NR2B) in the cat visual cortex and the effects of dark rearing. *Molecular Brain Research, 78*, 196–200.

Coghlan, V. M., Perrino, B. A., Howard, M., Langeberg, L. K., Hicks, J. B., Gallatin, W. M., & Scott, J. D. (1995). Association of protein kinase A and protein phosphatase 2B with a common anchoring protein. *Science, 267*, 108–111.

Corriveau, R. A., Huh, G. S., & Shatz, C. J. (1998). Regulation of class I MHC gene expression in the developing and mature CNS by neural activity. *Neuron, 21*, 505–520.

Czepita, D., Reid, S. M., & Daw, N. W. (1994). Effect of longer periods of dark-rearing on NMDA receptors in cat visual cortex. *Journal of Neurophysiology, 72*, 1220–1226.

Daw, N. W. (2003). Mechanisms of plasticity in the visual cortex. In L. M. Chalupa & J. S. Werner (Eds.), *The visual neurosciences* (pp. 126–145). Cambridge: MIT Press.

Daw, N. W., & Beaver, C. J. (2001). Developmental changes and ocular dominance plasticity in the visual cortex. *Keio Journal of Medicine, 50*, 192–197.

Daw, N. W., & Reid, S. M. (1996). Role of metabotropic glutamate receptors in the cat visual cortex during development. *Journale de Physiologie (Paris), 90*, 173–177.

Daw, N. W., Gordon, B., Fox, K. D., Flavin, H. J., Kirsch, J. D., Beaver, C. J., Ji, Q.-H., Reid, S. M., & Czepita, D. (1999). Injection of MK-801 affects ocular dominance shifts more than visual activity. *Journal of Neurophysiology, 81*, 204–215.

Daw, N. W., Videen, T. O., Parkinson, D., & Rader, R. K. (1985). DSP-4 (*N*-(2-chloroethyl)-*N*-ethyl-2-bromobenzylamine) depletes noradrenaline in kitten visual cortex without altering the effects of visual deprivation. *Journal of Neuroscience, 5*, 1925–1933.

Di Cristo, G., Berardi, N., Cancedda, L., Pizzorusso, T., Putignano, E., Ratto, G. M., & Maffei, L. (2001). Requirement of ERK activation for visual cortical plasticity. *Science, 292*, 2337–2340.

Dudek, S. M., & Bear, M. F. (1989). A biochemical correlate of the critical period for synaptic modification in the visual cortex. *Science, 246*, 673–675.

Fagiolini, M., & Hensch, T. K. (2000). Inhibitory threshold for critical-period activation in primary visual cortex. *Nature, 404*, 183–186.

Fagiolini, M., Fritschy, J.-M., Low, K., Mohler, H., Rudolph, U., & Hensch, T. K. (2004). Specific GABA$_A$ circuits for visual cortical plasticity. *Science, 303*, 1681–1683.

Fagiolini, M., Katagiri, H., Miyamoto, H., Mori, H., Grant, S. N., Mishina, M., & Hensch, T. K. (2003). Separable features of visual cortical plasticity revealed by *N*-methyl-D-aspartate receptor 2A signaling. *Proceedings of the National Academy of Sciences of the United States of America, 100*, 2854–2859.

Feldman, D., Sherin, J. E., Press, W. A., & Bear, M. F. (1990). *N*-methyl-D-aspartate-evoked calcium uptake by kitten visual cortex maintained in vitro. *Experimental Brain Research, 80*, 252–259.

Fischer, Q. S., Beaver, C. J., Yang, Y., Rao, Y., Jacobsdottir, K., Storm, D. R., McKnight, G. S., & Daw, N. W. (2004). Requirement for the RIIβ isoform of PKA, but not calcium stimulated adenylyl cyclase, in visual cortical plasticity. *Journal of Neuroscience, 24*, 9049–9058.

Fischer, Q. S., Yang, Y., Beaver, C. J., & Daw, N. W. (2004). Activation of mGluR1 receptors contributes to ocular dominance plasticity. *Society for Neuroscience Abstracts*, 154.9.

Fischer, Q. S., Yang, Y. P., Jakobsdottir, K. B., McKnight, G. S., & Daw, N. W. (2003). Type II PKA and its localization by AKAP150 is crucial for ocular dominance plasticity in mice. *Society for Neuroscience Abstracts, 29*, 37.9.

Fox, K. D., Sato, H., & Daw, N. W. (1989). The location and function of NMDA receptors in cat and kitten visual cortex. *Journal of Neuroscience, 9*, 2443–2454.

Fox, K. D., Daw, N. W., Sato, H., & Czepita, D. (1992). The effect of visual experience on development of NMDA receptor synaptic transmission in kitten visual cortex. *Journal of Neuroscience, 12*, 2672–2684.

Frank, M. G., Issa, N. P., & Stryker, M. P. (2001). Sleep enhances plasticity in the developing visual cortex. *Neuron, 30*, 275–287.

Fregnac, Y., Shulz, D., Thorpe, S., & Bienenstock, E. (1992). Cellular analogs of visual cortical epigenesis I. Plasticity of orientation selectivity II. Plasticity of binocular integration. *Journal of Neuroscience, 12*, 1280–1300.

Galuske, R. W., Kim, D.-S., Castren, E., & Singer, W. (2000). Differential effects of neurotrophins on ocular dominance plasticity in developing and adult visual cortex. *European Journal of Neuroscience, 12*, 3315–3330.

Gianfranceschi, L., Siciliano, R., Walls, J., Morales, B., Kirkwood, A., Huang, Z. J., Tonegawa, S., & Maffei, L. (2003). Visual cortex is rescued from the effects of dark rearing by overexpression of BDNF. *Proceedings of the National Academy of Sciences of the United States of America, 100*, 12486–12491.

Gillespie, D. C., Crair, M. C., & Stryker, M. P. (2000). Neurotrophin 4/5 alters responses and blocks the effect of monocular deprivation in cat visual cortex during the critical period. *Journal of Neuroscience, 20*, 9174–9186.

Gordon, B., Allen, E. E., & Trombley, P. Q. (1988). The role of norepinephrine in plasticity of visual cortex. *Progress in Neurobiology, 30*, 171–191.

Gordon, B., Daw, N. W., & Parkinson, D. (1991). The effect of age on binding of MK-801 in the cat visual cortex. *Developmental Brain Research, 62*, 61–67.

Gordon, J. A., Cioffi, D., Silva, A. J., & Stryker, M. P. (1996). Deficient plasticity in the primary visual cortex of alpha-calcium/calmodulin-dependent protein kinase II mutant mice. *Neuron, 17*, 491–499.

Gu, Q. (2002). Neuromodulatory transmitter systems in the cortex and their role in cortical plasticity. *Neuroscience, 111*, 815–835.

Gu, Q., & Singer, W. (1993). Effects of intracortical infusion of anticholinergic drugs on neuronal plasticity in kitten striate cortex. *European Journal of Neuroscience, 5*, 475–485.

Gu, Q., & Singer, W. (1995). Involvement of serotonin in developmental plasticity of kitten visual cortex. *European Journal of Neuroscience, 7*, 1146–1153.

Gu, Q., Liu, Y., & Cynader, M. S. (1994). Nerve growth factor-induced ocular dominance plasticity in adult cat visual cortex. *Proceedings of the National Academy of Sciences of the United States of America, 91*, 8408–8412.

Hanover, J. L., Huang, Z. J., Tonegawa, S., & Stryker, M. P. (1999). Brain-derived neurotrophic factor overexpression induces precocious critical period in mouse visual cortex. *Journal of Neuroscience, 19*, RC40.

Hata, Y., Tsumoto, T., & Stryker, M. P. (1999). Selective pruning of more active afferents when cat visual cortex is pharmacologically inhibited. *Neuron, 22*, 375–381.

Hensch, T. K., & Stryker, M. P. (1996). Ocular dominance plasticity under metabotropic glutamate receptor blockade. *Science, 272*, 554–557.

Hensch, T. K., Gordon, J. A., Brandon, E. P., McKnight, G. S., Iderzda, R. L., & Stryker, M. P. (1998). Comparison of plasticity *in vivo* and *in vitro* in the developing visual cortex of normal and protein kinase A R1β -deficient mice. *Journal of Neuroscience, 18*, 2108–2117.

Huang, Z. J., Kirkwood, A., Pizzorusso, T., Porciatti, V., Morales, B., Bear, M. F., Maffei, L., & Tonegawa, S. (1999). BDNF regulates the maturation of inhibition and the critical period of plasticity in mouse visual cortex. *Cell, 98*, 739–755.

Huber, K. M., Sawtell, N. B., & Bear, M. F. (1998). Effects of the metabotropic glutamate receptor antagonist MCPG on phosphoinositide turnover and synaptic plasticity in visual cortex. *Journal of Neuroscience, 18*, 1–9.

Huh, G. S., Boulanger, L. M., Du, M., Riquelme, P. A., Brotz, M., & Shatz, C. J. (2000). Functional requirement for class I MHC in CNS development and plasticity. *Science, 290*, 2155–2159.

Imamura, K., Kasamatsu, T., Shirokawa, T., & Ohashi, T. (1999). Restoration of ocular dominance plasticity mediated by adenosine 3′,5′-monophosphate in adult visual cortex. *Proceedings of the Royal Society of London. Series B. Biological sciences, 266*, 1507–1516.

Jin, X.-T., Beaver, C. J., Ji, Q.-H., & Daw, N. W. (2001). Effect of the group I metabotropic glutamate agonist DHPG on the visual cortex. *Journal of Neurophysiology, 86*, 1622–1631.

Kasamatsu, T., & Pettigrew, J. D. (1979). Preservation of binocularity after monocular deprivation in the striate cortex of kittens treated with 6-hydroxydopamine. *Journal of Comparative Neurology, 185*, 139–162.

Kasamatsu, T., & Shirokawa, T. (1985). Involvement of β -adrenoceptors in the shift of ocular dominance and monocular deprivation. *Experimental Brain Research, 59*, 507–514.

Kleinschmidt, A., Bear, M. F., & Singer, W. (1987). Blockade of "NMDA" receptors disrupts experience-dependent plasticity of kitten striate cortex. *Science, 238*, 355–358.

Kohara, K., Kitamura, A., Morishima, M., & Tsumoto, T. (2001). Activity-dependent transfer of brain-derived neurotrophic factor to postsynaptic neurons. *Science, 291*, 2419–2423.

Lee, H.-K., Barbarosie, M., Kameyama, K., Bear, M. F., & Huganir, R. L. (2000). Regulation of distinct AMPA receptor phosphorylation sites during bidirectional synaptic plasticity. *Nature, 405*, 955–959.

Lee, W. C. A., & Nedivi, E. (2002). Extended plasticity of visual cortex in dark-reared animals may result from prolonged expression of cpg15-like genes. *Journal of Neuroscience, 22*, 1807–1815.

Liao, D. S., Mower, A. F., Neve, R. L., Sato-Bigbee, C., & Ramoa, A. S. (2002). Different mechanisms for loss and recovery of binocularity in the visual cortex. *Journal of Neuroscience, 22*, 9015–9023.

Lin, M. H., Takahashi, M. P., Takahashi, Y., & Tsumoto, T. (1994). Intracellular calcium increase induced by GABA in visual cortex of fetal and neonatal rats and its disappearance with development. *Neuroscience Research, 20*, 85–94.

Lisman, J. E. (1989). A mechanism for the Hebb and the anti-Hebb processes underlying learning and memory. *Proceedings of the National Academy of Sciences of the United States of America, 86*, 9574–9578.

Lisman, J. E. (2001). Three Ca2+ levels affect plasticity differently: the LTP zone, the LTD zone and no man's land. *Journal of Physiology, 532*, 285.

Mataga, N., Fujushima, S., Condie, B. G., & Hensch, T. K. (2001). Experience-dependent plasticity of mouse visual cortex in the absence of the neuronal activity-dependent marker egr1/zif268. *Journal of Neuroscience, 21*, 9724–9732.

Mataga, N., Mizuguchi, Y., & Hensch, T. K. (2004). Experience-dependent pruning of dendritic spines in visual cortex by tissue plasminogen activator. *Neuron, 44*, 1031–1041.

Mataga, N., Nagai, R., & Hensch, T. K. (2002). Permissive proteolytic activity for visual cortical plasticity. *Proceedings of the National Academy of Sciences of the United States of America, 99*, 7717–7721.

McCormick, D. A., & Prince, D. A. (1987). Post-natal development of electrophysiological properties of rat cerebral cortical pyramidal neurons. *Journal of Physiology, 383*, 743–762.

Mower, A. F., Liao, D. S., Nestler, E. J., Neve, R. L., & Ramoa, A. S. (2002). cAMP/Ca2+ response element-binding protein function is essential for ocular dominance plasticity. *Journal of Neuroscience, 22*, 2237–2245.

Mower, G. D., & Kaplan, I. V. (2002). Immediate early gene expression in the visual cortex of normal and dark reared cats: differences between fos and egr-1. *Molecular Brain Research, 105*, 157–160.

Muller, C. M., & Griesinger, C. B. (1998). Tissue plasminogen activator mediates reverse occlusion plasticity in visual cortex. *Nature Neuroscience, 1*, 47–53.

Pham, T. A., Impey, S., Storm, D. R., & Stryker, M. P. (1999). CRE-mediated gene transcription in neocortical neuronal plasticity during the developmental critical period. *Neuron, 22*, 63–72.

Pham, T. A., Rubenstein, J. L. R., Silva, A. J., Storm, D. R., & Stryker, M. P. (2001). The CRE/CREB pathway is transiently expressed in thalamic circuit development and contributes to refinement of retinogeniculate axons. *Neuron, 31*, 409–420.

Pizzorusso, T., Medini, P., Berardi, N., Chierzi, S., Fawcett, J. W., & Maffei, L. (2002). Reactivation of ocular dominance plasticity in the adult visual cortex. *Science, 298*, 1248–1251.

Pizzorusso, T., Ratto, G. M., Putignano, E., & Maffei, L. (2000). Brain-derived neurotrophic factor causes cAMP response element-binding protein phosphorylation in the absence of calcium increases in slices and cultured neurons from rat visual cortex. *Journal of Neuroscience, 20*, 2809–2816.

Prasad, S. S., Kojic, L. Z., Li, P., Mitchell, D. E., Hachisuka, A., Sawada, J., Gu, Q., & Cynader, M. S. (2002). Gene expression patterns during enhanced periods of visual cortical plasticity. *Neuroscience, 111*, 36–42.

Ramoa, A. S., Mower, A. F., Liao, D., & Jafri, S. I. A. (2001). Suppression of cortical NMDA receptor function prevents development of orientation selectivity in the primary visual cortex. *Journal of Neuroscience, 21*, 4299–4309.

Ramoa, A. S., Paradiso, M. A., & Freeman, R. D. (1988). Blockade of intracortical inhibition in kitten striate cortex: effects on receptive field properties and associated loss of ocular dominance plasticity. *Experimental Brain Research, 73*, 285–296.

Rao, Y., Fischer, Q. S., Yang, Y., McKnight, G. S., LaRue, A., & Daw, N. W. (2004). Reduced ocular dominance plasticity and long-term potentiation in developing visual cortex of RIIα mutant mice. *European Journal of Neuroscience, 20*, 837–842.

Reid, S. M., Daw, N. W., Gregory, D. S., & Flavin, H. J. (1996). cAMP levels increased by activation of metabotropic glutamate receptors correlate with visual plasticity. *Journal of Neuroscience, 16*, 7619–7626.

Reiter, H. O., & Stryker, M. P. (1988). Neural plasticity without postsynaptic action potentials: less-active inputs become dominant when kitten visual cortical cells are pharmacologically inhibited. *Proceedings of the National Academy of Sciences of the United States of America, 85*, 3623–3627.

Renger, J. J., Hartman, K. N., Tsuchimoto, Y., Yokoi, M., Nakanishi, S., & Hensch, T. K. (2002). Experience-dependent plasticity without long-term depression by type 2 metabotropic glutamate receptors in developing visual cortex. *Proceedings of the National Academy of Sciences of the United States of America, 99*, 1041–1046.

Roberts, E. B., & Ramoa, A. S. (1999). Enhanced NR2A subunit expression and decreased NMDA receptor decay time at the onset of ocular dominance plasticity. *Journal of Neurophysiology, 81*, 2587–2591.

Roberts, E. B., Meredith, M. A., & Ramoa, A. S. (1998). Suppression of NMDA receptor function using antisense DNA blocks ocular dominance plasticity while preserving visual responses. *Journal of Neurophysiology, 80*, 1021–1032.

Sengpiel, F., & Kind, P. C. (2002). The role of activity in development of the visual system. *Current Biology, 12*, R818–R828.

Shatz, C. J., & Stryker, M. P. (1988). Prenatal tetrodotoxin infusion blocks segregation of retinogeniculate afferents. *Science, 242*, 87–89.

Shimegi, S., Fischer, Q. S., Yang, Y., Sato, H., & Daw, N. W. (2003). Blockade of cyclic AMP-dependent protein kinase does not prevent the reverse ocular dominance shift in the kitten visual cortex. *Journal of Neurophysiology, 90*, 4027–4032.

Silver, M. A., & Stryker, M. P. (2001). TrkB-like immunoreactivity is present on geniculocortical afferents in layer IV of kitten primary visual cortex. *Journal of Comparative Neurology, 436*, 391–398.

Silver, M. A., Fagiolini, M., Gillespie, D. C., Howe, C. L., Frank, M. G., Issa, N. P., Antonini, A., & Stryker, M. P. (2001). Infusion of nerve growth factor (NGF) into kitten visual cortex increases immunoreactivity for NGF, NGF receptors, and choline acetyltransferase in basal forebrain without affecting ocular dominance plasticity or column development. *Neuroscience, 108*, 569–585.

Taha, S., & Stryker, M. P. (2002). Rapid ocular dominance plasticity requires cortical but not geniculate protein synthesis. *Neuron, 34*, 425–436.

Taha, S., Hanover, J. L., Silva, A. J., & Stryker, M. P. (2002). Autophosphorylation of alpha CaMKII is required for ocular dominance plasticity. *Neuron, 36*, 483–491.

Trachtenberg, J. T., Trepel, C., & Stryker, M. P. (2000). Rapid extragranular plasticity in the absence of thalamocortical plasticity in the developing primary visual cortex. *Science, 287*, 2029–2031.

Wong, R. L., Meister, M., & Shatz, C. J. (1993). Transient period of correlated bursting activity during development of the mammalian retina. *Neuron, 11*, 923–938.

Yang, Y., Fischer, Q. S., & Daw, N. W. (2003). Inhibition mediated by $GABA_B$ receptors modulates ocular dominance plasticity in cat. *Society for Neuroscience Abstracts, 29*, 37.10.

Yang, Y., Fischer, Q. S., Zhang, Y., Baumgartel, K., Mansuy, I. M., & Daw, N. W. (2005). Reversible blockade of experience-dependent plasticity by calcineurin in mouse visual cortex. *Nature Neuroscience, 8*, 791–796.

Yang, C., Silver, B., Ellis, S. R., & Mower, G. D. (2001). Bidirectional regulation of mitochondrial gene expression during developmental neuroplasticity of visual cortex. *Biochemical and Biophysical Research Communications, 287*, 1070–1074.

Yang, S. N., Tang, Y. -G., & Zucker, R. S. (1999). Selective induction of LTP and LTD by postsynaptic $[Ca^{2+}]_i$ elevation. *Journal of Neurophysiology, 81*, 781–787.

Yang, C., Zheng, Y. T., Li, G. Y., & Mower, G. D. (2002). Identification of MUNC13-3 as a candidate gene for critical period neuroplasticity in visual cortex. *Journal of Neuroscience, 22*, 8614–8618.

Yuste, R. & Katz, L. C. (1991). Control of postsynaptic Ca++ influx in developing neocortex by excitatory and inhibitory neurotransmitters. *Neuron, 6*, 333–344.

12

Long-Term Potentiation and Long-Term Depression as Early Steps in Ocular Dominance Plasticity

Most investigators would consider long-term potentiation (LTP) and long-term depression (LTD) to be early steps in ocular dominance plasticity and in other plastic changes in the visual cortex. Long-term potentiation is the strengthening of a synapse that follows a high-frequency stimulus, which results in the postsynaptic potential produced by stimulation of the presynaptic cell getting larger. Long-term depression is the weakening of a synapse that follows a low-frequency stimulus that results in the postsynaptic potential getting smaller. Long-term potentiation and LTD have been extensively studied in both the hippocampus and visual cortex, so the mechanisms are fairly well understood.

Long-term potentiation can also be produced by stimulating the presynaptic cell to produce an excitatory postsynaptic potential (EPSP) in the postsynaptic cell, followed by stimulation of the postsynaptic cell to produce an action potential after an interval of 3 to 15 ms (Feldman, 2000). Similarly, LTD can be produced by stimulation of the postsynaptic cell followed by stimulation of the presynaptic cell after an interval of 0 to 100 ms. This is known as spike-timing LTP or LTD. Because the range of intervals that produces depression is long and the range of intervals that produces potentiation is short, firing that is not correlated between two inputs will lead to depression rather than potentiation. Thus, spontaneous activity from the deprived eye, which is not correlated with activity driven by the nondeprived eye, will lead to depression at the deprived-eye synapse and potentiation at the nondeprived eye synapse. Consequently, spike-timing LTD and LTP accounts neatly for what happens during monocular deprivation.

Long-term changes produced by various frequencies can be related to spike-timing long-term changes if additional assumptions are adopted (Sjostrom, Turrigiano, & Nelson, 2001). One assumption is that only the nearest-spike interactions are counted. Another is that spike interactions producing LTP win out over spike interactions producing LTD. At low frequencies of stimulation, the interval will be long, which will produce LTD rather than LTP. At high frequencies of stimulation, the interval will be short, and LTP will win out. This model has been used to fit the data from long-term spike-timing results to data from various constant frequencies of stimulation, and data from random firing in pairs of layer V neurons in the visual cortex. The predictions from the spike-timing results fit the results from various frequencies of stimulation and random firing very well.

Long-term potentiation can also be produced by coupling stimulation of the presynaptic neuron with depolarization of the postsynaptic neuron to 0 mV, and LTD by coupling stimulation of the presynaptic neuron with depolarization of the postsynaptic neuron to −50 mV. The hypothesis is that a small amount of calcium enters the cell at −50mV triggering a protein phosphatase cascade, and a large amount of calcium enters at 0 mV triggering a protein kinase cascade.

Interestingly, receptive field changes in the cortex can be produced by pairing stimulation of one eye with polarization of the cell; ocular dominance changes, orientation changes, and the distribution of ON and OFF responses can all be altered in this way (see Chapter 11; Fig. 12.1; Fregnac & Shulz, 1999). If stimulation of one eye is paired with depolarization of a cell in the

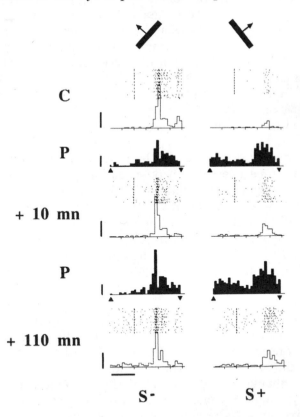

FIG. 12.1. Long-lasting modification of orientation preference when the nonpreferred stimulus (a horizontal bar moving upwards) is paired with depolarization of the cell and the preferred stimulus (a vertical bar moving to the right) is paired with hyperpolarization of the cell. Dots represent timing of action potentials from individual repeats of the stimulus. [Reprinted with permission from Fregnac, Y., & Shulz, D. E. (1999). *Journal of Neurobiology, 41*, 69–82.]

visual cortex, the preferred response of the cell will change to favor the eye being stimulated (ocular dominance) and the orientation of the stimulus used in the experiment. Pairing with hyperpolarization leads to changes that favor a stronger response to the nonstimulated eye and away from the orientation of the stimulus.

Here also the timing of the visual stimulation relative to the electrical stimulation is important (Schuett, Bonhoeffer, & Hubener, 2001). If the cortex is activated first visually then electrically, a shift that favors responding to the orientation of the visual stimulus is seen. If the cortex is activated first electrically then visually, the cell responds less well to the orientation of the visual stimulus. These effects occur primarily away from pinwheel centers, where the same preferred orientation occupies a relatively large area.

An underlying and usually unstated assumption is that LTP leads to the growth of synapses, and LTD leads to the retraction and elimination of synapses. This assumption needs to be proved by a direct experiment in which one watches an identified synapse, applies a high frequency stimulus to the presynaptic cell and sees the synapse grow, then applies a low frequency stimulus and sees the synapse retract. Assuming that the size of dendritic spines is related to the size of the synapses on them, then the size of synapses is indeed reduced by stimuli that produce LTD in the hippocampus (see Zhou, Homma, & Poo, 2004). In the visual system, spine motility is increased by monocular deprivation, while the average length, size of neck, and size of head are not changed (Oray, Majewska, & Sur, 2004). Presumably, some spines fed by afferents from the deprived eye are reduced in size and others fed by the nondeprived eye are increased in size, but this has not been proved directly.

Long-term potentiation and LTD are often stated to be a bidirectional process. This is a useful concept in that the early steps in both processes may involve the same substances, such as N-methyl-D-aspartate (NMDA) receptors and calcium. However, later steps involve different second messengers. Moreover, the formation of a synapse has to include the creation of a number of synaptic proteins, presumably under the control of one set of transcription factors, whereas the elimination of a synapse has to include the degradation of these proteins, which may be controlled by another set of transcription factors. Most current hypotheses suggest that there is a divergence of pathways controlled by different levels of intracellular calcium, with LTD leading to a low level of calcium which activates one set of second messengers and LTP leading to a high level of calcium which activates another set.

This separation of processes is illustrated particularly well by effects on the 1-amino-3-hydroxy-5-methyl-4-isoxazole propionic acid (AMPA) receptor GluR1 (Lee, Barbarosie, Kameyama, Bear, & Huganir, 2000). Phosphorylation of this receptor, leading to its activation at the postsynaptic density, is related to LTP, and dephosphorylation, leading to its inactivation, is related to LTD. The receptor can exist in three states: potentiated, normal. and depressed. Phosphorylation at serine 845 by protein kinase A (PKA) takes it from the depressed state to the normal one. Phosphorylation at serine 831 by calcium/calmodulin kinase II (CaMKII) takes it from the normal state to the potentiated one. Either protein phosphatase 1 or protein phosphatase 2A will take the receptor from the potentiated state to the normal state, or from the normal state to the depressed state. Thus, while phosphorylation of a single receptor is related to both LTP and LTD, the two processes have different phosphorylation sites and different mechanisms.

In ocular dominance plasticity, the elimination of synapses from the deprived eye comes before the growth of synapses from the nondeprived eye. Physiological recordings show that responses to the deprived eye can disappear over 12 h with little increase in responses from the nondeprived eye (Mioche & Singer, 1989). When the deprived eye is reopened and the nondeprived eye closed (reverse suture), responses to the newly closed eye disappear before responses to the newly opened eye appear. These results are confirmed by anatomical studies. After 4 days of monocular deprivation, geniculocortical terminals from the deprived eye are shrunken, with little change in the terminals from the nondeprived eye (Antonini & Stryker, 1993). Similarly, the early stages of monocular deprivation mimic LTD (Heynen, Yoon, Liu, Chung, Huganir, & Bear, 2003), and a decrease in the visually evoked response from the deprived eye is seen before an increase in the visually evoked response from the nondeprived eye (Frenkel & Bear, 2004). GluR1 is dephosphorylated at serine 845 in the contralateral cortex of rats after one eye is deprived for 24 h, but phosphorylation at serine 831 is not altered. Monocular deprivation also partially occludes LTD when subsequent attempts are made to induce this *in vitro*. All these results suggest that synapses from the deprived eye onto cells in the cortex have to be vacated before input from the nondeprived eye can occupy them.

It is tempting to suggest from these results that ocular dominance plasticity is most strongly related to LTD, and there are several cases where this is so. One example involves knockout of the RIIβ subunit of protein kinase A, where ocular dominance plasticity and LTD are absent, but LTP is present (Fischer, Beaver, Yang, Rao, Jacobsdottir, Storm, McKnight, & Daw, 2004). Another example involves knockout of the A kinase anchoring protein AKAP 79/150 which has a similar result (Fischer, Yang, Jakobsdottir, McKnight, & Daw, 2003). With knockout of the GABA synthesizing enzyme GAD65, ocular dominance plasticity and LTD are again both absent (Hensch, Fagiolini, Mataga, Stryker, Baekkeskov, & Kash, 1998; Choi, Morales, Lee, & Kirkwood, 2002). If protein kinase G inhibitors are used, the reverse occurs—ocular dominance plasticity and LTD are present, but LTP is absent (Beaver, Ji, Fischer, & Daw, 2001; Liu, Rao, & Daw, 2003).

Unfortunately, there are several counterexamples where ocular dominance plasticity is not related to LTD (see Table 12.1). Activation of the metabotropic glutamate receptor mGluR2 produces LTD, and mice mutant for mGluR2 do not have LTD, but do have ocular dominance plasticity (Renger, Hartman, Tsuchimoto, Yokoi, Nakanishi, & Hensch, 2002). Mice mutant for the RIβ subunit of PKA also lack LTD but have ocular dominance plasticity (Hensch, Gordon, Brandon, McKnight, Idzerda, & Stryker, 1998). Moreover, in mice mutant for the RIIα subunit of PKA, LTD is not significantly reduced, but ocular dominance plasticity is (Rao, Fischer, Yang, McKnight, LaRue, & Daw, 2004). Furthermore, application of BDNF produces LTP and blocks

TABLE 12.1. Correlation of Ocular Dominance Plasticity, Long-term Potentiation, and Long-term Depression

Treatment	Ocular dominance plasticity	Long-term potentiation	Long-term depression
PKA antagonist	Absent	Absent	Absent
NMDA antagonist	Absent	Absent	Absent
GAD65 knockout	Absent	Present	Absent
PKA RIIβ	Absent	Present	Absent
MAP kinase inhibitors	Absent	Absent	Not tested
PKA RIIα knockout	Reduced	Reduced	Present
AKAP150 knockout	Reduced	Present	Absent
PKA RIβ knockout	Present	Some forms absent	Absent
PKG antagonist	Present	Absent	Present
mGluR2 knockout	Present	Not tested	Absent
BDNF application/overexpression	Early	Increased	Reduced

LTD (Akaneya, Tsumoto, & Hatanaka, 1996; Akaneya, Tsumoto, Kinoshita, & Hatanaka, 1997), whereas overexpression of BDNF induces ocular dominance plasticity early (Hanover, Huang, Tonegawa, & Stryker, 1999). This suggests that the molecular mechanisms for ocular dominance plasticity and LTD are not always the same, nor are they the same for LTP.

The one general rule that does seem to apply is that if both LTP and LTD are abolished, then ocular dominance plasticity is also abolished. There are now two well-established examples of this rule using PKA antagonists and NMDA antagonists. The NMDA antagonist D-amino-phosphonovalerate (APV) has been known for some time to affect plasticity in the hippocampus, and it also abolishes ocular dominance plasticity in the visual cortex (Bear, Kleinschmidt, Gu, & Singer, 1990). This is a specific effect on plasticity and is not due simply to a reduction in the activity reaching the cortex (Daw, Gordon, Fox, Flavin, Kirsch, Beaver, Ji, Reid, & Czepita, 1999). D-Amino-phosphonovalerate also abolishes LTP (Artola & Singer, 1987) and LTD (Dudek & Bear, 1992). Another molecule known to be involved in plasticity in the hippocampus and *Drosophila* is PKA. Antagonists to PKA also abolish ocular dominance plasticity (Beaver et al., 2001), LTP, and LTD (Liu et al., 2003).

However, the ocular dominance plasticity results that have been cited so far are all results from recording a number of single cells from all layers of the visual cortex. The LTP and LTD results nearly all come from stimulation of layer IV with recordings of field potentials in layers II and III. The lack of correlation may therefore occur because there are different mechanisms of plasticity in different layers. To test this hypothesis, we decided to record single cells in cortical slices by making whole cell recordings in various layers, and stimulating in a way that mimicked the predominant flow of information in the cortex; that is, stimulating white matter for recordings in layer IV, layer IV for recordings in layers II and III, and layers II and III for recordings in layers V and VI (Lund & Boothe, 1975). As a first step, we compared

TABLE 12.2. Variation of Long-term Potentiation with Layer

Treatment	II/III	V	VI
Control	Potentiation 234 ± 13%	Potentiation 175 ± 9%	Potentiation 189 ± 9%
NMDA antagonist	No change 93 ± 4%	Depression 84 ± 2%	Potentiation 169 ± 4%
mGluR1 antagonist	Reduced potentiation 134 ± 4%	Reduced potentiation 134 ± 3%	No change 111 ± 3%
MGluR5 antagonist	Reduced potentiation 170 ± 2%	No change 103 ± 2%	Enhanced potentiation 309 ± 8%

the effects of the NMDA antagonist APV with those of various metabotropic glutamate receptor antagonists, bathing the whole slice with the antagonists because there is considerable information on the laminar distribution of these receptors (Reid & Daw, 1997; Wang, Jin & Daw, 1998; Beaver, Ji, & Daw, 1999; Jin, Beaver, Ji, & Daw, 2001).

The results for LTP elicited by theta burst stimulation are shown in Table 12.2 (Wang & Daw, 2003). Essentially, LTP in layers II and III depends on NMDA receptors and partially on the mGluR1 receptor. Long-term potentiation in layer V depends on NMDA receptors and mGluR5 and partially on mGluR1. Long-term potentiation in layer VI depends on mGluR1 but not on NMDA receptors, and the mGluR5 antagonist produces an enhanced potentiation.

The results for LTD elicited by low-frequency stimulation of 1 Hz for 10 min are shown in Table 12.3 (Rao & Daw, 2004). Essentially, LTD in layers II/III and V depends on NMDA receptors but not on mGluR receptors.

TABLE 12.3. Variation of Long-term Depression with Layer

Treatment	II/III	V	VI
Control	Depression 70 ± 5%	Depression 63 ± 7%	Depression 65 ± 7%
NMDA antagonist	No change 93 ± 6%	No change 103 ± 9%	Depression 77 ± 5%
mGluR antagonist	Depression 70 ± 3%	Depression 71 ± 7%	No change 94 ± 10%
GDP-β-S			Reduced depression 80 ± 5%
Group II mGluR antagonist			Depression 55 ± 8%
Group I mGluR antagonist			No change 93 ± 5%

241

*LONG-TERM
POTENTIATION
AND
LONG-TERM
DEPRESSION AS
EARLY STEPS IN
OCULAR
DOMINANCE
PLASTICITY*

Long-term depression in layer VI, on the other hand, depends on mGluR receptors, probably group I mGluRs, but not on NMDA receptors. Thus, for both LTP and LTD NMDA receptors play some role in layers II/III and V, but none in layer VI, whereas metabotropic glutamate receptors play a role in layer VI, but little in layers II/III and V.

The relationship between ocular dominance plasticity, LTP, and LTD is therefore complicated. It is clear that most comparisons so far have involved apples and oranges: ocular dominance plasticity measured in all layers compared with LTP and LTD measured with field potentials in layers II and III. However, it is hard to know how to make a direct comparison. There are different ways of eliciting LTP and LTD, as described above. Which should one use? Field potentials are commonly measured for LTP and LTD because the techniques are easy. It would be better to use whole-cell recordings with stimulation of a single input to that cell, but technically that is much more difficult, and how would one measure the corresponding ocular dominance plasticity? The best solution would seem to be to use ocular dominance plasticity itself to test mechanisms of ocular dominance plasticity, particularly because this is now easily done with knockout mice when available. However, this comment should not detract from all the experiments that have been done showing mechanisms of LTP plasticity that have subsequently also been shown to be mechanisms of ocular dominance plasticity.

References

Akaneya, Y., Tsumoto, T., & Hatanaka, Y. (1996). Brain-derived neurotrophic factor blocks long-term depression in rat visual cortex. *Journal of Neurophysiology, 76*, 4198–4201.

Akaneya, Y., Tsumoto, T., Kinoshita, S., & Hatanaka, Y. (1997). Brain-derived neurotrophic factor enhances long-term potentiation in rat visual cortex. *Journal of Neuroscience, 17*, 6707–6716.

Antonini, A., & Stryker, M. P. (1993). Rapid remodelling of axonal arbors in the visual cortex. *Science, 260*, 1819–1821.

Artola, A., & Singer, W. (1987). Long-term potentiation and NMDA receptors in rat visual cortex. *Nature, 330*, 649–652.

Bear, M. F., Kleinschmidt, A., Gu, Q., & Singer, W. (1990). Disruption of experience dependent synaptic modifications in striate cortex by infusion of an NMDA receptor antagonist. *Journal of Neuroscience, 10*, 909–925.

Beaver, C. J., Ji, Q. -H., & Daw, N. W. (1999). Effect of the Group II metabotropic glutamate agonist, 2R,4R-APDC, varies with age, layer and visual experience in the visual cortex. *Journal of Neurophysiology, 82*, 86–93.

Beaver, C. J., Ji, Q. -H., Fischer, Q. S., & Daw, N. W. (2001). cAMP-dependent protein kinase mediates ocular dominance shifts in cat visual cortex. *Nature Neuroscience, 4*, 159–163.

Choi, S. Y., Morales, B., Lee, H. K., & Kirkwood, A. (2002). Absence of long-term depression in the visual cortex of glutamic acid decarboxylase-65 knock-out mice. *Journal of Neuroscience, 22*, 5271–5276.

Daw, N. W., Gordon, B., Fox, K. D., Flavin, H. J., Kirsch, J. D., Beaver, C. J., Ji, Q. -H., Reid, S. M., & Czepita, D. (1999). Injection of MK-801 affects ocular dominance shifts more than visual activity. *Journal of Neurophysiology, 81*, 204–215.

Dudek, S. M., & Bear, M. F. (1992). Homosynaptic long-term depression in area CA1 of hippocampus and effects of N-methyl-D-aspartate receptor blockade. *Proceedings of the National Academy of Sciences of the United States of America, 89*, 4363–4367.

Feldman, D. E. (2000). Timing-based LTP and LTD at vertical inputs to layer II/III pyramidal cells in rat barrel cortex. *Neuron, 27*, 45–56.

Fischer, Q. S., Beaver, C. J., Yang, Y., Rao, Y., Jacobsdottir, K., Storm, D. R., McKnight, G. S., & Daw, N. W. (2004). Requirement for the RII isoform of PKA, but not calcium stimulated adenylyl cyclase, in visual cortical plasticity. *Journal of Neuroscience, 24*, 9049–9058.

Fischer, Q. S., Yang, Y. P., Jakobsdottir, K. B., McKnight, G. S., & Daw, N. W. (2003). Type II PKA and its localization by AKAP150 is crucial for ocular dominance plasticity in mice. *Society for Neuroscience Abstracts, 29*, 37.9.

Fregnac, Y., & Schulz, D. E. (1999). Activity-dependent regulation of receptive field properties of cat area 17 by supervised Hebbian learning. *Journal of Neurobiology, 41*, 69–82.

Frenkel, M. Y., & Bear, M. F. (2004). How monocular deprivation shifts ocular dominance in visual cortex of young mice. *Neuron, 44*, 1–20.

Hanover, J. L., Huang, Z. J., Tonegawa, S., & Stryker, M. P. (1999). Brain-derived neurotrophic factor overexpression induces precocious critical period in mouse visual cortex. *Journal of Neuroscience, 19*, RC40.

Hensch, T. K., Fagiolini, M., Mataga, N., Stryker, M. P., Baekkeskov, S., & Kash, S. F. (1998). Local GABA circuit control of experience-dependent plasticity in developing visual cortex. *Science, 282*, 1504–1508.

Hensch, T. K., Gordon, J. A., Brandon, E. P., McKnight, G. S., Idzerda, R. L., & Stryker, M. P. (1998). Comparison of plasticity *in vivo* and *in vitro* in the developing visual cortex of normal and protein kinase A R1β -deficient mice. *Journal of Neuroscience, 18*, 2108–2117.

Heynen, A. J., Yoon, B. -J., Liu, C. -H., Chung, H. J., Huganir, R. L., & Bear, M. F. (2003). Molecular mechanism for loss of visual cortical responsiveness following brief monocular deprivation. *Nature Neuroscience, 6*, 854–862.

Jin, X. -T., Beaver, C. J., Ji, Q. -H., & Daw, N. W. (2001). Effect of the group I metabotropic glutamate agonist DHPG on the visual cortex. *Journal of Neurophysiology, 86*, 1622–1631.

Lee, H. -K., Barbarosie, M., Kameyama, K., Bear, M. F., & Huganir, R. L. (2000). Regulation of distinct AMPA receptor phosphorylation sites during bidirectional synaptic plasticity. *Nature, 405*, 955–959.

Liu, S., Rao, Y., & Daw, N. W. (2003). Roles of protein kinase A and protein kinase G in synaptic plasticity in the visual cortex. *Cerebral Cortex, 13*, 864–869.

Lund, J. S., & Boothe, R. G. (1975). Interlaminar connections and pyramidal neuron organisation in the visual cortex, area 17, of the macaque monkey. *Journal of Comparative Neurology, 159*, 305–334.

Mioche, L., & Singer, W. (1989). Chronic recordings from single sites of kitten striate cortex during experience-dependant modifications of receptive field properties. *Journal of Neurophysiology, 62*, 185–197.

Oray, S., Majewska, A., & Sur, M. (2004). Dendritic spine dynamics are regulated by monocular deprivation and extracellular matrix degradation. *Neuron, 44*, 1021–1030.

Rao, Y., & Daw, N. W. (2004). Layer variations of long-term depression in rat visual cortex. *Journal of Neurophysiology, 92*, 2652–2658.

Rao, Y., Fischer, Q. S., Yang, Y., McKnight, G. S., LaRue, A., & Daw, N. W. (2004). Reduced ocular dominance plasticity and long-term potentiation in developing visual cortex of RIIα mutant mice. *European Journal of Neuroscience, 20*, 837–842.

Reid, S. M., & Daw, N. W. (1997). Activation of metabotropic glutamate receptors has different effects in different layers of cat visual cortex. *Visual Neuroscience, 14*, 83–88.

Renger, J. J., Hartman, K. N., Tsuchimoto, Y., Yokoi, M., Nakanishi, S., & Hensch, T. K. (2002). Experience-dependent plasticity without long-term depression by type 2 metabotropic glutamate receptors in developing visual cortex. *Proceedings of the National Academy of Sciences of the United States of America, 99*, 1041–1046.

Schuett, S., Bonhoeffer, T., & Hubener, M. (2001). Pairing-induced changes of orientation maps in cat visual cortex. *Neuron, 32*, 325–337.

Sjostrom, P. J., Turrigiano, G. G., & Nelson, S. B. (2001). Rate, timing and cooperativity jointly determine cortical synaptic plasticity. *Neuron, 32*, 1149–1164.

Wang, X.-F., & Daw, N. W. (2003). Long-term potentiation varies with layer in rat visual cortex. *Brain Research, 989*, 26–34.

Wang, X.-F., Jin, X.-T., & Daw, N. W. (1998). The effect of ACPD on the responses to NMDA and AMPA varies with layer in slices of rat visual cortex. *Brain Research, 812*, 186–192.

Zhou, Q., Homma, K. J., & Poo, M. -M. (2004). Shrinkage of dendritic spines associated with long-term depression of hippocampal synapses. *Neuron, 44*, 749–757.

13

Deprivation Myopia and Emmetropization

In Chapter 6 it was established that the eyeball grows in most people to be the correct size for the image to be in focus on the retina. This process is called *emmetropization* and it is very precise, requiring a tolerance of 2% in matching eye length to focal length. Many infants are born hyperopic and become emmetropic by 2 to 3 years of age. Some are born emmetropic and become myopic with age; that is, their eyeballs are too large for the power of the lens and the cornea, so that the image falls in front of the retina. A few are born myopic and this is a condition that needs to be reversed before reaching young adulthood because the eyeball can grow, but it cannot shrink.

The process of emmetropization requires a focused image on the retina. This point was underlined by a passing observation made by Hubel, Wiesel, and LeVay (1975) in their work on monocular deprivation. In addition to the effects of monocular deprivation on the visual cortex, they discovered that the eyeball of the deprived eye was longer than normal (Fig. 13.1). The difference in length was over 1 mm and the coating of the eyeball (sclera) on the posterior surface was thinned (Wiesel & Raviola, 1977). The effect was greater in young animals and persisted for years after opening the eye again. When both eyes were closed, elongation of the eyeball was found in both eyes. Elongation of the eyeball depended on the diffusion of the image by the lid suture, rather than some mechanical effect of the lid suture on the eyeball, because the eyeballs were the same size when an animal with one eye closed was reared in the dark (Raviola & Wiesel, 1985). Thus, the focused image on the retina stops the eyeball from growing beyond the appropriate size. Disruption of emmetropization by diffusion of the image on the retina is called *form-deprivation myopia*.

A diffused image also causes myopia in humans. The largest study compared 73 patients with a variety of binocular visual abnormalities that prevented a clear image on the retina to 12,000 normal subjects (Rabin, van Sluyters, & Malach, 1981). The patients with binocular abnormalities were significantly more myopic (Fig. 13.2). Seven patients with monocular visual anomalies were also more myopic in the affected eye. Another study

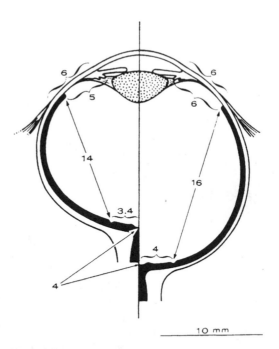

FIG. 13.1. Measurements illustrating the effects of neonatal lid fusion on various eye dimensions. Normal eye on the left, deprived eye on the right. The temporal halves of each retina are shown. Measurements in millimeters. Eyelids sutured from 2 weeks to 18 months of age. [Reprinted with permission from Wiesel, T. N., & Raviola, E. (1977). *Nature, 266*, 66–68. Copyright 1977 MacMillan Magazines Limited.]

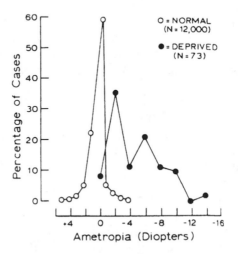

FIG. 13.2. Refractive error in normal and binocularly deprived eyes. The distribution of ametropia in binocularly deprived subjects is based on data from the more hyperopic of each subject's two eyes. [Reprinted with permission from Rabin, J., et al. (1981). *Investigative Ophthalmology and Visual Science, 20*, 561–564.]

compared a pair of twins, one of whom had a congenital lens opacity (Johnson, Post, Chalupa, & Lee, 1982). The eyeball was 2 mm longer in the deprived eye of that twin, while the eyeballs of the normal twin differed by less than 0.2 mm. While various different theories have been proposed to account for these results, the consensus today is that the important factor in emmetropization is a clear image on the retina.

Control of emmetropization involves communication of signals from the retina to the growing wall of the eyeball. Form-deprivation myopia occurs in chicks and *Macacca mulatta* after the optic nerve is cut (Troilo, Gottlieb, & Wallman, 1987; Wildsoet & Pettigrew, 1988; Raviola & Wiesel, 1985), and in chicks and tree shrews when signals are prevented from reaching the central nervous system by blocking activity in retinal ganglion cells (Norton, Essinger, & McBrien, 1994; McBrien, Moghaddam, Cottriall, Leech, & Cornell, 1995). Thus, some signals affecting growth of the eyeball must emanate within the retina from bipolar or amacrine cells; signals from ganglion cells going to the central visual system are not necessary.

A dramatic illustration of local control is provided by experiments in chicks wearing translucent occluders placed so that the image is blurred on *part* of the retina (Wallman, Gottlieb, Rajaram, & Fugate-Wentzek, 1987). The sclera grows so that the part of the eyeball with a diffused image becomes myopic (the eyeball is elongated), while the part of the eyeball with a clear image remains emmetropic (Fig. 13.3). Refraction also varies from one part of the retina to another in normal animals. For example, in pigeons the upper part of the eyeball, which looks at the ground, is myopic in comparison with the lower part of the eyeball, which looks at more distant objects (Fitzke, Hayes, Hodos, Holden, & Low, 1985). Local control of the size of the eyeball provides a mechanism to keep different parts of the retina in focus for objects at different distances, where the animal habitually looks at objects at different distances in different parts of the field of view.

Form-deprivation myopia implies a process of emmetropization, but does not prove it. For proof, one needs to show that the system becomes emmetropic after it is disturbed. Emmetropization as an active process is most easily studied in chicks because their eyes show substantial growth over the first few weeks of life. Eyes covered with a negative lens grow more than usual, and eyes covered with a positive lens grow less than usual (Schaeffel, Glasser, & Howland, 1988; Irving, Sivak, & Callender, 1992). When the lenses are taken off, the reverse occurs. Moreover, chicks that are reared with translucent occluders to produce form-deprivation myopia become emmetropic after the occluders are removed (Troilo, 1990; see Fig. 13.4). In all cases, the growth of the eyeball tends to compensate for the treatment so that the image becomes focused on the retina.

There is a critical period for these changes in eye length, just as there is for the effects of visual deprivation in the visual cortex. This has been most carefully studied in the tree shrew, where the eyeball has a rapid period of growth between birth and 4 weeks of age, followed by slower growth to 10 weeks of age (Siegwart & Norton, 1998). The susceptibility to myopia in response to form deprivation is highest at 5 to 8 weeks of age, but there is still some susceptibility at 10 to 13 weeks, after the eyeball normally stops growing (Fig. 13.5).

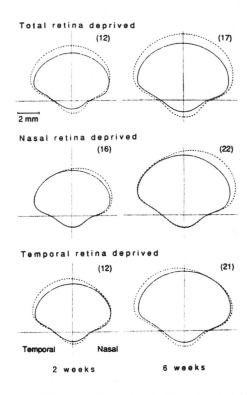

FIG. 13.3. Effect on the shape of the eye of form-deprivation of part of the retina. When the nasal retina is deprived, this part of the eyeball grows, and when the temporal retina is deprived, that part of the eyeball grows. *Solid lines* show normal eyeballs and *interrupted lines* deprived eyeballs. Results represent the average of a number of eyeballs, with the numbers given in parentheses. [Reprinted with permission from Wallman, J., et al. (1987). *Science, 237,* 73–77. Copyright 1987 AAAS.]

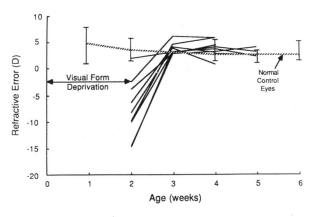

FIG. 13.4. Recovery from form-deprivation myopia in chicks. Myopia was induced by 2 weeks of visual form deprivation with translucent occluders. After the occluders were removed, the chicks became emmetropic within 1 to 3 weeks. [From Troilo, D. (1990). *Myopia and the control of eye growth (CIBA Found. Symp. 155)* (pp. 89–102). Copyright © 1990. Reprinted by permission of John Wiley & Sons, Inc.]

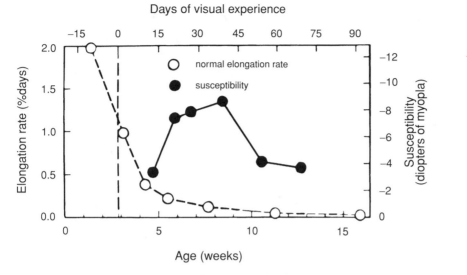

FIG. 13.5. Normal elongation rate and susceptibility to induced myopia in tree shrews. Reprinted from Siegwart, J. T., & Norton, T. T. (1998). *Vision Research, 38*, 3505–3515. Copyright 1998, with permission from Elsevier.]

Similar results are found in another primate, the marmoset (Troilo, Nickla, & Wildsoet, 2000). This agrees with results in humans, where the percentage of myopic schoolchildren increases most rapidly between 7 and 15 years of age.

Two compensatory changes in the shape of the eyeball have been shown to produce emmetropization in the chick. One is an overall change in the length of the eyeball. The other is a change in the thickness of the layer of vascular tissue between the retina and the sclera, called the *choroid*. When the choroid thickens, it pushes the retina forward, which can compensate for the elongation of the eyeball that occurs in form-deprivation myopia (Fig. 13.6). In hyperopia, the choroid thins and the retina moves back to compensate. Compensation for lack of focus in chicks involves first a change in the thickness of the choroid, followed by a change in the length of the eyeball, during which the choroid tends to revert to its original thickness (Wallman, Wildsoet, Xu, Gottlieb, Nickla, Marran, Krebs, & Christensen, 1995; see Fig. 13.7).

Given that a focused image can have a local effect on the growth of the eyeball, what might be the mechanism? First, there must be a cell in the retina that can detect the difference between a focused image and an image that is diffused or out of focus. This cell then needs to release some substance, perhaps a neurotransmitter, and the amount of the substance released must be quite different for a focused image compared with an unfocused one. The substance or transmitter then needs to diffuse to the choroid or sclera without being taken up by cells along the way, or broken down by enzymes. Finally, there needs to be a mechanism whereby the substance or neurotransmitter affects the growth of the choroid and sclera.

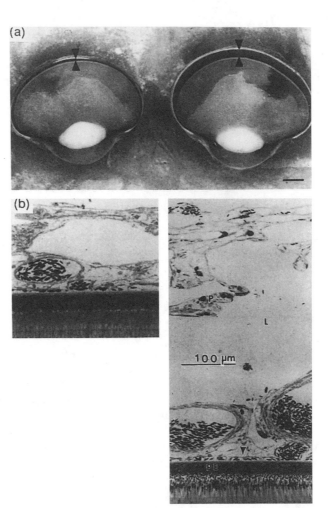

FIG. 13.6. Choroidal expansion in eyes recovering from myopia induced by form-deprivation. (a) Unfixed hemisected eyes. *Arrows* indicate choroidal boundaries. (b) Sections of the posterior eye wall. Abbreviations: Ch, choroid, delimited by *arrows*; L, lacuna; R, retina. [Reprinted from Wallman, J., et al. (1995). *Vision Research, 35*, 37–50. Copyright 1995, with permission from Elsevier.]

How the direction of blur is detected is an unresolved question (for review, see Wallman & Winawer, 2004). Chromatic aberration may play a role through the detection of the focus of blue wavelengths, which normally focus in front of the retina, versus red wavelengths, which normally focus behind it. However, raising animals in monochromatic light does not prevent compensation for spectacle lenses, so this is not the only cue. Possibly other aberrations—astigmatism, spherical aberration and coma—might together provide a cue. Accommodation (much accommodation in hyperopic eyes and little in myopic eyes) might also provide a cue over time, but would not account for local growth of part of the eyeball. It seems likely that multiple cues are employed, so that elimination of one of them brings the others into play (Wildsoet, Howland, Falconer, & Dick, 1993).

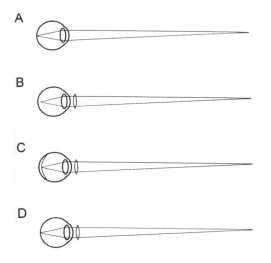

FIG. 13.7. Effect of thickness of choroid on refraction. (A) Image in focus on the retina in a young chick; (B) a positive lens places the image in front of the retina; (C) the choroid thickens to move the retina forward, and the image into focus again; (D) the optics of the eyeball change as it grows, and the choroid thins again to its original width.

In looking for substances that may carry the signal from the neural retina to the choroid and sclera, an important issue is finding substances whose expression levels have the same sign as changes in the eye, that is, increase with myopic changes (plus sign) and decrease with hyperopic changes (minus sign) or vice versa. In the chick model of myopia, two such substances are currently known: glucagon and retinoic acid. Glucagon is found in one class of amacrine cells. Activity in these cells, assayed by the immediate early gene ZENK (egr-1), is suppressed by minus lenses and form deprivation, which lead to ocular elongation, and is enhanced by plus lenses and termination of form deprivation, which suppress ocular elongation (Fischer, McGuire, Schaeffel, & Stell, 1999). A glucagon agonist inhibits myopia development and a glucagon antagonist inhibits hyperopia development (Feldkaemper & Schaeffel, 2002; Vessey, Leneses, Rushforth, Hruby, & Stell, 2005). Moreover, retinal glucagon content decreases after minus lens treatment and choroidal glucagon content increases after plus lens treatment. These effects are specific to proglucagon-derived peptides, as opposed to secretin-related peptides (Vessey, Rushforth, & Stell, 2005). Thus, glucagon could represent an early step along the pathway that prevents ocular elongation.

While retinoic acid changes in opposite directions under opposite signs of defocus, the situation is complicated by the fact that the retinal and choroidal changes are in opposite directions, at least in chicks. In the retina, the level of retinoic acid is associated with increased elongation of the eyeball, from experiments in the guinea pig (McFadden, Howlett, & Mertz, 2004) and chicks (Seko, Shimizu, & Tokoro, 1998). In line with this, inhibition of retinoic acid synthesis also inhibits elongation of the eyeball from form deprivation (Bitzer, Feldkaemper, & Schaeffel, 2000). On the other hand, in the choroid spectacle lenses that elongate the eyeball lead to a decrease in retinoic acid and those that halt eye-growth lead to an increase in retinoic acid (Mertz & Wallman, 2000). In line with these findings, application of retinoic acid to cultured sclera at physiological concentrations produces an inhibition of proteoglycan production, implying that the choroidal level of retinoic acid affects the sclera with the correct sign (Mertz & Wallman, 2000). Curiously, feeding retinoic acid to guinea pigs results in rapid eye elongation (McFadden et al., 2004). Clearly, further experiments are needed to clarify these results. Although all experiments point to retinoic acid as a bidirectional factor associated with eye elongation, it is unclear how increases in the retina are related to decreases in the choroid, and the nature of the reactions by which retinoic acid affect the sclera. What is also missing is data in which the endogenous retinoic acid is depleted, then exogenous retinoic acid is applied, to test whether it has the predicted action.

Other factors are associated with eyeball changes but are not bidirectional. One is the retinal neurotransmitter dopamine. Retinal dopamine levels are reduced in form-deprivation myopia (Stone, Lin, Laties, & Iuvone, 1989). Dopamine agonists partially reduce form-deprivation myopia and dopamine antagonists enhance it (Stone et al., 1989; Schaeffel, Bartmann, Hagel, & Zrenner, 1995; Schmid & Wildsoet, 2004). Moreover, the ablation of dopamine amacrine cells with 6-hydroxydopamine blocks the development of form-deprivation myopia (Li, Schaeffel, Kohler, & Zrenner, 1992). However, the time course of the changes in dopamine and rate of ocular elongation do not tally well (see Wallman & Winawer, 2004). Thus, the exact role of dopamine and its relationship to the bidirectional factors glucagon and retinoic acid remain to be worked out.

Another factor is the neurotransmitter acetylcholine acting through muscarinic receptors. The muscarinic antagonist atropine reduces the rate of myopic progression in children and form-deprivation myopia in monkeys (see Wallman & Winawer, 2004). Acetylcholine acts at many sites in the eye, including the neural retina, retinal pigment epithelium, choroids, and ciliary body. A retinal site of action seems unlikely for a variety of reasons, in particular because ablation of acetylcholine amacrine cells and retinal muscarinic receptors does not abolish form-deprivation myopia, although atropine is still effective (Fischer, Miethke, Morgan, & Stell, 1998). An effect through the action of acetylcholine on accommodation is also unlikely because atropine also acts on myopia in chicks, where there is no effect on accommodation (see Wallman & Winawer, 2004), and the M1 antagonist pirenzepine affects myopia but not accommodation in tree shrews (Cottriall & McBrien, 1996). The failure of many nonspecific or M1-specific antagonists to inhibit myopia, together with the high concentrations required for the antagonists that do have an effect, raises the possibility that the agents may act through a nonmuscarinic mechanism (Luft, Ming, & Stell, 2003).

Thus, there are many experiments that still need to be done to understand local control of eye growth. We need to know what the complete sequence of biochemical reactions is; which of the substances that have so far been investigated are part of this sequence of reactions and which affect the reactions, but are not part of the sequence; whether the signal goes directly from the retina to the sclera, or the signal affects the choroid first, with the choroid in turn

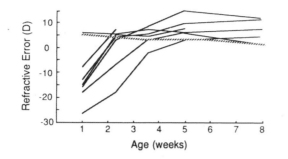

FIG. 13.8. Recovery from form-deprivation myopia overshoots the normal level in chicks with the optic nerve sectioned. Eyes were covered with translucent occluders for the first week. When occluders were taken off, recovery occurred over 1 to 3 weeks; however, all chicks had become hyperopic by the end of 5 weeks. [From Troilo, D. (1990). *Myopia and the control of eye growth (CIBA Found. Symp. 155)* (pp. 89–102). Copyright © 1990. Reprinted by permission of John Wiley & Sons, Inc.]

affecting the sclera; the role of the retinal pigment epithelium as an intermediary; and whether the sequence of reactions is the same in emmetropization and form-deprivation myopia.

While emmetropization uses local cues within the eyeball, it does involve the central nervous system as well. All chicks can recover from form-deprivation myopia when their eyes are opened again, but the emmetropization is more accurate with an intact optic nerve than with the optic nerve sectioned (Troilo, 1990; Wildsoet & Wallman, 1995; see Fig. 13.8). Moreover, amblyopia, which is a cortical defect, may cause hyperopia. Some early evidence on this point came from Lepard (1975), who showed that the difference in refraction between normal and amblyopic eyes in strabismic amblyopes continues to increase for some time after the amblyopia develops (see Fig. 6.7). Monkeys with amblyopia produced by strabismus, or by blurred vision from a −10D lens in one eye, also become hyperopic, and the hyperopia develops after the amblyopia (Kiorpes & Wallman, 1995).

Emmetropization in primates is more complicated than in chicks. There is less room for the eyeball to grow; consequently, compensation may occur for a small amount of anisometropia, but not for a large amount (Hung, Crawford, & Smith, 1994). Indeed, rearing with −10D lenses, for which a larger eyeball would compensate, actually leads to a smaller one (Smith, Hung, & Harwerth, 1994). This may have occurred because contact lenses rather than spectacles were used. Alternatively, the primate visual system might interpret a large amount of hyperopia incorrectly. Interestingly, Nathan, Kiely, Crewther, and Crewther (1985) found that refractive errors in children that affect primarily the fovea result in hyperopia, while refractive errors that affect primarily the periphery result in myopia. Perhaps the brain interprets the lack of well-focused images in the amblyopic eye as evidence of myopia, and therefore reduces elongation to compensate, producing hyperopia (see Kiorpes & Wallman, 1995).

The state of accommodation can also affect the whole process. There is a level of tonic accommodation that varies among individuals. A high level of tonic accommodation is found in corrected hyperopes, and a comparative lack of tonic accommodation in late-onset myopes, as compared with emmetropes (McBrien & Millodot, 1987). It could be that the eyeball adjusts to the level of tonic accommodation found in different individuals. People with a high level of accommodation would tend to have the image focused in front of the retina, leading to compensation with a small eyeball, and people with a low level of accommodation would tend to have the image focused behind the retina, leading to a large eyeball.

Form-deprivation myopia is different from the other types of visual deprivation discussed in earlier chapters, in that it involves signals within the retina. Amblyopia from strabismus, anisometropia and monocular deprivation, and meridional amblyopia from astigmatism, all involve changes that occur primarily in the visual cortex. Moreover, the mechanisms are different for amblyopia and form-deprivation myopia. So far, glucagon, retinoic acid, dopamine, and acetylcholine have been implicated in form-deprivation myopia, while glutamate receptors, calcium, second messengers, and protein kinases and phosphatases have been implicated in visual cortex changes.

At the functional level, there is a clear interaction between the two processes. Form-deprivation leads to myopia, other optical changes can lead to hyperopia, and amblyopia can also lead to hyperopia in the long run. At the same time, hyperopia can lead to strabismus, which can lead to amblyopia. Moreover, myopia can lead to loss of contrast sensitivity. This emphasizes again the complexity of the visual system, and the interactions between its various components. The whole system is delicately balanced as it grows, and a deficit in any one of the components can lead to deficits in the others. We saw in earlier chapters how this is true in sensory and motor components of the system in the development of binocular vision. This chapter points out how it is also true in optical and sensory components of the system in the development of correct focus on the retina.

References

Bitzer, M., Feldkamper, M., & Schaeffel, F. (2000). Visually induced changes in components of the retinoic acid system in fundal layers of the chick. *Experimental Eye Research, 70*, 97–106.

Cottriall, C. L., & McBrien, N. A. (1996). The M1 muscarinic antagonist pirenzepine reduces myopia and eye enlargement in the tree shrew. *Investigative Ophthalmology and Visual Science, 37*, 1368–1379.

Feldkaemper, M., & Schaeffel, F. (2002). Evidence for a potential role of glucagon during eye growth regulation in chicks. *Visual Neuroscience, 19*, 755–766.

Fischer, A. J., McGuire, J. J., Schaeffel, F., & Stell, W. K. (1999). Light and focus-dependent expression of the transcription factor ZENK in the chick retina. *Nature Neuroscience, 2*, 706–712.

Fischer, A. J., Miethke, P., Morgan, I. G., & Stell, W. K. (1998). Cholinergic amacrine cells are not required for the progression and atropine-mediated suppression of form-deprivation myopia. *Brain Research, 794*, 48–60.

Fitzke, F. W., Hayes, B. P., Hodos, W., Holden, A. L., & Low, J. C. (1985). Refractive sectors in the visual field of the pigeon eye. *Journal of Physiology, 369*, 33–44.

Hubel, D. H., Wiesel, T. N., & LeVay, S. (1975). Functional architecture of area 17 in normal and monocularly deprived macaque monkeys. *Cold Spring Harbor Symposia on Quantitative Biology, 40*, 581–589.

Hung, L. F., Crawford, M. J., & Smith, E. L. (1994). Spectacle lenses alter eye growth and the refractive status of young monkeys. *Nature Medicine, 1,* 761–765.

Irving, E. L., Sivak, J. G., & Callender, M. G. (1992). Refractive plasticity in the developing chick eye. *Ophthalmic Physiological Optics, 12,* 448–456.

Johnson, C. A., Post, R. B., Chalupa, L. M., & Lee, T. J. (1982). Monocular deprivation in humans: a study of identical twins. *Investigative Ophthalmology, 23,* 135–138.

Kiorpes, L., & Wallman, J. (1995). Does experimentally-induced amblyopia cause hyperopia in monkeys? *Vision Research, 35,* 1289–1298.

Lepard, C. W. (1975). Comparative changes in the error of refraction between fixing and amblyopic eyes during growth and development. *American Journal of Ophthalmology, 80,* 485–490.

Li, X. X., Schaeffel, F., Kohler, K., & Zrenner, E. (1992). Dose-dependent effects of 6-hydroxydopamine on deprivation myopia, electroretinograms, and dopaminergic amacrine cells in chickens. *Visual Neuroscience, 9,* 483–492.

Luft, W. A., Ming, Y., & Stell, W. K. (2003). Variable effects of previously untested muscarinic receptor antagonists on experimental myopia. *Investigative Ophthalmology and Visual Science, 44,* 1330–1338.

McBrien, N. A., & Millodot, M. (1987). The relationship between tonic accommodation and refractive error. *Investigative Ophthalmology and Visual Science, 28,* 997–1004.

McBrien, N. A., Moghaddam, H. O., Cottriall, C. L., Leech, E. M., & Cornell, L. M. (1995). The effects of blockade of retinal cell action potentials on ocular growth, emmetropization and form deprivation myopia in young chicks. *Vision Research, 35,* 1141–1152.

McFadden, S. A., Howlett, M. H. C., & Mertz, J. R. (2004). Retinoic acid signals the direction of ocular elongation in the guinea pig eye. *Vision Research, 44,* 643–653.

Mertz, J. R., & Wallman, J. (2000). Choroidal retinoic acid synthesis: a possible mediator between refractive error and compensatory eye growth. *Experimental Eye Research, 70,* 519–527.

Nathan, J., Kiely, P. M., Crewther, S. G., & Crewther, D. P. (1985). Disease-associated visual image degradation and spherical refractive errors in children. *American Journal of Optometry and Physiological Optics, 62,* 680–688.

Norton, T. T., Essinger, J. A., & McBrien, N. A. (1994). Lid-suture myopia in tree shrews with retinal ganglion cell blockade. *Visual Neuroscience, 11,* 143–154.

Rabin, J., Van Sluyters, R. C., & Malach, R. (1981). Emmetropization: a vision dependent phenomenon. *Investigative Ophthalmology, 20,* 561–564.

Raviola, E., & Wiesel, T. N. (1985). An animal model of myopia. *New England Journal of Medicine, 312,* 1609–1615.

Schaeffel, F., Glasser, A., & Howland, H. C. (1988). Accomodation, refractive error and eye growth in chickens. *Vision Research, 28,* 639–657.

Schaeffel, F., Bartmann, M., Hagel, G., & Zrenner, E. (1995). Studies on the role of the retinal dopamine/melatonin system in experimental refractive errors in chickens. *Vision Research, 35,* 1247–1264.

Schmid, K. L., & Wildsoet, C. F. (2004). Inhibitory effects of apomorphine and atropine and their combination on myopia in chicks. *Optometry and Vision Science, 81,* 137–147.

Seko, Y., Shimizu, M., & Tokoro, T. (1998). Retinoic acid increases in the retina of the chick with form deprivation myopia. *Ophthalmic Research, 30,* 361–367.

Siegwart, J. T., & Norton, T. T. (1998). The susceptible period for deprivation-induced myopia in tree shrew. *Vision Research, 38,* 3505–3515.

Smith, E. L., Hung, L. F., & Harwerth, R. S. (1994). Effects of optically induced blur on the refractive status of young monkeys. *Vision Research, 34,* 293–301.

Stone, R. A., Lin, T., Laties, A. M., & Iuvone, P. M. (1989). Retinal dopamine and form-deprivation myopia. *Proceedings of the National Academy of Sciences of the United States of America, 86,* 704–706.

Troilo, D. (1990). Experimental studies of emmetropization in the chick. In G. R. Bock & K. Widdows (Eds.), *Myopia and the control of eye growth (CIBA Found. Symp. 155)* (pp. 89–102). Chichester, UK: Wiley.

Troilo, D., Gottlieb, M. D., & Wallman, J. (1987). Visual deprivation causes myopia in chicks with optic nerve section. *Current Eye Research, 6,* 993–999.

Troilo, D., Nickla, D. L., & Wildsoet, C. F. (2000). Form deprivation myopia in mature common marmosets (*Callithrix jacchus*). *Investigative Ophthalmology and Visual Science, 41,* 2043–2049.

Vessey, K. A., Leneses, K. A., Rushforth, D. A., Hruby, V. J., & Stell, W. K. (2005). Glucagon receptor agonists and antagonists affect the growth of the chick eye: A role for glucagonergic regulation of emmetropization? *Investigative Ophthalmology and Visual Science*, in press.

Vessey, K. A., Rushforth, D. A., & Stell, W. K. (2004). Pro-glucagon-derived peptides that prevent form-deprivation myopia in chicks: towards identifying endogenous peptides that promote emmetropization. *Investigative Ophthalmology and Visual Science, 45 Suppl.*, 1231.

Wallman, J., & Winawer, J. (2004). Homeostasis of eye growth and the question of myopia. *Neuron., 43*, 447–468.

Wallman, J., Gottlieb, M. D., Rajaram, V., & Fugate-Wentzek, L. (1987). Local retinal regions control local eye growth in chicks. *Science, 237*, 73–77.

Wallman, J., Wildsoet, C. F., Xu, A., Gottlieb, M. D., Nickla, D. L., Marran, L., Krebs, W., & Christensen, A. M. (1995). Moving the retina: choroidal modulation of refractive state. *Vision Research, 35*, 37–50.

Wiesel, T. N., & Raviola, E. (1977). Myopia and eye enlargement after neonatal lid fusion in monkeys. *Nature, 266*, 66–68.

Wildsoet, C. F., & Pettigrew, J. D. (1988). Experimental myopia and anomalous eye growth patterns unaffected by optic nerve section in chickens: evidence for local control of eye growth. *Clinical Vision Sciences, 3*, 99–107.

Wildsoet, C. F., & Wallman, J. (1995). Choroidal and scleral mechanisms of compensation for spectacle lenses in chicks. *Vision Research, 35*, 1175–1194.

Wildsoet, C. F., Howland, H. S., Falconer, S., & Dick, K. (1993). Chromatic aberration and accommodation: their role in emmetropization in the chick. *Vision Research, 33*, 1593–1063.

Glossary

AC/A Ratio This ratio represents the amount of convergence that occurs for a specific amount of accommodation. In normal people, if one refocuses from an object at 10 feet away to an object at 3 feet away, the amount of convergence is appropriate so that the object at 3 feet will fall on corresponding parts of the retinas. This is a normal AC/A ratio. Some people may converge too much (a high AC/A ratio) and some people may converge too little (a low AC/A ratio). See *Near Response*.

Accommodation Change in the shape of the lens to focus images at different distances on the retina. Contraction of the circular ciliary muscle around the margin of the lens makes the lens more convex to focus nearby objects. Relaxation of the ciliary muscle and tension in the zonule fibers that support the lens makes the lens flatter to focus objects far away.

Acuity The ability to detect fine detail. It is tested in a doctor's office by asking the subject to read a line of letters (Snellen acuity). Somebody who can read a line at 20 ft (6 m) that a person with normal adult acuity can read at 60 ft (18 m) is said to have an acuity of 20/60 or 6/18, which is one third of normal. People with acuity of less than 20/200 (10% of normal) after correction of their optics are legally blind.

Acuity can also be tested with a grating of black and white lines of equal width. The subject is asked to detect the orientation of the lines in the grating, compared with a uniform grey area of the same shape and overall luminance. The limit of acuity is the finest grating that can be detected. The result is expressed in cycles/degree, where one cycle is the width of one black plus one white line, and one calculates how many cycles can be detected in 1° of arc from the point of view of the observer. Most people can see 30 cycles/degree and this is equivalent to a Snellen acuity of 20/20.

Another test that can be used with some people who cannot read is the Landolt C. The letter C is arranged in one of four orientations. The subject is asked to detect whether the gap in the C is on the left, right, top, or bottom, and the size of the C is reduced until the subject can no longer detect the position of the gap.

Adaptation This word has been used to describe a large variety of phenomena. In general, it means that the state of the visual system changes to become more or less sensitive to some class of stimuli.

Light adaptation is the process of becoming used to a higher level of illumination so that one is most sensitive to objects near this level of illumination. While the visual system is able to respond over 12 log units of brightness, at any one time the system only responds to 2 log units. For objects that are not colored, the brightest object is white, an object 2 log units less bright than this is black, and in between are shades of grey. Light adaptation occurs rapidly, in seconds, or less for moderate changes of illumination.

Dark adaptation is the process of becoming more sensitive to dim objects. It is determined by the percentage of molecules of the rod photopigment, rhodopsin, that are bleached. Bleached molecules send signals up the visual pathway that are equivalent to a background of light so that an object that is much dimmer than this background cannot be seen. Rhodopsin regenerates with a slow time course—the time constant is about 15 min—so that one cannot see clearly in very dim light until 30 to 45 min have passed.

Light and dark adaptation depend on processes that occur in the retina. Cells at higher levels of the system can adapt to more complicated stimuli. See *After-Effects.*

Afferents Axons that come into the nucleus or area being described.

After-Effects After-effects occur because of adaptation of cells at higher levels of the visual system. The best known are probably the direction selective after-effects. In the waterfall phenomenon, after staring at a waterfall, the bank nearby will appear to move upward. In the spiral after-effect, after staring at the center of a rotating spiral, when the rotation stops it will appear as though the spiral is rotating in the opposite direction. These after-effects are due to adaptation of direction-selective cells in the visual cortex.

Another example is the tilt after-effect. In the tilt after-effect, the subject stares at a set of lines tilted to the left for a few minutes, then transfers his/her attention to a set of vertical lines. The vertical lines appear to be tilted to the right for a short while.

Anisometropia A difference in focus for the two eyes so that when one eye accommodates for an object to be in focus on the retina of that eye, the object is out of focus for the retina of the other eye. Anisometropia is a problem because accommodation is consensual: that is, the two eyes accommodate together and cannot accommodate separately in normal people.

Anomalous Retinal Correspondence If the connections between one of the retinas and some part of cortex are rewired during development so that the fovea of one eye, and some point that is not the fovea in the other eye, project to the same place in the cortex, then the subject has anomalous retinal correspondence. This occurs in strabismus, but rarely, because it requires that the angle of strabismus be constant (comitant) over a substantial period of time so that the new connections can be established.

Aphakia This is the absence of a lens in the eye. It occurs in cataract, when the lens is taken out. There are three resulting optical problems. First, the eye needs an additional lens to focus (a contact lens or spectacles), but this leads to images that are different sizes on the retina if the additional lens is outside the eyeball. Second, another lens is required to avoid the difference in magnification, unless an intraocular lens implant is used. Third, the eye cannot accommodate.

Astigmatism A cylindrical component in the optics of the eye so that when lines in one orientation are in focus, lines along the orthogonal orientation are out of focus.

Binocular Fusion For images that fall on corresponding points of the two retinas, the images will be fused into a single perception in the visual cortex. There can be a small mismatch, and the images will still be fused. For example, an object that is further away than the plane of fixation will fall on noncorresponding points of the two retinas, but it will be seen as single and distant. See *Panum's Fusional Area.*

Blob This is the term for areas in layers III and II of primate striate cortex that stain heavily for cytochrome oxidase, which is a marker for increased metabolic activity. The blobs are in the center of ocular dominance columns and contain a high percentage of color-coded cells.

Cataract A lens that is cloudy. Cataracts are most frequently found in old people, but they can also be congenital. There are a variety of causes, such as rubella (German measles). If the cloudiness is confined to the center of the lens, then a clear image can be obtained through the edge of the lens. When the cataract covers the whole lens, the image on the retina is diffused.

Channels A term used by psychophysicists to describe properties that are handled in a parallel fashion. For example, there are channels for dealing with red, as opposed to green, and yellow, as opposed to blue.

Choroid A layer of vascular tissue between the sclera and pigment epithelium.

Comitant Strabismus A form of strabismus where the eyes move together so that there is a fairly constant angle between the direction of view of the two eyes. Congenital esotropia is usually comitant.

Contrast Sensitivity Sensitivity to contrast is a measure of the minimum contrast that can be seen. Generally speaking, an object can be detected if it differs from the background by more than 1%. However, this depends on the size of the object and the overall illumination. Contrast sensitivity is generally measured with gratings where both spatial frequency and contrast can be varied. It is usually expressed as

$$\frac{L_{max} + L_{min}}{L_{max} - L_{min}}$$

where L_{max} is the luminance of the lighter stripes and L_{min} is the luminance of the darker stripes. Thus, the contrast sensitivity for a 1% difference in luminance is $\sim$200.

Cortical Plate As the cerebral cortex develops, young cells migrate out from the ventricular zone through the subventricular and intermediate zones to form the cortical plate. The cortical plate consists of cells that have reached their final destination, and cells migrating through, until all layers of the cortex are formed.

Crowding A letter is less visible when part of a row of letters than when presented by itself. This is a form of masking, with some differences. For the distinction between masking and crowding, see Pelli, Palomares, and Majaj (2004).

Cue Various aspects of the image may be used to detect a perception. For example, stereopsis, motion parallax, shading, and superposition may all be used to determine the perception of depth, and these are called cues to depth perception.

Dichoptic Masking The image in one eye suppresses, or masks, the image in the other.

Diplopia Diplopia is double vision. It is usually binocular, occurring with strabismus when the image in the crooked eye is not suppressed. In rare cases of anomalous retinal correspondence, it can be monocular. In these cases, the new fixation point in the crooked eye is connected to central vision in the cortex, the original connections still exist, and the signals traveling down the original connections are not suppressed.

Disparity Disparity occurs when an image falls on noncorresponding parts of the two retinas. It happens whenever there is an object at a different distance from the object being fixated. For objects nearer than the fixation point, the lines of sight from the two eyes cross each other between the eyes and the plane of fixation. This is called crossed disparity. For an object further than the fixation point, the lines of sight from the two eyes do not cross each other, and this is called uncrossed disparity.

Eccentricity The field of view comprises the fixation point and an area out to approximately 90° away from the fixation point. Eccentricity is a measure of distance away from the fixation point in the field of view, usually expressed in degrees of angle. It can also be the distance from the fovea in the retina.

Efferents Axons that leave the nucleus or area being considered.

Electroretinogram (ERG) This is a measure of the sum of all the electrical activity in the retina measured from electrodes outside the retina. In humans, it can be measured between an electrode placed on the sclera and an electrode placed on the skin. There are several components of the ERG: the **a** wave, coming from photoreceptors; the **b** wave, coming from cells in the inner nuclear layer, and summed by the Muller cells, which are the glial cells of the retina; and the **c** wave, coming from the pigment epithelium.

Emmetropia The visual state where images are in focus on the retina.

Esotropia Strabismus where one eye turns inward. It can be congenital, probably from a variety of causes that remain to be pinned down. It can occur in young children from hyperopia and in older children also from a variety of causes.

Exotropia Strabismus where one eye turns outward.

Fixation The process of looking directly at an object. In normal people, this means that the image of the object falls on the foveas of the two eyes. Because images that are stationary on the retina disappear (because signals in the visual cortex are transient), the process of fixation actually involves slow eye movements away from the object, with small fast movements (microsaccades) that tend to bring the image back to the fovea.

FPL   Forced-choice preferential looking technique. An infant faces two displays. An observer looks at the infant from behind a screen and is forced to record whether the infant is looking at the left display or the right display. If the records from the observer show that the infant looks at one display more than the other on more than 75% of the observations, the infant is said to be able to discriminate between the displays. Some criterion level other than 75% may be chosen.

Fusion   See *Binocular Fusion.*

GABA   Gamma-aminobutyric acid, the primary inhibitory neurotransmitter of the cerebral cortex.

Gabor Patch   A circular patch filled with a grating whose contrast decreases towards the edge of the patch.

Glutamate   The primary excitatory neurotransmitter of the cerebral cortex.

Grating Acuity   See *Acuity.*

Habituation   When a stimulus is presented repeatedly, the response may decrease. If it does, this is called habituation. Habituation is particularly noticeable in the response from cells in the visual cortex in young animals. Sometimes one may have to wait several seconds between stimuli if each response to the stimulus is to be as large as the first.

Hypercolumn   The cortex is organized in a columnar fashion: that is, cells on a line perpendicular to the surface of the cortex tend to have similar properties. There are columns in primary visual cortex in primates for ocular dominance, orientation and color, organized around the blobs, which are primarily for color. Thus, there is a small module, approximately 1 mm × 1 mm, which analyses a small area of the field of view for all these parameters. This module is called a hypercolumn. Next door will be another hypercolumn, analyzing a neighboring part of the field of view. The size of a hypercolumn tends to be constant as one moves across the cortex. However, the area of field of view that it analyses increases with eccentricity (the distance from the fovea). Near the fovea, a hypercolumn analyses approximately 0.3° of the field of view, and 20° away from the fovea, a hypercolumn analyses 1.5° of the field of view. Thus, the part of the visual field that falls on the fovea is analyzed in greater detail than the rest of the visual field.

Hyperopia   Where the image is consistently behind the retina because the eyeball is too small for the focusing power of the cornea and lens and there is not enough accommodative power in the system to overcome this. It can be corrected with convex lenses.

Hypertropia   Strabismus where the deviating eye looks upward.

Hypotropia   Strabismus where the deviating eye looks downward.

Incomitant Strabismus   Strabismus where one eye moves and the other moves much less, or not at all. An obvious example occurs when the muscle that moves the eye outward is paralyzed.

Increment Threshold   Measurement of the smallest increment in luminance that can be seen against a background. This depends on the size of the object, just as contrast sensitivity depends on spatial frequency.

Knock-out mice Mice with a mutation that knocks out a specific protein.

LTD Long-term depression. This is a long-term change in the efficacy of transmission across a synapse as a result of low frequency stimulation of the input to the synapse.

LTP Long-term potentiation. This is a long-term change in the efficacy of transmission across a synapse as a result of high-frequency stimulation of the input to the synapse. Long-term potentiation is believed to underlie some forms of memory, primarily because it is a prominent phenomenon in the hippocampus, and people with lesions of the hippocampus have deficits in short-term memory.

Masking The visibility of an object can be decreased by an object placed beside it (spatial masking) or by another object seen after it (temporal masking). For example, if a letter is flashed on the screen followed a moment later by a circle around it, the letter may not be seen. Similarly, letters in a line are less visible than a letter by itself (the crowding phenomenon). Both temporal and spatial masking occur in people with normal vision.

Meridional Amblyopia The form of amblyopia that occurs with astigmatism. Lines oriented along the axis of good vision are less visible than lines oriented along the orthogonal axis, if the astigmatism is maintained and not corrected for several years before the age of 7.

Metabotropic Glutamate Receptors Glutamate receptors that affect the cell through second messengers rather than through channels.

Microsaccade A small saccadic eye movement made to keep the image near the fovea during the process of fixation.

Myopia The eyeball is too long for the power of the cornea and the lens so that the image is consistently focused in front of the retina.

Near Response This term is used to refer to the three things that occur when the eyes refocus on a near object: the lens accommodates, the eyes converge, and the pupil contracts.

NMDA Receptors A type of glutamate receptor that is voltage dependent so that it amplifies the response in the postsynaptic cell multiplicatively.

Nystagmus Nystagmus is a jerky movement of the eyes. In normal people, nystagmus can be stimulated by an environment moving around the person [optokinetic nystagmus (OKN)] or by activation of the vestibular system (vestibular nystagmus). In these two cases, there is a slow movement of the eyes designed to keep the image stationary on the retina, followed by a saccadelike fast movement to bring the eyes back to a central position. Nystagmus can also be pathological in patients who have amblyopia and lose good fixation. In this case, the nystagmus is usually a slow wandering of the eyes from side to side (pendular nystagmus), rather than an alternation of slow and fast movements.

Object Color Constancy Objects tend to appear the same color under different sources of illumination. For example, a blue sweater will appear blue in both tungsten light and daylight, and a yellow sweater will appear yellow in both those sources of illumination, even though tungsten light is yellowish and daylight is bluish.

Octave When acuity is tested, a difference of a factor of two is known as an octave.

Ocular Dominance Histogram   A sample of cells is evaluated for ocular dominance (whether it is driven more by the contralateral eye or more by the ipsilateral eye according to a 7- point scale: 1, contralateral only; 7, ipsilateral only; 4, equally driven by both eyes; 2 and 6, strongly dominated by one eye; 3 and 5, weakly dominated by one eye), and a histogram is formed from the results.

Ocular Dominance Plasticity   Where one eye is closed for a period of time and the ocular dominance histogram is found to be shifted.

OKN   See *Nystagmus.*

Orientation Bias Cells   Cells that respond to movement of a bar perpendicular to its length for all orientations but have a response that is significantly different for one orientation compared with the orthogonal orientation.

Orthotropia   The two eyes look in the same direction and the image of the object being fixated falls on the foveas of the two retinas.

Panum's Fusional Area   Images falling on noncorresponding parts of the two retinas can be fused, presumably by the cells in the visual cortex that are sensitive to disparity. However, there is a limit: The area in one eye that can be fused with a point in the other is known as Panum's fusional area. It is approximately 15' wide near the fovea and gets larger with eccentricity. Images falling outside Panum's area will produce diplopia if not suppressed.

Parallel Processing   This term refers to different aspects of visual perception being processed in parallel with each other. For example, there are cells that respond to objects brighter than the background and cells that respond to objects darker than the background, among bipolar and ganglion cells in the retina, cells in the lateral geniculate nucleus, and simple cells in the visual cortex. The two types of signal are separated from each other after processing by the photoreceptors, and do not come together again until the visual cortex is reached. Thus, there is little interaction between the two types of signal along the way.

Perimetry   Measurement of the boundaries of the field of view by bringing an object in from the periphery until it can be seen.

Phoria   The eyes have a tendency to look in different directions, but this can be overcome by fixating on an object.

Plasticity   The state of a part of the nervous system may be altered by signals impinging on that part. The ability for this alteration to occur is called plasticity.

Prospective Study   A study where a population is investigated for factors that may affect a disease or condition, starting before the onset of the disease or condition.

Protein Kinases   Proteins that phosphorylate another protein.

Protein Phosphatases   Proteins that dephosphorylate another protein.

Pursuit Eye Movements   Also known as smooth pursuit eye movements. These occur when the eyes are following an object. The eyes cannot move smoothly unless there is an object to be followed. If a person is asked to move their eyes smoothly from one point to another, what actually happens is a series of saccades. Smooth pursuit eye movements are essentially fixation on a moving object.

Quantum Catch   The number of quanta of light caught by a photoreceptor compared with the number of quanta falling on the photoreceptor. The quantum catch depends on the length of the photoreceptor, whether the light comes in parallel to the photoreceptor or at an angle, the density of pigment, how much of the pigment is bleached, and how the inner segment of the photoreceptor funnels light into the outer segment.

Radial Glia   Glial cells that extend from the ventricular surface underneath the cerebral cortex to the pial surface above it. As cells migrate from the ventricular surface to their final position in the cortex, they climb up the radial glia.

Receptive Field   The area of visual field or retina over which a cell can be activated, directly or indirectly.

Reflection Spectrum   One can measure the percentage of light reflected by an object for each wavelength in the visible spectrum. This is the reflection spectrum of the object. Red objects reflect red wavelengths (620–700 nm), green objects reflect green wavelengths (520–560 nm), and blue objects reflect blue wavelengths (420–480 nm). The light that reaches the eye from an object is the product of the wavelengths emitted by the source of illumination and the reflection spectrum of the object. Generally speaking, the color of an object in a multicolored scene is predicted better by its reflection spectrum than by the composition of wavelengths that reach the eye from it. Thus, object color constancy occurs.

Refraction   The process of measuring the optics of the eye for correction with spectacles or contact lenses.

Resolution Limit   The limit of the finest detail that can be seen; that is, the limit of acuity.

Retrospective Study   A study where a population is investigated for factors that may affect a disease or condition, starting after the onset of the disease or condition. Bias is much more likely in a retrospective study than in a prospective study, and data from the time before the disease or condition started may not be reliable.

Reverse Suture   The eyelids of one eye are sutured closed for a period, then opened, and the eyelids of the other eye are sutured closed.

Rivalry   Different images fall on the two retinas and the image perceived alternates between the two. For example, if horizontal lines fall on the left retina and vertical lines fall on the right retina, the perceived image will alternate between horizontal and vertical lines.

Saccade   A fast eye movement designed to move the line of sight to a new and interesting object in the periphery of the field of view. Saccadic eye movements are ballistic, that is, once one is started it cannot be interrupted, and a period of 200 ms is necessary before another one can be started. Large saccadic eye movements are very fast—up to 800° per second.

Saturation Discrimination   Discrimination of a color from a more or less saturated color of the same hue, that is, how much white needs to be added or subtracted before one can notice the difference.

Sclera   The outside coat of the eyeball.

Scotoma   A blind spot caused by a lesion in the visual pathways. A lesion of the retina or optic nerve will affect one eye only so the scotoma will be monocular. A lesion of the optic tract, lateral geniculate nucleus, optic radiations, or visual cortex will affect both eyes so the scotoma will be binocular. See Figure 2.3.

Sign-Conserving Synapse and Sign-Reversing Synapse With a sign-conserving synapse, the response in presynaptic and postsynaptic cells has the same sign. If the presynaptic cell is hyperpolarized, then the postsynaptic cell will be also. If the presynaptic cell is depolarized so will the postsynaptic cell. Because excitation is often represented by a plus sign and inhibition by a minus sign, cells are said to have the same sign. At a sign-reversing synapse, hyperpolarization of the presynaptic cell leads to depolarization of the postsynaptic cell and depolarization of the presynaptic cell leads to hyperpolarization of the postsynaptic cell. The transmitter at sign-conserving synapses is excitatory, and the transmitter at sign-reversing synapses is inhibitory. For hyperpolarization in the presynaptic cell to act on the postsynaptic cell, there has to be spontaneous activity and continuous release of transmitter at the synapse.

The terminology has arisen because photoreceptors hyperpolarize in response to light. Thus, depolarizing bipolar cells are excited by light but inhibited by the transmitter released from photoreceptors because the hyperpolarized photoreceptors depolarize the bipolar cell across the sign-reversing synapse between them. It is easier to say that depolarizing bipolar cells are excited by light through a sign-reversing synapse than to say that they are excited by light through an inhibitory synapse.

Simultaneous Color Contrast The tendency for an object surrounded by a different color to take on a color opposite to the surroundings. Thus, a grey spot in a red surround tends to look greenish, in a green surround reddish, in a blue surround yellowish, and in a yellow surround bluish.

Snellen Acuity See *Acuity*.

Spatial Frequency The periodicity of a periodic object such as a grating. Expressed in terms of cycles/degree. See *Contrast Sensitivity*.

Spatial Uncertainty Uncertainty about the location of an object. This can be tested by asking a subject to line up an object between two other objects above and below it (see Fig. 8.3); by asking a subject to place objects equidistant on various sides of a marker in the center (see Fig. 8.13); and by vernier stimuli (see Fig. 3.7).

Spectral Sensitivity Sensitivity to various different wavelengths compared with each other. In the dark-adapted state, the spectral sensitivity curve follows the sensitivity of the rod pigment rhodopsin. In the light-adapted state, it follows the envelope of the curves for the red-absorbing and green-absorbing cone pigments, with a smaller contribution from the blue-absorbing cone pigment.

Stereopsis Three-dimensional vision. Stereoscopic depth perception depends on disparity. The cells in the visual cortex that are sensitive to crossed disparity detect near objects and lead to a perception of nearness and possibly convergent eye movements. The cells sensitive to uncrossed disparity detect far objects. Stereoscopic acuity, like vernier acuity, is much better than grating acuity. Observers with very good stereoscopic vision can discriminate two objects that are 0.02 in. apart in depth at a distance of 6 ft. This corresponds to 2″ of arc from the point of view of the observer.

Strabismus Strabismus is when the two eyes look in different directions. Colloquially known as cross-eyed, or squint.

Subplate Cells Subplate cells are cells found below the cortical plate during development. They are generated before cells that are destined to end up in layers II to VI of the cortex. Most of them die soon after birth. The remnant are called interstitial cells.

Successive Color Contrast If one stares at an object for a period of time, the next object observed afterward will be tinged with the complementary color. For example, looking at grey after staring at red will make the grey appear greenish, and so on.

Suppression Term used to refer to suppression of the image in one eye by the image in the other eye. It is the visual system's mechanism to avoid diplopia. Suppression can be alternating, as in binocular rivalry or alternate fixation by an exotrope, or it can be continual suppression of one eye by the other, as in suppression of the image in the amblyopic eye by the straight eye in congenital esotropes.

Teller Acuity Cards Cards with gratings of various spatial frequencies printed on them used to test acuity in infants and children by the forced-choice preferential looking technique.

Temporal Frequency This term is usually applied to a grating where the stripes are flickered between black and white; that is, the white stripes become black and the black stripes become white several times a second. The rate of flicker can be increased until the flicker is no longer noticed. The frequency at which this happens depends on the contrast of the stimulus. Consequently one can construct a temporal sensitivity curve, just as one constructs a contrast sensitivity curve for spatial frequency.

Tilt After-Effect See *After-Effects*.

Transcription Factor A factor that controls the expression of a gene or group of genes.

Tropia The eyes point in different directions.

VEP Visually evoked potential. This is measured from electrodes placed on the scalp over the visual cortex. To get much of a potential, one needs a stimulus that will activate lots of cells in the visual cortex in synchrony with each other. One stimulus commonly used is a checkerboard, with the squares on the checkerboard flickering between black and white.

Vergence Eye movements by which the eyes look at objects at different distances—convergence for nearby objects, and divergence for objects far away. These are slow eye movements. They are conjugate, in the sense that the eyes move together (all eye movements—saccades, smooth pursuit eye movements and vergence movements—are conjugate).

Vernier Acuity This is the ability to detect a break in a line. It can be measured with a grating, as shown in Figure 3.7, or a single line that is essentially one line in that figure. Vernier acuity is approximately 10% of grating acuity: while grating acuity is 2′ of arc in normal people, vernier acuity is 12″ of arc.

Waiting Period When afferents from the lateral geniculate nucleus to the visual cortex (and from other parts of thalamus to other parts of cortex) reach the subplate underneath their target, they wait there for a period of time before turning upwards to their final position. This is the waiting period.

Index

Entries in the glossary are referred to with the letter g

AC/A ratio, 60, 115, 255g
Accommodation, 255g
  development of, 60
  relationship with convergence, 115
  role in myopia, 251–252
Acetylcholine and form-deprivation myopia
    249–250
Acuity, 255g
  in anisometropia, 146–148
  away from the fovea, 147–148,
    161–163
  development of, 34–36, 93–95, 101
  in strabismus, 150–151, 160
Adaptation, 256g
Adult
  plasticity in, 175–176
Afferents, 256g
After-effects, 256g
A kinase anchoring protein
  and LTP, 238–239
  and visual plasticity, 222
Albino animals and humans
  errors at chiasm 68–70
Amblyopia, 1, 113, 145–165
  cells responsible for, 136–137
  meridional amblyopia, 119–121
  recovery from, 181–183
  stimulus deprivation amblyopia, 147–148,
    155
Anisometropia, 119, 145–148, 256g
  critical period for, 180
  effect on cells in lateral geniculate and
    cortex, 134–135
Anomalous retinal correspondence, 117–118,
    150, 163
  location in visual cortex, 138–139
Aphakia, 256g
Astigmatism, 119–121, 257g

Axons
  development of, 65
  retraction and sprouting of terminals, 82–84,
    130–131

Binocular deprivation, 104, 131–132
Binocular function, 183
  loss of, 135–136
Binocular fusion, 257g
Binocular summation, 55
  in strabismus, 162–163
Blobs, 257g
  development of, 81
Border distinctness, 159

Calcium
  and LTP, 237–238
  and visual plasticity, 219–221
Calcium/calmodulin-dependent protein
    kinase
  and LTP, 238–239
  and visual plasticity, 199–200, 219–221
Cataract, 2, 121–123, 257g
  critical period for effects of, 178–180
Cell death, 82
Cell types
  P, M, X, Y, and W, 15–16, 40, 94
    in monocular deprivation, 128
  simple, complex and hypercomplex,
    21–22
Channels, 257g
Chemoaffinity hypothesis, 65
Chiasm. See Optic chiasm
Chondroitin sulfate proteoglycans
  and visual plasticity 235
Choroid, 257g
  changes in myopia and hyperopia,
    247–248

Color vision, 7
  double opponent cells, 22–25
  object color constancy, 22–25, 260g
  opponent color cells, 22–25
  simultaneous color contrast, 22–24
Columns in cerebral cortex, 76, 81–82
Comitant strabismus. *See* Strabismus
Competition 188
  in anisometropes, 148
  as a mechanism in plasticity, 130, 198–199
Contour integration
  development of, 44
Contrast sensitivity, 257g
  in anisometropia, 148
  in astigmatism, 122
  development of, 36–40, 93
  in myopia, 124–125
  in strabismus, 136–137, 151–154
Convergence. *See* Vergence
Corpus callosum
  development of, 83–84
Cortical plate, 76, 77, 257g
Counting features, 159
CREB and visual plasticity, 223, 227
Critical periods, 169–189
  comparison in cat, monkey and human, 170
  comparison for amblyopia, binocular
    function and stereopsis in strabismus,
    183
  at higher levels of visual system, 173
  for parvocellular and magnocellular systems,
    174
  in anisometropia, 180
  in strabismus, 180
Crowding phenomenon, 153–156, 258g
  role in visual plasticity, 204, 221–222
Cytochrome oxidase blobs, 19–21, 257g

Dark adaptation, 41, 256g
Dark rearing
  as a criterion for factors associated with
    visual plasticity, 204
  effect on development, 102–106
  effect on NMDA receptors, 211–214
  effect on visual plasticity, 175, 204
Dendrites
  development of, 84
2–deoxyglucose technique, 99
Depth perception, 21–22
  development of, 47–49
Depolarization of neuron
  and plasticity, 210–211
Dichoptic masking, 258g
Diplopia, 117, 258g
Direction sensitivity
  cellular mechanisms for, 25
  critical period for, 173–174

deprivation, 132–134
  development of, 43–44
  perception of in amblyopes, 159
Disparity, 16–17, 258g
  development of, 102
Distorted sampling, 158
Divergence. *See* Vergence
Dopamine
  role in form-deprivation myopia,
    249–250
Double Vision. *See* Diplopia

Eccentricity, 258g
  acuity at various eccentricities, 150–151
Efferents, 258g
Electrical activity
  role in development 68–70, 75
  role in plasticity, 197, 208–210
Electroretinogram (ERG), 34, 258g
Emmetropia, 258g
  emmetropization, 243
ERK and visual plasticity, 222, 227
Esotropia, 113, 258g
  accommodative, 114–115, 118–119
  congenital, 117–119
Exotropia, 113, 118–119, 258g
Extrastriate pathway, 9
Eyeball, growth of, 121–124
Eye movements
  development of, 56–60
  input to lateral geniculate from, 68
  pursuit, or smooth pursuit, 58–59, 68, 261g
  saccades, 56–58, 262g

Feedback factors
  in visual plasticity, 200–201
Field of view
  development of, 44–45
  monocular segment, acuity in amblyopes,
    148–150
  periphery in amblyopes, 161–163
Fine detail, perception of, 13–14
Fixation, 31, 258g
  development of 59
  point of fixation in strabismus, 150–151
Forced-choice preferential looking technique
    (FPL), 33–34, 258g
Form-deprivation myopia, 243–245

GABA in visual plasticity, 214–217, 259g
Gabor patch, 44, 150, 259g
Ganglion cells, 14
"Gating" control of plasticity, 202
Glucagon and experimental myopia, 249
Grating acuity. *See* Acuity
Growth-associated proteins in plasticity,
    202–204

Growth factors
    and LTP, 239–240
    role in visual plasticity, 217–219, 226

Habituation, 92, 259g
Hebb postulate, 71, 198–199
Hierarchical processing, 22–26
Hippocampus, 4
Hubel, David, 4, 127
Hypercolumn, 19–21, 259g
Hyperopia, 114, 259g
    at birth, 123–124
Hypertropia, 113, 259g
Hypotropia, 113, 259g

Illusions
    Ponzo illusion, 7–8
Immediate early genes and visual plasticity,
    223–234
Immune system molecules and visual
    plasticity, 227
Incomitant strabismus. *See* Strabismus
Increment threshold, 259g

"Knock-out" mice and visual plasticity, 207,
    260g

Lateral geniculate nucleus, 8, 14–17
    development of, 68–70, 94–96
Lateral inhibition
    development of, 94–95
Long-term depression, 235–241, 260g
Long-term potentiation, 235–241, 260g
    and visual plasticity, 235–241

Masking, 260g
Meridional amblyopia, 119–121, 260g
Metabotropic glutamate receptors, 260g
    and LTP, 238–239
    and visual plasticity, 204, 214–215
Microsaccade, 31, 260g
Modulatory pathways (acetylcholine,
    noradrenaline and serotonin)
    effect on lateral geniculate nucleus, 16–17
    in visual plasticity, 201–202, 225–226
Molecular cues to development, 66–81
Molyneux's question, 1–2
Monocular deprivation, 127–132
    and competition, 130
    critical period for, 170–177
    effect on myopia, 243–245
Movement, 25
    asymmetry in movement perception with
        esotropia, 186–187
    perception of in amblyopes, 159
    preference for movement in the nasal
        direction, 116–117

Myopia, 123–124, 245–247, 260g
    form-deprivation myopia, 243–245

Nature-nurture controversy, 2–3, 91, 102, 104
Near response, 260g
Neural disarray, 158
NMDA receptors, 260g
    and LTP, 237
    in visual plasticity, 202–204, 211–214
Nystagmus, 260g
    in esotropes, 115, 116

Object color constancy, 260g
Octave, 260g
Ocular dominance, 18–19, 19–21, 261g
    in binocular deprivation, 104
    segregation of columns, 81–82
        correlation with onset of stereopsis, 52–54
    in monocular deprivation, 129–130
Ocular dominance plasticity, 207, 261g
Optic chiasm, misrouting in, 68–70, 115
Optics of eye
    in newborn human, 32
    in animals, 92, 98
Optokinetic nystagmus (OKN), 32, 34, 60, 261g
    asymmetry in, 60, 116
Orientation sensitivity, 19–21
    cellular mechanisms for, 105–106
    critical period for, 174
    deprivation, 132–134
    development of, 43–44, 91, 97–102, 105–106
Orthotropia, 49, 55, 261g

Panum's fusional area, 49, 261g
Parallel processing, 21–22, 261g
Patching, 4, 181
Patterns, perception of, 45, 47
Perimetry, 261g
Phoria, 261g
Photoreceptors, 12, 16
    and development of acuity, 35–36
    and development of contrast sensitivity,
        36–40
Pinwheels, 20
    development of, 81
Plasticity, 261g
Preferential looking technique. *See*
    Forced-choice preferential looking
    technique
Pretectum, 8, 9–10, 11
Prospective study, 261g
Protein kinase A
    and LTP, 238–239
    and visual plasticity, 221–222
Protein kinases C and G and visual plasticity,
    223–234
    and LTP, 238–239

Protein synthesis
  and visual plasticity, 223–225
Pulvinar, 9, 11
Pupil, 11

Quantum catch, 262g

Radial glia, 77, 262g
Receptive fields, 12–14, 262g
  in binocular deprivation, 104–106
  in peripheral field of view, 163
    development of, 94–106
Reeler mouse, 81
Reflection spectrum, 7, 262g
Refraction, 262g
Resolution limit, 262g
Retina, 10–16
  development of, 66–67, 93–96
  waves of activity in, 71–72
Retinoic acid and experimental myopia,
    249–250
Retrospective study, 262g
Reverse suture, 130–132, 178, 262g
Rivalry, 262g

Saccades. *See* Eye movements
Saturation discrimination, 262g
Sclera, 262g
  changes in form-deprivation myopia,
    247–248
Scotoma, 262g
Shape discrimination, 159
Sign-conserving and sign-reversing synapses,
    12–14, 263g
Simultaneous color contrast, 22–24, 263g
Sleep and visual plasticity, 225
Snellen acuity. *See* acuity
Spatial distortions
  in strabismus, 151–152
Spatial frequency channels, 40, 263g
Spatial localization
  in anisometropes, 148, 155
Spatial uncertainty, 263g
  in strabismus, 157–158
Spectral sensitivity, 40–41, 263g
Stereopsis, 50–52, 263g
  correlation with segregation of ocular
    dominance columns, 52–54
  correlation with peak of critical period for
    monocular deprivation, 174
  development in cat and monkey, 52–54
  development of crossed cf. uncrossed, 51–52

development in man, 50–52
  pre- and post-stereoptic periods, 55
  in strabismus, 135–136, 184–185
Strabismus, 3–4, 113–119, 150–153, 264g
  comitant, 117, 135–136, 257g
  experimental in animals, 135–141
  incomitant, 117, 135–136, 259g
Subplate cells, 75, 77–78, 79, 264g
Successive color contrast, 264g
Superior Colliculus, 8
  topography in, 73–74
Suppression of vision in one eye, 117–119 ,
    160, 264g
  mechanisms, 139
Suprachiasmatic nucleus, 8
Synapses
  development of, 84–85

Tangential projections in visual cortex, 78–79
Teller acuity cards (TAC), 264g
Temporal frequency, 264g
Temporal resolution
  development of, 94–95
Tilt after-effect, 256g
  as a test for binocularity in strabismus,
    162–163, 183
Tissue plasminogen activator and visual
    plasticity, 225
Topographic organization, 8
  development of, 72–74
  in amblyopia, 145
Transcription Factor, 264g
Tropia, 264g

Undersampling, 158

Ventricular zone, 75
Vergence, 31, 47, 115, 264g
  development of, 60
Vernier acuity, 264g
  in anisometropia, 148
  development of, 41–43
  in strabismus, 156–157
Visual cliff, 47–48
Visual cortex, 9–11, 16–22
  columnar organization, 18–22
  development of, 74–82, 96–102
Visual evoked potential (VEP), 32, 34, 264g
  in esotropes, 115

"Waiting period," 77, 264g
Wiesel, Torsten, 4, 127